T0297812

Download Your Included Ebook Today!

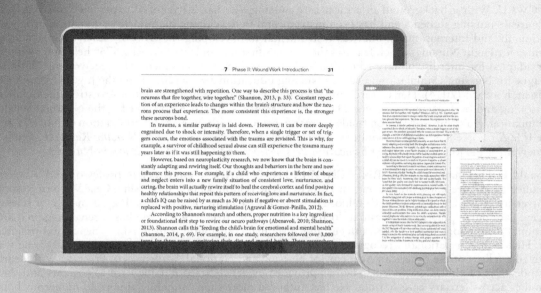

Your print purchase of *Handbook of Clinical Nursing: Pediatric and Neonatal Nursing* **includes an ebook download** to the device of your choice—increasing accessibility, portability, and searchability!

Download your ebook today at http://spubonline.com/pedandneo and enter the access code below:

1CLCKGYNR

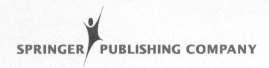

SPC

Celeste M. Alfes, DNP, MSN, RN, CNE, CHSE-A, is associate professor and director of the Center for Nursing Education, Simulation, and Innovation at the Frances Payne Bolton School of Nursing, Case Western Reserve University (CWRU) in Cleveland, Ohio. She earned a bachelor of science in nursing (University of Akron), master of science in nursing (University of Akron), and doctor of nursing practice at CWRU. With a background in critical care nursing, she has 20 years of experience teaching baccalaureate nursing students and has been instrumental in developing high-fidelity simulation programs nationally and internationally. She was instrumental in developing the Dorothy Ebersbach Academic Center for Flight Nursing, which features the nation's first high-fidelity Sikorsky S76® helicopter simulator adapted for interdisciplinary education and crew resource management. She received the National League for Nursing's Simulation Leader in Nursing Education award (2012) and the Joyce Griffin-Sobel Research award (2014). Her research incorporates interprofessional simulations to strengthen clinical reasoning and performance outcomes. Dr. Alfes currently serves as a reviewer for the National Science Foundation, is a coinvestigator on funded research projects with the Laerdal Foundation of Norway and the U.S. Air Force Research Laboratory, is on the editorial board of *Applied Nursing Research*, and is a reviewer for the journals *Nursing Education Perspectives* and *Clinical Simulation in Nursing*.

Ronald L. Hickman, Jr., PhD, RN, ACNP-BC, FNAP, FAAN, is an associate professor and a board-certified acute care nurse practitioner at Frances Payne Bolton School of Nursing, Case Western Reserve University (CWRU) in Cleveland, Ohio. He earned a bachelor of arts in biology, a master of science (acute care nurse practitioner), and a doctorate in nursing from CWRU. He received regional and national distinctions for his commitment and sustained contributions to nursing science and practice. Dr. Hickman is a nationally recognized nurse scientist and advanced practice nurse. In 2015, he was elected a fellow of the American Academy of Nursing and National Academies of Practice. With nearly two decades of clinical experience, he has provided evidence-based nursing care to patients and their families across tertiary care settings. He has authored more than 50 publications and numerous book chapters with a clinical focus, and serves as a contributing editor for the *American Journal of Critical Care*. As an associate editor of *A Guide to Mastery in Clinical Nursing*, Dr. Hickman's clinical expertise in the management of patients requiring life-sustaining care in emergency departments and intensive care units is highlighted in the book's content regarding emergency and critical care, medical–surgical, and nurse anesthesia care.

Joyce J. Fitzpatrick, PhD, MBA, RN, FAAN, FNAP, is Elizabeth Brooks Ford Professor of Nursing, Frances Payne Bolton School of Nursing, Case Western Reserve University (CWRU) in Cleveland, Ohio, where she was the dean from 1982 through 1997. She is also an adjunct professor, Department of Geriatrics, Ichan School of Medicine, Mount Sinai Hospital, New York, New York. She earned a bachelor of science in nursing (Georgetown University), an MS in psychiatric–mental health nursing (The Ohio State University), a PhD in nursing (New York University), and an MBA at CWRU. She was elected a fellow of the American Academy of Nursing (AAN; 1981) and a fellow in the National Academies of Practice (1996). She received the *American Journal of Nursing* Book of the Year award 20 times. Dr. Fitzpatrick received the American Nurses Foundation Distinguished Contribution to Nursing Science award for sustained commitment and contributions to the development of the discipline (2002). She was a Fulbright Scholar at University College Cork, Cork, Ireland (2007–2008), and was inducted into the Sigma Theta Tau International Research Hall of Fame (2014). In 2016, she was named a Living Legend of the AAN. Dr. Fitzpatrick's work is widely disseminated in nursing and health care literature; she has authored or edited more than 300 publications, including more than 80 books. She even served as a coeditor of the *Annual Review of Nursing Research* series, volumes 1 to 26, and she currently edits the journals *Applied Nursing Research*, *Archives of Psychiatric Nursing*, and *Nursing Education Perspectives*, the official journal of the National League for Nursing.

Handbook of Clinical Nursing: PEDIATRIC AND NEONATAL NURSING

Celeste M. Alfes, DNP, MSN, RN, CNE, CHSE-A

Ronald L. Hickman, Jr., PhD, RN, ACNP-BC, FNAP, FAAN

Joyce J. Fitzpatrick, PhD, MBA, RN, FAAN, FNAP

EDITORS

Elizabeth Zimmermann, DNP, MSN, RN, CHSE (Pediatric)

Marguerite DiMarco, PhD, RN, CPNP, FAAN (Pediatric)

Amy Bieda, PhD, RN, APRN, PNP- BC, NNP- BC (Neonatal)

Content Editors

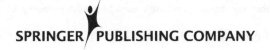

SPRINGER / PUBLISHING COMPANY

Springer Publishing Company, LLC
11 West 42nd Street
New York, NY 10036
www.springerpub.com

Acquisitions Editor: Joseph Morita
Compositor: Newgen KnowledgeWorks
ISBN: 978-0-8261-3033-4
ebook ISBN: 978-0-8261-3642-8

18 19 20 21 22 / 5 4 3 2 1

Extracted from *A Guide to Mastery in Clinical Nursing: The Comprehensive Reference*

The author and the publisher of this Work have made every effort to use sources believed to be reliable to provide information that is accurate and compatible with the standards generally accepted at the time of publication. Because medical science is continually advancing, our knowledge base continues to expand. Therefore, as new information becomes available, changes in procedures become necessary. We recommend that the reader always consult current research and specific institutional policies before performing any clinical procedure. The author and publisher shall not be liable for any special, consequential, or exemplary damages resulting, in whole or in part, from the readers' use of, or reliance on, the information contained in this book. The publisher has no responsibility for the persistence or accuracy of URLs for external or third-party Internet websites referred to in this publication and does not guarantee that any content on such websites is, or will remain, accurate or appropriate.

Library of Congress Cataloging-in-Publication Data
Names: Alfes, Celeste M., editor. | Hickman, Ronald, editor. | Fitzpatrick, Joyce J., 1944- editor.
Title: Handbook of clinical nursing. Pediatric and neonatal nursing / Celeste M. Alfes,
  Ronald L. Hickman, Jr., Joyce J. Fitzpatrick, editors.
Other titles: Pediatric and neonatal nursing | Contained in (work): Guide to mastery in clinical nursing.
Description: New York, NY : Springer Publishing Company, LLC, [2018] | Extracted from
  A guide to mastery in clinical nursing : the comprehensive reference / Joyce J. Fitzpatrick,
  Celeste M. Alfes, Ronald Hickman, editors. 2018. | Includes bibliographical references.
Identifiers: LCCN 2017059924| ISBN 9780826130334 (paper back) | ISBN 9780826136428 (ebook)
Subjects: | MESH: Pediatric Nursing | Neonatal Nursing
Classification: LCC RT41 | NLM WY 159 | DDC 610.73—dc23
LC record available at https://lccn.loc.gov/2017059924

Contact us to receive discount rates on bulk purchases.
We can also customize our books to meet your needs.
For more information please contact: sales@springerpub.com

Printed in the United States of America.

Contents

NEONATAL NURSING

Contributors

Celeste M. Alfes, DNP, MSN, RN, CNE, CHSE-A
Associate Professor
Director, Center for Nursing Education, Simulation, and Innovation
Frances Payne Bolton School of Nursing
Case Western Reserve University
Cleveland, Ohio

Nanci M. Berman, MSN, RN
Assistant Professor
Lorain County Community College
Elyria, Ohio

Amy Bieda, PhD, RN, APRN, PNP-BC, NNP-BC
Assistant Professor
Director, BSN Program
Lead Faculty, Neonatal Nurse Practitioner Program
Frances Payne Bolton School of Nursing
Case Western Reserve University
Cleveland, Ohio

Julia E. Blanchette, BSN, RN, CDE
PhD Student
Frances Payne Bolton School of Nursing
Case Western Reserve University
Cleveland, Ohio

Sheila Blank, MSN, RN
Licensed School Nurse
Clinical Instructor
Bitonte College of Health and Human Services
Department of Nursing
Youngstown State University
Youngstown, Ohio

Mary Ann Blatz, DNP, RN, RNC-NIC, IBCLC
Advanced Practice Nurse
NICU Nursing Research and Development
Neonatal Intensive Care Unit
Rainbow Babies and Children's Hospital
University Hospitals Cleveland Medical Center
Cleveland, Ohio

Pamela Harris Bryant, DNP, RN, CRNP, AC-PC
Pediatric Nurse Practitioner
Assistant Professor
School of Nursing
University of Alabama at Birmingham
Birmingham, Alabama

Valerie Cachat, MSN, RN, CPNP
Nurse Practitioner
Sickle Cell Anemia Center
Rainbow Babies and Children's Hospital
University Hospitals Cleveland Medical Center
Cleveland, Ohio

Michelle Calabretta, MSN, RN, CPNP-AC
Certified Pediatric Nurse Practitioner
Department of Pediatric Orthopaedics
University Hospitals Cleveland Medical Center
Cleveland, Ohio

Emily Canitia, MSN, RN, CPNP-AC/PC
Pediatric Nurse Practitioner
Pediatric Orthopedic Surgery
Rainbow Babies and Children's Hospital
University Hospitals Cleveland Medical Center
Cleveland, Ohio

Beverly Capper, MSN, RN, RNC-NIC
Assistant Director
BSN Program
Frances Payne Bolton School of Nursing
Case Western Reserve University
Cleveland, Ohio

Kerry D. Christy, CPNP AC/PC, MSN, BSN, RN
Pediatric Surgery Nurse Practitioner
Rainbow Babies and Children's Hospital
University Hospitals Cleveland Medical Center
Cleveland, Ohio

Christopher J. Contino, DNP, RN, ENP-C, FNP-BC, CEN, CRN
Emergency Nurse Practitioner
Atlantic Emergency Associates
Atlantic City, New Jersey

Christine Horvat Davey, BSPS, BSN, RN
PhD Student
Frances Payne Bolton School of Nursing
Case Western Reserve University
Cleveland, Ohio

Charlene M. Deuber, DNP, RN, NNP-BC, CPNP
Neonatal Nurse Practitioner
Newborn Care at Einstein Montgomery Medical Center
Children's Hospital of Philadelphia
East Norriton, Pennsylvania

Tina Di Fiore, MSN, RN
Clinical Nurse Specialist
Office of Advanced Practice Nursing
Cleveland Clinic Children's Hillcrest Hospital
Cleveland, Ohio

Marguerite DiMarco, PhD, RN, CPNP, FAAN
Associate Professor
Frances Payne Bolton School of Nursing
Case Western Reserve University
Cleveland, Ohio

Mary Alice Dombrowski, DNP, MSN, RN
Certified Family Nurse Practitioner
Department of Pediatric Gastroenterology, Hepatology, and Nutrition
Rainbow Babies and Children's Hospital
University Hospitals Cleveland Medical Center
Cleveland, Ohio

Donna A. Dowling, PhD, RN
Professor
Frances Payne Bolton School of Nursing
Case Western Reserve University
Cleveland, Ohio

Sherita K. Etheridge, MSN, RN, CPNP-PC
Nursing Instructor
Family, Community, and Health Systems
University of Alabama at Birmingham
Birmingham, Alabama

Paula Forsythe, MSN, RN
Clinical Nurse Specialist Neonatal Services
Neonatology Department
Rainbow Babies and Children's Hospital
University Hospitals Cleveland Medical Center
Cleveland, Ohio

Laurine Gajkowski, ND, RN, CPN
Instructor of Pediatric and Community Health Nursing
Frances Payne Bolton School of Nursing
Case Western Reserve University
Cleveland, Ohio
Staff Nurse
Rainbow Babies and Children's Hospital
University Hospitals Cleveland Medical Center
Cleveland, Ohio

Michael D. Gooch, DNP, RN, ACNP-BC, FNP-BC, ENP-BC, ENP-C, CFRN, CTRN, TCRN, CEN, NREMT-P
Assistant Professor of Nursing
Vanderbilt University School of Nursing
Flight Nurse
Vanderbilt University Medical Center's LifeFlight
Emergency Nurse Practitioner
TeamHealth Faculty
Middle Tennessee School of Anesthesia
Nashville, Tennessee

Melanie Gibbons Hallman, DNP, RN, CRNP, CEN, FNP-BC
Instructor/Nurse Practitioner
School of Nursing
University of Alabama at Birmingham
Birmingham, Alabama

Rae Jean Hemway, MPA, BSN, RNC-NIC
Director of Pediatric Nursing
New York–Presbyterian Hospital
New York, New York

Michelle A. Janas, MSN, RN, CPN
Advanced Clinical Nurse Coordinator
Pediatric Orthopedics
Rainbow Babies and Children's Hospital
University Hospitals Cleveland Medical Center
Cleveland, Ohio

Jennifer Johntony, MSN, RN, CPNP-AC/PC
Pediatric Nurse Practitioner
The Congenital Heart Collaborative
Rainbow Babies and Children's Hospital
University Hospitals Cleveland Medical Center
Cleveland, Ohio

Helene M. Lannon, MSN, RN, APRN, NNP-BC
Neonatal Nurse Practitioner
Neonatal Intensive Care Unit
Pediatrix Medical Group of Nevada at Sunrise Children's Hospital
Las Vegas, Nevada

Jane F. Marek, DNP, MSN, RN
Assistant Professor
Frances Payne Bolton School of Nursing
Case Western Reserve University
Cleveland, Ohio

Kathleen Maxwell, MSN, RN, CNS, CNP
Family Nurse Practitioner
Pediatric Neurology
Rainbow Babies and Children's Hospital
University Hospitals Cleveland Medical Center
Cleveland, Ohio

Steadman McPeters, DNP, RN, CRNP, CPNP-AC, RNFA
Assistant Professor
Director of Clinical Graduate Program Subspecialty Tracks and Dual Option & Acute
  Care Pediatric Nurse Practitioner Specialty Track Coordinator
Department of Family, Community, and Health Systems
School of Nursing
University of Alabama at Birmingham
Birmingham, Alabama

Anne M. Modic, BSN, RN, BC-NNP
Neonatal Nurse Practitioner/Department of Neonatology
Rainbow Babies and Children's Hospital
University Hospitals Cleveland Medical Center
Cleveland, Ohio

Lamon Norton, DNP, RN, FNP, ACNP
Managing Partner
UEE Health Care Consulting Emergency Nurse Practitioner
Faculty
Samford University
Homewood, Alabama

Sharon Perry, MSN, RN, CPNP, CPN
Nurse Practitioner
Pediatric Gastroenterology, Hepatology, and Nutrition
Rainbow Babies and Children's Hospital
University Hospitals Cleveland Medical Center
Cleveland, Ohio

Karla Phipps, MSN, RN, APRN, NNP-BC
Neonatal Nurse Practitioner
Rainbow Babies and Children's Hospital
University Hospitals Cleveland Medical Center
Cleveland, Ohio

Breanne M. Roche, MSN, RN, CPNP, CPHON
Pediatric Nurse Practitioner
Rainbow Babies and Children's Hospital
University Hospitals Cleveland Medical Center
Cleveland, Ohio

Suzanne Rubin, DNP, MPH, RN, CRNP-P
Nursery Pediatric Nurse Practitioner
Johns Hopkins Hospital
Baltimore, Maryland

Donna M. Schultz, DNP, RN, APRN, NNP-BC
Neonatal Nurse Practitioner
Mednax Medical Group
Baylor University Medical Center & The Tots Clinic
Dallas, Texas

Barbara Greitzer Slone, MS, MPH, RN, CPNP
Chief Nurse Practitioner
Neonatal Intensive Care Unit
Department of Pediatrics
New York University Winthrop Hospital
Mineola, New York

Tedra S. Smith, DNP, RN, CRNP, CPNP-PC, CNE
Assistant Professor
School of Nursing
University of Alabama at Birmingham
Birmingham, Alabama

Patricia M. Speck, DNSc, APN, APRN, FNP-BC, DF-IAFN, FAAFS, FAAN
Professor and Coordinator
Advanced Forensic Nursing Department of Family, Community, & Health Systems
School of Nursing
University of Alabama at Birmingham
Birmingham, Alabama

Mary F. Terhaar, DNSC, RN, ANEF, FAAN
Associate Dean for Academic Affairs
Arline H. and Curtis F. Garvin Professor
Frances Payne Bolton School of Nursing
Case Western Reserve University
Cleveland, Ohio

Ke-Ni Niko Tien, MSN, RN, APRN, NNP-BC
Nurse Practitioner
Neonatal Intensive Care Unit
Cleveland Clinic
Cleveland, Ohio

Rachel Tkaczyk, MSN, RN, CPNP-AC/PC-BC
Pediatric Nurse Practitioner
Assistant Clinical Professor
Drexel University
Philadelphia, Pennsylvania

Mary Variath, MSN, RN
Instructor
Frances Payne Bolton School of Nursing
Case Western Reserve University
Cleveland, Ohio

Karen Vosper, BSN, RN, CPN
Advanced Clinical Nurse
Cystic Fibrosis Center
Cleveland, Ohio

Rosanna P. Watowicz, PhD, RD, LD
Assistant Professor
Department of Nutrition
School of Medicine
Case Western Reserve University
Cleveland, Ohio

Rachael Weigand, MSN, RN, CPN P-PC
Nurse Practitioner
Heart Center
Akron Children's Hospital
Brecksville, Ohio

Elizabeth Wirth-Tomaszewski, DNP, RN, CRNP, CCRN, ACNP-BC, ACNPC
Assistant Clinical Professor and Track Director
Adult Gerontology Acute Care Nurse Practitioner Program
College of Nursing and Health Professions
Drexel University
Philadelphia, Pennsylvania

Shannon Courtney Wong, MSN, RN, CPNP
Instructor
Frances Payne Bolton School of Nursing
Case Western Reserve University
Cleveland, Ohio

Jodi Zalewski, MSN, RN, CPNP-AC
Pediatric Nurse Practitioner
The Congenital Heart Collaborative
University Hospitals Cleveland Medical Center
Cleveland, Ohio

Jenelle M. Zambrano, DNP, RN, CNS, CCNS, CCRN
Director, Professional Practice and Development
Fountain Valley Regional Hospital and Medical Center
Fountain Valley, California

Elizabeth Zimmermann, DNP, MSN, RN, CHSE
Instructor of Pediatric and Community Health Nursing
Frances Payne Bolton School of Nursing
Case Western Reserve University
Cleveland, Ohio

Preface

Many transitions can occur for registered nurses as they decide to move from one clinical practice area to another. This handbook is designed for the generalist registered nurse who may be transitioning to the pediatric or neonatal clinical setting and wants to know the primary clinical problems that nurses may encounter. The *Handbook of Clinical Nursing: Pediatric and Neonatal Nursing* has selected clinical topics curated by Dr. Elizabeth Zimmermann, Dr. Marguerite DiMarco, and Dr. Amy Bieda. These content editors identified expert clinicians in their fields to author entries for this comprehensive compendium of pediatric and neonatal clinical nursing content, which is included in *A Guide to Mastery in Clinical Nursing: The Comprehensive Reference* for individuals across the life span. No prior work of this nature has been published as a pediatric and neonatal reference handbook. The objective is to provide detailed information on the most important pediatric and neonatal topics in clinical nursing practice for both new registered nurses and those transitioning to a new clinical area. Each clinical content area includes the key clinical nursing problems that would be encountered in generalist nursing practice. For each clinical problem, there is an overview of the clinical problem, pertinent clinical background, clinical aspects for the nurse (assessment; nursing interventions, management, and clinical implications; and outcomes), and a summary. Key references are provided for each entry, including both classic references and current citations from clinical and research literature.

In summary, this handbook has particular relevance to several groups of nurses. Nurse faculty will find it useful as a synopsis for clinical problems encountered in pediatric and neonatal nursing. Clinicians transitioning to new clinical areas will have a ready resource for key clinical problems they may encounter in the pediatric or neonatal clinical area. And, importantly, newly licensed registered nurses will find this handbook an invaluable reference for the delivery of safe, quality, family-centered care of their pediatric and neonatal patients.

Celeste M. Alfes
Ronald L. Hickman, Jr.
Joyce J. Fitzpatrick

Celeste M. Alfes

Guide to Mastery in Pediatric and Neonatal Nursing

Pediatric and neonatal nurses of all levels dedicate themselves to promoting optimal physical, mental, and social well-being of neonates, infants, children, and adolescents. Nursing as a profession advocates to protect and support children of all ages to provide the highest level of quality family-centered care, which is evidence based and equitable.

This comprehensive resource is composed of 50 alphabetized entries designed for the beginning nurse practitioner, practicing nurse, or nursing student, and is divided into two sections: Pediatric Nursing and Neonatal Nursing. Each concise entry features essential and relevant information written by experienced nurse practitioners, clinicians, and faculty on the conditions, disorders, and pathologic processes commonly seen in the neonatal and pediatric inpatient and outpatient settings. Novice and expert nurses will find entries that provide a concise overview and background; clinical aspects; assessment; nursing interventions, treatment, and management; and outcomes of the clinical condition.

We anticipate that students and practicing nurses alike will find this resource to be an invaluable reference for the delivery of safe, quality, family-centered care of pediatric and neonatal patients.

Pediatric Nursing

Christopher J. Contino
Celeste M. Alfes

Overview

Abdominal pain is a common problem in children. Although most children with acute abdominal pain have self-limited conditions, the pain may be indicative of a surgical or medical emergency (Leung & Sigalet, 2003). Abdominal pain in children is a complicated complaint in the emergency care setting. The chief complaint of abdominal pain comprises approximately 5% to 10% of emergency department visits annually (Kendall & Moreira, 2016). Although many cases of abdominal pain are not life threatening, there are a multitude of causes that may require emergent intervention from emergency room nurses.

Background

Abdominal pain comprises a significant portion of emergency department visits annually (Kendall & Moreira, 2016). Although abdominal pain affects all patient populations, there are key demographics that may have a more significant course, and include the elderly aged 65 years and older, and immunocompromised patients, such as individuals living with HIV. Individuals from these at-risk populations have disproportionately higher rates of mortality and morbidity compared to younger adults with a functioning immune system. In the emergency department, nurses usually are the first point of contact for the patient, and it is important that they are able to recognize life-threatening emergencies and care for the patient appropriately (Cole, Lynch, & Cugnoni, 2006).

The abdomen can be broadly divided into four quadrants: right upper, left upper, right lower, and left lower. Additionally, the epigastric area, just under the xiphoid process, is a key area for assessment. Understanding the location of pain may help in determining the cause of the origin of the pain. Right-upper quadrant pain may be because of cholecystitis, hepatitis, or ulcers. Left-upper quadrant pain may involve the spleen or stomach. Right-lower quadrant pain may be appendicitis or diverticulitis, and left-lower quadrant pain may be from colitis, or diverticulitis. Depending on the gender of the patient, lower abdominal pain can stem from genitourinary processes such as ectopic pregnancy and pelvic inflammatory disease in the female, or testicular disease in the male patient. Diffuse abdominal pain can be from a multitude of causes (Penner, Fishman, & Majumdar, 2016).

Pediatric patients with abdominal pain pose a challenge with diagnosis and may vary widely with age. In the infant through toddler years, patients may not be able to adequately describe their pain. Many of the differential diagnoses remain salient; however, in the very young infant, consider pyloric stenosis, intussusception, Hirschsprung's disease, and Meckel's diverticulitis. Pediatric patients may become dehydrated faster than adults, so fluid balance is key. Also, pediatric patients can cardiovascular compensate longer than adults; however, when the decompensation occurs, it happens rapidly. To assess a pediatric patient frequently and thoroughly, keep a high index of suspicion for serious disease.

In the pediatric population, gastroenteritis is the most common cause of abdominal pain. Viruses such as rotavirus, Norwalk virus, adenovirus, and enterovirus are the most frequent causes of abdominal pain. The most common bacterial agents include *Escherichia coli*, Yersinia, Campylobacter, Salmonella, and Shigella (Leung & Sigalet, 2003).

Appendicitis is the most common surgical condition in children who present with abdominal pain. Approximately one in 15 pediatric patients develop appendicitis. Lymphoid tissue or a fecalith obstructs the appendiceal lumen, the appendix becomes distended, and then ischemia and necrosis may develop. Patients with appendicitis classically present with vague, visceral, and poorly localized, periumbilical pain. Within 6 to 48 hours from onset, the pain becomes parietal as the overlying peritoneum becomes inflamed; the pain then becomes well localized and constant in the right iliac fossa (Leung & Sigalet, 2003).

Clinical Aspects

ASSESSMENT

A thorough history is required when evaluating children with abdominal pain to identify the most likely cause. An initial history and evaluation followed by a physical examination and a reassessment of certain points of the history should be conducted to narrow the list of suspicious etiologies (Leung & Sigalet, 2003). Children who are unable to verbalize typically present with late symptoms of disease and children up to the teenage years have a poor sense of onset or location of pain. A classic sequence of shifting pain usually occurs with appendicitis and any child with pain that localizes to the right-lower quadrant should be suspected of having appendicitis (Leung & Sigalet, 2003). Moreover, inquiry into the location, timing of onset, character, severity, duration, and radiation of pain is very important but must be viewed in the context of the child's age. Any abnormalities during the initial evaluation should be addressed immediately, and only after this should further assessment be performed.

Once it has been established that the patient is otherwise stable, a thorough history and physical examination may commence. All patients should receive a thorough SAMPLE history. This includes signs and symptoms, allergies, medications, past illnesses, last oral intake, and events leading up to the present illness. The patient's pain should be characterized utilizing the OPQRST mnemonic, which evaluates onset, provocative and palliative factors, quality, radiation, site or location, associated signs and symptoms, and time. With abdominal pain, the location of pain may help to narrow the differential diagnosis although it should not be relied on as many etiologies of abdominal pain can vary from patient to patient. The character and nature of it can also help to narrow the diagnosis. There are three main types of pain described as visceral, somatic, and referred. Visceral pain is typically described as dull and unable to localize, and usually originates from solid organs and the walls of hollow organs. Somatic pain is usually described as sharp and can be localized, and is usually caused by inflammation ischemia or peritoneal irritation. Referred pain is pain that is felt at a location distant from its originating source. This is a key concept to remember as several potentially life-threatening disease processes may be felt as abdominal pain but do not originate in the abdominal area; a key example of this would be myocardial ischemia presenting as epigastric pain.

NURSING INTERVENTIONS, MANAGEMENT, AND IMPLICATIONS

Initial nursing interventions should include ensuring that airway, breathing, and circulatory status are adequate and secure. All undifferentiated abdominal pain in patients should have nothing by mouth in the case that surgery may be necessary. Pediatric patients are at high risk for dehydration and should have intravenous access secured early, preferably with a large-bore intravenous (IV) catheter in the antecubital space. This is important should fluid resuscitation be necessary; additionally many diagnostic imaging modalities require this for IV contrast administration. The nurse should prepare to obtain diagnostic samples of blood and urine. Local protocol should dictate when and how to obtain the samples. Laboratory evaluation should be tailored to the individual patient to avoid unnecessary testing; however, in some clinical settings, there are established nursing protocols and these should dictate the nurse's plan of care.

OUTCOMES

When discussing any clinical disease process, it is important to discuss outcomes. Regarding abdominal pain, the main outcome in the emergency department setting is rapid exclusion of life-threatening causes of pain that require emergency intervention. This includes timely diagnosis, early consultation with specialists including surgery, and collaboration with ancillary departments. Pain control is also a significant outcome measure (Kendall & Moreira, 2016). Once an appropriate physical examination has been conducted, pain control should be a priority. Pain should be assessed and reassessed frequently by utilizing a developmentally appropriate pediatric pain scale (Ball, Bindler, Cowen, & Shaw, 2017). The ultimate outcome is to reduce mortality and morbidity.

Summary

Abdominal pain is a common complaint in the emergency department, with a wide variety of potential causes. Although a large portion of pediatric patients with abdominal pain do not have a specific cause of their pain, there are a few disease processes that are immediately life threatening. It is crucial that emergency department nurses can recognize the spectrum of possible causes of pain, be able to recognize unstable or ill patients, and institute appropriate interventions. The key to most abdominal pain complaints is a thorough history and physical examination, with assistance from appropriate laboratories and imaging as necessary.

Ball, J., Bindler, R., Cowen, K., & Shaw, M. (2017). *Principles of pediatric nursing: Caring for children*. Hokoben, NJ: Pearson.

Cole, E., Lynch, A., & Cugnoni, H. (2006). Assessment of the patient with acute abdominal pain. *Nursing Standard, 20*(39), 67–75.

Kendall, J. L., & Moreira, M. E. (2016). Evaluation of the adult with abdominal pain in the emergency department. In R. Hockberger & J. Grayzel (Eds.), *UpToDate*. Retrieved from https://www.uptodate.com/contents/evaluation-of-the-adult-with -abdominal-pain-in-the-emergency-department

Leung, A. K. C., & Sigalet, D. L. (2003). Acute abdominal pain in children. *American Family Physician, 67*(11), 2321–2327.

Penner, R. M., Fishman, M. B., & Majumdar, S. R. (2016). Evaluation of the adult with abdominal pain. In A. Auerbach, M. Aronson, & D. J. Sullivan (Eds.), *UpToDate*. Retrieved from https://www.uptodate.com/contents/evaluation-of-the -adult-with-abdominal-pain

■ ACUTE RENAL FAILURE

Christine Horvat Davey

Overview

Acute renal failure (ARF), also known as "acute kidney injury" (AKI), is a reversible acute decline in renal function with rapid onset (Devarajan, 2017). The most extensively used and standardized definitions for pediatric ARF are pediatric RIFLE (pRIFLE; risk for renal dysfunction, injury to the kidney, failure of kidney function, loss of kidney function, and end-stage renal disease), Acute Kidney Injury Network (AKIN), and kidney disease improving global outcomes (KDIGOs) classifications (Sutherland et al., 2015). ARF is marked by a decrease in glomerular filtration rate, an inability of the kidneys to regulate fluid and electrolyte homeostasis as well as an increase in serum creatinine and blood urea nitrogen levels (Andreoli, 2009). The exact incidence of pediatric ARF is unknown. Nursing care of pediatric patients with ARF focuses on determination and treatment of the underlying cause of ARF along with early medical management.

Background

The incidence of ARF is rising in relation to increased use of advanced medical technology for children who are critically ill or experience chronic conditions (Devarajan, 2017). Worldwide, one in three children experience ARF during an occurrence of hospitalization (Susantitaphong et al., 2013). Pediatric ARF can arise from multiple causes with clinical manifestations that range from minimal elevation in serum creatinine to anuric renal failure (Devarajan, 2017).

The pathophysiology behind an acute kidney insult is classified into three phases: development, extension, and resolution. During the development phase, a kidney insult leads to injury and may be subclinical (Hayes, 2017). Repair processes commence during the extension phase. Adaptive repair results in correction of the renal structure without long-term consequence (Hayes, 2017). Maladaptive repair often results in change of renal structure and in turn reduced kidney function (Hayes, 2017). Net result of renal injury and repair are represented in the extension phase (Hayes, 2017). Overall, renal recovery results from adaptive repair whereas progression leads to change in kidney function and/or structure that can be detected by histopathology, imaging studies, or biomarkers (Basile et al., 2016).

Diagnosis of ARF is based on characteristic signs and symptoms: edema, decreased urine output, hematuria, hypertension, and laboratory results. Diagnosis of ARF by laboratory results is based on serum creatinine levels. Normal serum creatinine level for an infant is 0.2 to 0.4 mg/dL, 18 to 35 µmol/L (Devarajan, 2017). Diagnostic use of serum creatinine levels can present issues. ARF serum creatinine is an insensitive and delayed measure of decreased kidney function as serum creatinine may not increase until a 50% or higher reduction in glomerular filtration rate is present (Andreoli, 2009; Devarajan, 2017). Additionally, if dialysis is initiated as a treatment, serum creatinine levels cannot be measured accurately. An abnormal urinalysis can also indicate ARF. Although individuals with prerenal ARF may display a normal urinalysis, urinalysis is most often used to determine the underlying cause of ARF. Regardless of the limitations posed by serum creatinine levels in the diagnosis of ARF, it is presently the best laboratory test for diagnosis in pediatrics.

The risk of ARF is highest among children cared for in an intensive care unit (Devarajan, 2017). Pediatric patients requiring critical care or dialysis have the highest ARF mortality rates (Sutherland et al., 2015). Several key factors can contribute to ARF in pediatrics: hypoxia, ischemia, acute injury, or illness. Nephrotoxic-induced ARF is often related to hospitalization as hospitalization poses increased risk for exposure to medications that are nephrotoxic (Sutherland et al., 2013). In addition to the environmental factors, there may be genetic risk factors for ARF. Several candidate polymorphisms have shown an association with ARF (Andreoli, 2009).

ARF causes can be classified in several ways. The most widely used mechanism for classification are the three major categories based on anatomic location of the primary injury: prerenal, intrinsic renal, and postrenal disease. Prerenal disease is caused by reduced renal perfusion because of hypovolemia (bleeding, gastrointestinal, urinary, or cutaneous losses), or decline of effective circulation (septic shock, heart failure, or cirrhosis) (Devarajan, 2017). Prerenal is considered the most common form of pediatric ARF. In prerenal, glomerular filtration rate is reduced, but renal tubular function remains intact in prerenal disease (Devarajan, 2017). Intrinsic renal or intrarenal disease is most commonly caused by sepsis, nephrotoxins, prolonged hypoperfusion, or severe glomerular diseases. Structural damage to the renal parenchyma occurs in intrinsic renal disease. Postrenal disease or obstructive ARF is most commonly a result of congenital or acquired anatomic obstructions of the lower urinary tract (Devarajan, 2017).

A less used approach to classification of ARF is based on clinical setting or circumstance and urine output. Hospital-acquired ARF is often multifactorial and often associated with multiple organ failure (Devarajan, 2017). Hospital-acquired ARF greatly complicates clinical outcomes. Community-acquired ARF is often the result of a single primary insult, most often volume depletion, but is regularly reversible (Devarajan, 2017). Measurement of urine output can be used, but presence of normal urine output does not exclude ARF. The ability to classify the cause of ARF can lead to early and targeted medical interventions.

Clinical Aspects

ASSESSMENT

As soon as the diagnosis of ARF is suspected or determined, further assessment is dedicated to identifying the underlying cause. This evaluation includes an accurate record of an individual's physical assessment, medical history, and laboratory data. The physical assessment should focus on signs and symptoms related to alterations in renal function. These assessment findings include decreased or no urine output, edema, hematuria, and/or hypertension (Devarajan, 2017).

NURSING INTERVENTIONS, MANAGEMENT, AND IMPLICATIONS

Nursing responsibilities include accurate blood pressure measurement and assessment for edema or volume depletion, which is indicated by dry mucous membranes, decreased skin turgor, tachycardia, orthostatic falls in blood pressure, and decreased peripheral perfusion. Assessment of recent weight gain, signs of systemic disease such as rash or joint disease, palpation of enlarged kidneys, an indication of renal vein thrombosis and an enlarged bladder, which may indicate urethral obstruction, are also important (Devarajan, 2017).

An accurate medical history is essential, as there is often a known etiologic factor that predisposes the child to ARF. These factors include heart failure, shock, or a preceding streptococcal infection seen in patients with poststreptococcal glomerulonephritis (Devarajan, 2017). Laboratory data to monitor when assessing for alterations in renal function include elevation of serum creatinine and/or blood urea nitrogen levels, abnormal urinalysis, hyperkalemia, hyponatremia, or less often hypernatremia, high anion gap (metabolic acidosis), hypocalcemia, and/or hyperphosphatemia. Renal imaging can also be performed or, on rare occasions, a kidney biopsy may be conducted to determine the underlying cause. Usage of an accurate physical assessment, medical history, and laboratory data can facilitate initiation of proper and timely nursing care that can positively impact patient outcomes.

Nursing care of pediatric patients with ARF should focus on treatment of ARF and prevention of long-term sequelae. Priority nursing care includes monitoring of vital signs, maintenance of proper blood pressure, accurate measurement of intake and output, maintenance of electrolyte and nutrition balance, and determination of the underlying cause of ARF. If necessary, initiation of hemodialysis, peritoneal dialysis, continuous renal reperfusion therapy (CRRT), monitoring of laboratory data, and psychological support for the family unit should be initiated.

OUTCOMES

Evidence-based nursing practice should focus on treatment of ARF and prevention of long-term sequelae. Early determination of ARF based on signs, symptoms, and laboratory data as well as prompt correction of the underlying cause facilitate positive outcomes. In addition to correction of the underlying cause of ARF, effective management of signs, symptoms, and treatment options, which can include hemodialysis, peritoneal dialysis, and CRRT are required. Effective nursing care outcomes should result in correction of ARF without long-term sequelae (Hayes, 2017).

Summary

The incidence of pediatric ARF is expected to increase, and therefore, it is important to recognize the early signs and symptoms of the condition. Early detection and medical management can facilitate positive outcomes and decreased incidence of long-term sequelae.

Andreoli, S. P. (2009). Acute kidney injury in children. *Pediatric Nephrology, 24*(2), 253–263. doi:10.1007/s00467-008-1074-9

Basile, D., Bonventre, J., Mehta, R., Nangaku, M., Unwin, R., Rosner, M., . . . Ronco, C. (2016). Progression after AKI: Understanding maladaptive repair processes to predict and identify therapeutic treatments. *Journal of the American Society of Nephrology, 27*(3), 687–697. doi:10.1681/ASN.2015030309

Devarajan, P. (2017). Acute kidney injury in children: Clinical features, etiology, evaluation, and diagnosis. In T. Mattoo (Ed.). *UpToDate.* Retrieved from https://www.uptodate.com/contents/acute-kidney-injury-in-children-clinical-features-etiology-evaluation-and-diagnosis

Hayes, W. (2017). Stop adding insult to injury—Identifying and managing risk factors for the progression of acute kidney injury in children. *Pediatric Nephrology, 32*(12), 2235–2243. doi:10.1007/s00467-017-3598-3

Susantitaphong, P., Cruz, D., Cerda, J., Abulfaraj, M., Alqahtani, F., Koulouridis, I., & Jaber, B. L. (2013). World incidence of AKI: A meta-analysis. *Clinical Journal of the American Society of Nephrology, 8*(9), 1482–1493. doi:10.2215/CJN.00710113

Sutherland, S. M., Byrnes, J., Kothari, M., Longhurst, C., Dutta, S., Garcia, P., & Goldstein, S. (2015). AKI in hospitalized children: Comparing the pRIFLE, AKIN, and KDIGO definitions. *Clinical Journal of the American Society of Nephrology, 10*(4), 554–561. doi:10.2215/CJN.01900214

Sutherland, S. M., Ji, J., Sheikhi, F. H., Widen, E., Tian, L., Alexander, S., & Ling, X. B. (2013). AKI in hospitalized children: Epidemiology and clinical associations in a national cohort. *Clinical Journal of the American Society of Nephrology, 8*(10), 1661–1669. doi:10.2215/CJN.00270113

■ APPENDICITIS

Kerry D. Christy

Overview

Acute appendicitis is one of the primary causes of abdominal pain in children and a leading contributor to the emergency department visits worldwide. A thorough assessment and examination must be conducted to distinguish appendicitis from other diseases that could cause acute abdominal pain. Once identified, attentive monitoring for potential complications preoperatively and postoperatively will ensure patient safety.

Background

Butler (2015) defines acute appendicitis as the inflammation of the appendix, which is a blind-ending pouch that arises where the small and large intestine meet (cecum). Although appendicitis has been treated for more than 300 years, the cause is still not entirely known (Rentea, St. Peter, & Snyder, 2016). In most cases, it is presumed that luminal obstruction by stool may incite the process; alternatively, a neoplasm, parasite, or lymphocyte proliferation may induce the appendix to swell (Rentea et al., 2016). The obstruction leads to inflammation and decreased blood flow to the appendix with subsequent bacterial overgrowth (Brown, 2014). This progression generates an inflammatory exudate on the surface of the appendix, which locally irritates the perineum (peritonitis) causing symptoms classic to appendicitis (Butler, 2015). Appendicitis can be described in three categories: simple acute appendicitis, gangrenous appendicitis, or complicated perforated appendicitis. Acute appendicitis is the inflammation of the appendix while gangrene suggests a microscopic perforation or discoloration of the appendix (Pennington & Burke, 2015). Appendiceal perforation is described by Butler (2015) as having generalized peritonitis and formation of an abscess or phlegmon.

The lifetime risk of getting appendicitis in the Western world is about 7% (Pennington & Burke, 2015). The U.S. incidence is one per 1,000 (Rentea et al., 2016), but geographical differences have been reported (Bhangu, Søreide, Di Saverio, Assarsson, & Drake, 2015). The incidence of acute appendicitis typically peaks in the summer months. It most often occurs between the ages of 10 and 19 years, and males have a slightly higher prevalence (Bhangu et al., 2015). It has been found that up to 40% of children who present with appendicitis have perforated appendix (Tian, Heiss, Wulkan, & Raval, 2015). Children are often unable to specify their symptoms or location of pain when it occurs, delaying the evaluation and allowing time for perforation to occur. Fortunately, overall mortality with appendicitis is low in the United States and only slightly higher in low- and middle-income countries (Bhangu et al., 2015). The key to treating appendicitis is to have an accurate assessment and timely intervention. This is how nursing plays a large role in the management of appendicitis.

Clinical Aspects

ASSESSMENT

Nurses are most often the first line of evaluation both preoperatively and postoperatively, so knowing the pertinent symptoms, risk factors, and complications of appendicitis are key for a positive outcome. Beginning with a thorough primary assessment in triage and asking the relevant questions to both the patient and his or her caregiver leads to an accurate diagnosis. The assessment of symptoms, including timing and location, as well as nausea, vomiting, anorexia, diarrhea or constipation, fevers, chills, or sepsis is critical. A hallmark symptom of appendicitis is the gradual onset of diffuse abdominal pain most often starting around the umbilicus (Bishop & Carter, 2013). With time, often just a few hours, the diffused abdominal pain will worsen and localize to the right-lower quadrant where the appendix is located. Any moving, walking, jumping, and even riding in the car may exacerbate the pain. Patients with acute appendicitis will be in pain, but they often do not appear ill, and the pain will not improve with time until perforation occurs. Following the perforation, peritonitis develops, and patients may become febrile, tachycardic, hypotensive, and septic (Brown, 2014).

A thorough assessment rules out other conditions that can mimic appendicitis. Make sure to assess any signs of a streptococcal infection as well as flank or urinary pain that could be caused by a urinary tract infection (Bishop & Carter, 2013). A primary indicator of appendicitis during physical examination is tenderness at McBurney's point—tenderness on the right side of the abdomen one third along a line between the superior iliac spine and umbilicus. Involuntary guarding is often associated with palpation of this area. Three other key findings that suggest peritoneal and pelvic irritation are a positive Rovsing sign, Psoas sign, and Obturators sign. All these findings support a diagnosis that there is peritoneal and pelvic irritation, but do not definitively diagnose appendicitis.

Although physical findings can be helpful in pinpointing a diagnosis, laboratory tests as well as imaging confirm appendicitis. A complete blood count (CBC) with differential and C-reactive protein (CRP) are most often drawn and an elevated white blood cell count with a left shift and elevated CRP are found to be associated with appendicitis (Bishop & Carter, 2013). These labs are also important for postoperative monitoring of perforated appendicitis and also for antibiotic management (Brown, 2014). Radiographic tests used to diagnose appendicitis include ultrasound and CT. Ultrasound, while useful, is often operator specific as well as limited by the location of the appendix (Bishop & Carter, 2013). A CT scan with intravenous and oral contrast is much more accurate and can identify the location of the appendix as well as findings of appendicitis such as inflammation, wall thickening, fat stranding, or abscess formation.

NURSING INTERVENTIONS, MANAGEMENT, AND IMPLICATIONS

Once a diagnosis of appendicitis has been made, there are four main nursing diagnoses that correlate with appendicitis that must be considered both pre- and postoperatively. Those are deficient fluid volume, acute pain, risk for infection, and deficient knowledge of the parent and/or patient. Preoperatively, these patients should have nothing by mouth (NPO) and be given intravenous (IV) fluids as they are frequently dehydrated. Resuscitation is vital before the administration of anesthesia and can be given with a fluid bolus of an isotonic solution followed by the maintenance of IV fluids. If children do not have appendicitis, rather have viral gastroenteritis, these fluids often improve their symptoms and again help confirm a diagnosis (Bishop & Carter, 2013). Postoperatively, it is important to continue intravenous hydration while awaiting return of bowel function. Adequate hydration can be evaluated by monitoring urine output. If urine output is around 1 mL/kg/hr with a normal specific gravity, there is adequate hydration.

Administration of pain medication before definitive diagnosis will not completely mask the symptoms of appendicitis and if a thorough exam is done, the diagnosis can still be made. Postoperatively, pain assessment is the key as it can mark the progression of healing and alert to a complication such as the formation of an abscess if pain is not improving or new pain is noted. Pain control can be managed by distraction techniques, ice, or analgesics such as morphine sulfate or Toradol while NPO, and oral pain meds when taking a diet (Bishop & Carter, 2013).

If the decision is made to go to the operating room, broad-spectrum antibiotics should also be administered preoperatively. Antibiotics administered before surgery have shown a reduction in wound infections as well as abscess formation (Bishop & Carter, 2013). Postoperatively, antibiotics are often given for 24 hours for acute appendicitis; however, perforated appendicitis often requires a longer duration of broad-spectrum antibiotics to prevent wound infections and abscess formation (Brown, 2014). The American Pediatric Surgical Association is now recommending that antibiotic therapy be based on clinical criteria, such as down-trending labs and no fever, rather than a set, standard time frame (Brown, 2014). The surgery may be done either way laparoscopically or open; however, frequent inspection of the wounds must be performed. Identifying any erythema, drainage, or tenderness could indicate a wound infection and may warrant prolonged antibiotic coverage (Bishop & Carter, 2013).

Families of pediatric patients with an appendicitis can be overwhelmed with the abundance of information they receive from medical teams. As a nurse, it is important to identify if there is deficient knowledge or lack of recall of information received and help to relieve any anxiety or answer questions the family may have. Postoperatively, nurses must educate the family about wound care, management of surgical wound dressings, appropriate bathing timeframe, and symptoms to look for at home that warrant a call to the surgeon.

OUTCOMES

From preoperative to postoperative care, nursing plays a role in preventing potential complications, promoting overall comfort, and reducing anxiety through patient and family education. Through the team efforts of both the nursing staff and the surgical team, patients with appendicitis can have shorter hospitalizations with positive outcomes.

Summary

Acute appendicitis is one of the most common pediatric conditions that require emergent surgery. Signs and symptoms of appendicitis often mimic those of other conditions so it is vital that the nursing staff be educated on hallmark signs, such as fevers, nausea, vomiting, and right-lower quadrant pain, to diagnose appendicitis. From preoperative to postoperative care, nursing plays a role in preventing potential complications, promoting overall comfort, and reducing anxiety through patient and family education. Through the team efforts of both the nursing staff and the surgical team, patients with appendicitis can have shorter hospitalizations with positive outcomes.

Bhangu, A., Søreide, K., Di Saverio, S., Assarsson, J. H., & Drake, F. T. (2015). Acute appendicitis: Modern understanding of pathogenesis, diagnosis, and management. *Lancet, 386*(10000), 1278–1287. doi:10.1016/s0140-6736(15)00275-5

Bishop, C. A., & Carter, M. E. (2013). Appendicitis. In N. T. Browne, L. M. Flanigan, C. A. McComiskey, & P. Pieper (Eds.), *Nursing care of the pediatric surgical patient* (3rd ed., pp. 407–415). Burlington, MA: Jones & Bartlett.

Brown, R. L. (2014). Appendicitis. In M. M. Ziegler, R. G. Azizkhan, D. von Allmen, & T. R. Weber (Eds.), *Operative pediatric surgery* (2nd ed., pp. 613–631). New York, NY: McGraw-Hill.

Butler, K. L. (2015). Acute appendicitis. In K. L. Butler & M. Harisinghani (Eds.), *Acute care surgery: Imaging essentials for rapid diagnosis* (pp. 79–86). New York, NY: McGraw-Hill.

Pennington, E. C., & Burke, P. A. (2015). Appendix. In G. M. Doherty (Ed.), *Current diagnosis & treatment: Surgery* (14th ed., pp. 651–656) New York, NY: McGraw-Hill.

Rentea, R. M., St. Peter, S. D., & Snyder, C. L. (2016). Pediatric appendicitis: State of the art review. *Pediatric Surgery International, 33*(3), 269–283. doi:10.1007/s00383-016-3990-2

Tian, Y., Heiss, K. F., Wulkan, M. L., & Raval, M. V. (2015). Assessment of variation in care and outcomes for pediatric appendicitis at children's and non-children's hospitals. *Journal of Pediatric Surgery, 50*, 1185–1892. doi:10.1016/J.JPEDSURG.2015.06.012

■ ASTHMA

Laurine Gajkowski

Overview

Asthma is a common chronic inflammatory disorder of the large and small airways. Varying degrees of airflow obstruction occur due to bronchial muscle constriction, edema of the tracheobronchial mucosa, and increased mucous secretions. Susceptible children have intermittent respiratory symptoms, such as wheezing, dyspnea, and cough, especially at night. In the United States, 6.3 million children or 8.6% of those younger than 18 years have a diagnosis of asthma (Clarke, Ward, & Schiller, 2016). It poses a burden on the affected children, the parents, and the community. Children with asthma can experience a decreased quality of life because of impairment of daily activities, emergency department visits, and school absences (Miadich, Everhart, Borschuk, Winter, & Fiese, 2015). Childhood asthma is associated with high rates of school absenteeism (Cicutto, Gleason, & Szefler, 2014), and exacerbations or "flare-ups" of symptoms are the leading cause of pediatric hospital admissions in the United States (Sylvester & George, 2014). Nurses provide acute care to these children in hospitals when the level of respiratory compromise is too severe to be managed at home. Nursing interventions in outpatient settings such as schools and clinics are aimed at assisting the child and family to assume responsibility for asthma management.

Background

According to Global Initiative for Asthma (GINA), asthma is characterized by chronic airway inflammation. It is defined by the history of respiratory symptoms such as wheeze, shortness of breath, chest tightness, and cough that vary over time and in intensity, together with variable expiratory airflow limitation (GINA, 2016). Asthma is a complex disease caused by an interplay of many genetic and environmental factors. "Atopy, the genetic predisposition for the development of an immunoglobulin E (IgE)-mediated response to common aeroallergens, is the strongest identifiable predisposing factor for developing asthma" (NAEPP, 2007, p. 11). Other risk factors include intrauterine exposures (cigarette smoke, inadequate nutrition, and stress), prematurity, viral respiratory infections in early childhood, early antibiotic use, obesity, acetaminophen use, emotional stress, and air pollution (Woodruff, Bhakta, & Fahy, 2016). A hygiene hypothesis suggests that the increasing prevalence of allergies and asthma may be related to modern society's emphasis on cleanliness, which leads to reduced early exposure to pathogens in children. There have been many theories about possible primary prevention strategies for the development of asthma, but none of them has been proven by existing evidence (Beasley, Semprini, & Mitchell, 2015).

The prevalence and severity of asthma are highest in certain vulnerable populations. According to the National Health Interview Survey, "For children under age 15 years, the sex-adjusted percentage by race and ethnicity (of children) who had an asthma episode in the past 12 months was 3.7% for Hispanic children, 3.5% for non-Hispanic White children, and 9.1% for non-Hispanic Black children" (Clarke et al., 2016, p. 99). This variability in prevalence, morbidity, and mortality may be attributable to many factors, including access to culturally competent health care, exposure to inflammatory agents such as air pollution in urban environments, coping with psychosocial stress, and exposure to substandard housing problems such as mold and roaches (Gruber et al., 2016).

Ongoing research in genetics and immunology is increasing our knowledge about the development of asthma. Once a child has developed this condition, ongoing inflammatory exposures seem to increase the risk of exacerbations and lead to progressive loss of pulmonary function. A range of indoor and outdoor allergens, as well as viral infections, food, medicine (beta-blockers, aspirin, or other nonsteroidal anti-inflammatory drugs [NSAIDs]), exercise, psychological stress, and weather changes may trigger a child's asthma symptoms. Common indoor triggers include secondhand smoke, dust mites, mold, rodents, cockroaches, fragrances, chemical particulate matter, and pet dander. Common outdoor allergens include ozone, pollen, and air pollution (U.S. Environmental Protection Agency [EPA], Indoor Environments Division, Office of Air and Radiation, 2015).

Initially, the diagnosis of asthma is based on the child's physical examination, history of respiratory symptoms, and pulmonary function test (spirometry). The most common spirometry measurement is the child's forced expiratory volume in 1 second (FEV_1), and it is reported as a percentage of the predicted value for the child's height and age. This measurement can demonstrate impaired airflow and airway hyper-responsiveness. The child's clinical response to inhaled and oral medications is also considered in classifying the child's asthma severity. The "Classification of Asthma Severity in Children" was written in the *2007 National Asthma Education and Prevention Program (NAEPP)* by the National Heart, Lung, and Blood Institute of the National Institutes of Health (2007). Symptom-based definitions are used to classify the severity as "intermittent," "mild persistent," "moderate persistent," or "severe persistent." A child classified with the mildest form, "intermittent asthma," has symptoms 2 or fewer days per week, has no nighttime awakenings, requires use of a rescue inhaler 2 or fewer days per week for symptom control, and has a normal FEV_1 between exacerbations. In contrast, a child with the most severe form, "severe persistent asthma," has symptoms throughout the day, nighttime awakenings every night, uses a rescue inhaler several times daily, has extremely limited activity, uses oral corticosteroids two or more times per year, and has an FEV_1 fewer than 60% predicted.

Clinical Aspects

The typical presentation of a child during an acute asthma episode is ill and uncomfortable, with rapid, labored respirations and a fatigued look from an ongoing struggle to breathe. Coughing, nasal flaring, intercostal retractions, and accessory muscle use may be observed along with complaints of chest tightness. The expiratory phase is prolonged. On auscultation, wheezing is heard on expiration and/or inspiration unless the episode is so severe that a "silent chest" develops because of extremely poor air exchange. The child prefers to sit in an upright position, leaning forward in the tripod position. If the episode progresses to hypoxia, the child becomes wide-eyed, agitated, and confused or suddenly quiet as ventilation becomes ineffective. Episodes that fail to respond to medications, oxygen therapy, and hydration (acute severe asthma, also called *status asthmaticus*) can lead to death from respiratory failure, so the child must be immediately moved to and treated in the intensive care unit.

ASSESSMENT

The pediatric nurse begins with a respiratory assessment that includes color, respiratory rate, heart rate, level of consciousness, quality of breath sounds, ability to speak in sentences rather than single words, presence of abnormal findings that indicate impaired gas exchange (wheezing, nasal flaring, retractions, grunting, accessory muscle use, head bobbing), and pulse oximetry measurement. The pediatric nurse must compare the child's heart and respiratory rate to the normal ranges based on the child's age. Tachypnea, tachycardia, and SpO_2 fewer than 92% indicate hypoxemia. In addition to a respiratory assessment, the nurse must determine the child's fluid status based on the child's weight, intake and output, and skin turgor. Once the child's condition is stable, the nurse can assess the child's developmental and psychosocial concerns, as well as the family's home asthma management history, using the Childhood Asthma Control Test (C-ACT) and the GINA (2016).

NURSING INTERVENTIONS, MANAGEMENT, AND IMPLICATIONS

During the acute phase of an asthma exacerbation, the pediatric nurse focuses on the child's risk for respiratory failure. Nursing interventions that eliminate the risk for respiratory failure include ongoing monitoring of breathing, supporting respiratory functioning (positioning, oxygen administration, hydration), and medication administration. Two categories of medications are commonly used to treat asthma: control and quick relief. Control medications are used on a daily basis to prevent an exacerbation. These include inhaled long-acting beta$_2$-agonists (LABAs), inhaled corticosteroids (ICSs), oral leukotriene receptor antagonists (LTRAs), and others. Quick-relief medications are used when needed for asthma flare-ups. These include inhaled short-acting beta$_2$-agonists (SABAs), oral corticosteroids, and inhaled anticholinergics. These medications are ordered according to the child's asthma-severity classification. Nursing care often follows a standardized asthma care pathway that outlines a sequence for assessments and interventions to be used for hospitalized children. Studies have shown that the use of clinical pathways has decreased the patient length of stay and lowered the cost of treatment. Unfortunately, pathway use has not been shown to reduce hospital readmission rates (Sylvester & George, 2014). Support of parental participation in the hospitalized child's care is often essential for the child's overall sense of well-being.

At every health encounter, asthma education for self-management is a priority. Each member of the interprofessional team, including the bedside nurse, hospitalist, respiratory therapist, primary care provider, asthma specialist, and school nurse, develops a partnership with the patient and family. Supportive, open communication among all team members helps to build trust and alleviate misconceptions. Parents may be instructed to keep a symptom diary to help identify triggers. Asthma control is achieved through avoidance of triggers, adherence to prescribed controller and maintenance therapy, and the family's ability to recognize symptoms and respond appropriately to them. Families may need help to view asthma management from a prevention perspective instead of viewing it from a crisis perspective (Archibald, Caine, Ali, Hartling, & Scott, 2015). Any child diagnosed with asthma should be provided with an individualized written asthma action plan that spells out specific guidelines for daily management when the child is symptom free (green zone), when the child's symptoms begin to increase (yellow zone), and when emergency care is indicated (red zone; GINA, 2016). The pediatric nurse ensures that the child and/or caregivers have a clear understanding of their Asthma Home Management Plan. When caring for a child, it is especially important to educate about the correct use of inhaler devices and give the child an opportunity to perform a return demonstration. Parents need information about ways to reduce allergens at home, such as encasing the child's mattress and pillow to control dust mites, or reducing molds by lowering humidity.

OUTCOMES

The expected outcome of quality nursing care for the child asthma patient is successful self-management through avoidance of triggers, early recognition and treatment with rescue medications, and compliance with an individualized asthma action plan that maintains daily control of symptoms.

Summary

Because there is no cure for asthma, the care of children with asthma should focus on successful home management to control symptoms. Nurses must be knowledgeable about the pathophysiology of asthma, prevention and management of exacerbations, and principles of health-maintenance education, and play a critical role in providing comprehensive family-centered asthma education that promotes a sense of shared responsibility.

Archibald, M. M., Caine, V., Ali, S., Hartling, L., & Scott, S. D. (2015). What is left unsaid: An interpretive description of the information needs of parents of children with asthma. *Research in Nursing & Health, 38*(1), 19–28. doi:10.1002/nur.21635

Beasley, R., Semprini, A., & Mitchell, E. A. (2015). Risk factors for asthma: Is prevention possible? *Lancet, 386*(9998), 1075–1085. doi:10.1016/S0140-6736(15)00156-7

Cicutto, L., Gleason, M., & Szefler, S. J. (2014). Establishing school-centered asthma programs. *Journal of Allergy and Clinical Immunology, 134*(6), 1223–1230. doi:10.1016/j.jaci.2014.10.004

Clarke, T. C., Ward, B. W., & Schiller, J. S. (2016). Early release of selected estimates based on data from the January–March 2016 National Health Interview Survey. Retrieved from https://www.cdc.gov/nchs/data/nhis/earlyrelease/earlyrelease201609.pdf

Global Initiative for Asthma. (2016). Global strategy for asthma management and prevention (2016 update). Retrieved from http://ginasthma.org/wp-content/uploads/2016/04/GINA-2016-main-report_tracked.pdf

Gruber, K. J., McKee-Huger, B., Richard, A., Byerly, B., Raczkowski, J. L., & Wall, T. C. (2016). Removing asthma triggers and improving children's health: The asthma partnership demonstration project. *Annals of Allergy, Asthma & Immunology, 116*(5), 408–414. doi:10.1016/j.anai.2016.03.025

Miadich, S. A., Everhart, R. S., Borschuk, A. P., Winter, M. A., & Fiese, B. H. (2015). Quality of life in children with asthma: A developmental perspective. *Journal of Pediatric Psychology, 40*(7), 672–679. doi:10.1093/jpepsy/jsv002

National Heart, Lung, and Blood Institute. (2007). National Asthma Education Prevention Program: Expert panel report 3: Guidelines for the diagnosis and management of asthma. Retrieved from http://www.nhlbi.nih.gov/files/docs/guidelines/asthgdln.pdf

Sylvester, A. M., & George, M. (2014). Effect of a clinical pathway on length of stay and cost of pediatric inpatient asthma admissions: An integrative review. *Clinical Nursing Research, 23*(4), 384–401. doi:10.1177/1054773813487373

U.S. Environmental Protection Agency, Indoor Environments Division, Office of Air and Radiation. (2015). Asthma facts. EPA-402-F-04-019. Retrieved from https://www.epa.gov/sites/production/files/2015-10/documents/asthma_fact_sheet_eng_july_30_2015_v2.pdf

Woodruff, P. G., Bhakta, N. R., & Fahy, J. V. (2016). Asthma: Pathogenesis and phenotypes. In V. C. Broaddus (Ed.), *Murray and Nadel's textbook of respiratory medicine* (6th ed., pp. 713–730). Philadelphia, PA: Elsevier Saunders.

■ AUTISM SPECTRUM DISORDER

Sheila Blank
Celeste M. Alfes

Overview

Autism spectrum disorder (ASD) is a neurodevelopmental disorder that can affect a child developmentally, neurologically, and socially. They may communicate, interact, behave, and learn in ways that are different from others. ASD has a wide range of symptoms, behaviors, developmental and social delays that can range from gifted to severely challenged. Some people with ASD require a lot of help in their daily lives; others require less. For this reason, autism truly is an individual disorder.

ASD has been affecting children for the past century but within the last 10 years at an increasingly rapid rate, increasing 123% from 2002 to 2010 (Centers for Disease Control and Prevention [CDC], 2016). Autism does not discriminate based on race, ethnicity, or socioeconomic groups. Autism is gender-specific affecting males 4.5 times more likely (1 in 42) than females. Children who have a sibling with ASD are at a higher risk of being diagnosed with ASD. In 2013, the *Diagnostic and Statistical Manual of Mental Disorders* (5th ed.; *DSM-5*; American Psychiatric Association, 2013) grouped the diagnosis of autism together with Asperger's syndrome, childhood disintegrative disorder, Rett syndrome, and pervasive developmental disorders not otherwise specified (PDD-NOS; American Psychiatric Association, 2013). Asperger's syndrome is a higher functioning form of autism. Childhood disintegrative disorder is when the child begins to develop normally meeting each developmental milestone on time until the age of 3 or 4 years; then the child begins regressing, losing language, motor or social skills they may have previously learned. Rett syndrome is a severe brain disorder where a child begins to develop normally in early life, but between 6 and 18 months of age, changes in the normal patterns of mental and social development begin. Pervasive developmental disorder affects communication and socialization.

Background

ASD is a neurodevelopmental disorder that affects intellect, communication, and socialization with an unknown cause. Much research has been done in the search for a cause and the only common theme is that much more research needs to be conducted. Research in a variety of areas indicates that the cause is multifaceted. Researchers alluded to genetics and environmental factors with a possible connection to ASD but nothing concrete has emerged (NINDS, 2016).

The CDC established red flag indicators, which can be detected in children with ASD as early as infancy and up to about the age of 3 years. Red flag indicators focus on areas of socialization, communication, development, and behaviors. Some indicators include lack of meeting developmental milestones at the appropriate age such as head lagging, delay of speech, and no cooing or babbling within the first 6 months of age. Infants are usually social by gesturing, smiling, or turning of the head when their name is called; however, if ASD is suspected, infants develop a flat affect and lack socialization (CDC, 2016). As the child grows, other indicators can include aggression, tantrums, social isolation, lack of eye contact, and speech delays. About 25% to 30% of children with ASD have some words at 12 to 18 months of age but may lose them as they grow older. By the age of 3 or 4 years, a child with ASD may demonstrate no eye contact, very noticeable speech delays, repetitive words or phrases (echolalia), or total lack of speech. About 40% of the children with ASD do not talk at all. These children may demonstrate developmental delays, gross motor or fine motor movement delays. Children with ASD may become socially isolated and use self-play, which leads to inappropriate play. They do not understand or use pretend play. Repetitive movements such as hand flapping, turning, bouncing, spinning, and toe-walking are seen. Aggression and injurious behaviors may increase as the child grows.

Clinical Aspects

ASSESSMENT

ASD can be diagnosed as early as 18 months of age but more commonly by the age of 3 or 4 years. Diagnosis is difficult because not all children develop at the same pace. If delays are noticed, children with delays will be monitored more closely than a normally developing child and may be referred for further testing. Physicians can perform a modified checklist for autism in toddlers as early as 16 to 30 months. The checklist is a screening tool that can indicate if further testing is necessary. The checklist is a series of questions about developmental growth. If a child fails two or more of the critical items, then a referral should be made for further testing. The referral is made to a developmental specialist and a multidisciplinary team is formed. The team includes a psychologist, neurologist, psychiatrist, and speech therapist and they perform a variety of neurological assessments, in-depth cognitive testing, language testing, and hearing testing. Direct observation of the child in a variety of settings and a thorough history provided by the parents are crucial in the diagnosis process.

Sensory disturbances can affect behaviors and increase anxiety in an individual with ASD, which will cause difficulty in gathering necessary health information to provide appropriate care. Touch, increased sounds, textures, smells, and overly bright rooms are all sensory stimuli that can affect individuals with ASD. Nurses are taught the art of compassion and the appropriate use of touch when caring for any patient, but nurses need to realize when caring for a patient with ASD that this art may have negative effects. The best way to approach a patient with ASD is to take it slow, with no time restraints, but persistence is needed. The nurse needs to establish a working rapport with the patient before gathering assessment information. A brief preference assessment is a tool used to find individual favorites that can be used as reinforcers. A reinforcer is an object, food, computer game, movie, or television show that the patient likes and should be used to reinforce positive behavior (Cooper, Heron, & Heward, 2006). By reinforcing positive behavior, the nurse begins to establish a comfort level with the patient.

NURSING INTERVENTIONS, MANAGEMENT, AND IMPLICATIONS

Providing nursing care for children with ASD can be a difficult task. Children with ASD communicate, learn, and socialize differently than typically developing children. The lack of understanding of verbal and nonverbal language makes it difficult for children to communicate effectively and may lead to increased stress (Prelock & Nelson, 2012). Children with ASD are easily distracted; therefore, communication needs to be concise and focused directly to the individual. Effective communication needs to be delivered slowly, softly, and in short sentences. This method allows time for the patient to understand and process information. A communication board or picture exchange communication system (PECS) can be used to express an individual's needs and wants during a hospital stay or physician visit and can be customized for each patient to promote individual communication.

Health care visits or hospital stays can be difficult for individuals with ASD because of ineffective communication, sensory issues, understanding expectations, and general feelings of fear and anxiety (Prelock & Nelson, 2012). Children with ASD are very rigid in their daily routines and do not handle change well. Caregivers need to plan for health care visits and explain to individuals with ASD what to expect at each visit. Picture books or story books can be developed and read to the individual to promote understanding of what will be done at each visit and increase comfort level that can produce more accurate results during each visit. Role modeling is another technique that can be used to demonstrate what to expect at physician appointments and hospital stays, and the testing that needs to be done.

OUTCOMES

As shown throughout the literature, children diagnosed with ASD grow up and transition into adulthood. Numerous schools are available for children with ASD up until middle school years. A smaller number of high schools are available as the children grow and then education seems to drift off. Children with ASD need continued education to manage behaviors, learn, socialize, and communicate appropriately, and we need to continue that into the high school area and into young adult and adulthood.

Summary

Children with ASD lack socialization and communication, and have cognitive and developmental delays. Research has found that early diagnosis by age 3 or 4 years and intervention help some children with ASD better manage their behaviors and learn ways to cope with their deficits in an attempt to live a more typical life. To date, researchers have not been able to determine a concrete cause for ASD. With the increased numbers of children being diagnosed, efforts to improve the lives of children affected with ASD are needed.

American Psychiatric Association. (2013). *Diagnostic and statistical manual of mental disorders* (5th ed.). Arlington, VA: American Psychiatric Publishing.

Centers for Disease Control and Prevention. (2016). Autism spectrum disorder (ADS): Data and statistics. Retrieved from http://www.cdc.gov/ncbddd/autism/data.html

Cooper, J. O., Heron, T. E., & Heward W. L. (2006). *Applied behavior analysis* (2nd ed.). Upper Saddle River, NJ: Prentice Hall.

National Institute of Neurological Disorders and Stroke. (2016). Autism spectrum disorder fact sheet. Retrieved from http://www.ninds.nih.gov/disorders/autism/detail_autism.htm

Prelock, P. J., & Nelson N. W. (2012). Language and communication in autism: An integrated view. *Pediatric Clinics of North America, 59*(1), 129–145. doi:10.1016/j.pcl.2011.10.008

■ BRONCHIOLITIS RESPIRATORY SYNCYTIAL VIRUS

Shannon Courtney Wong

Overview

Bronchiolitis occurs when a viral or bacterial infection invades the lower respiratory tract, causing inflammation and obstruction of the bronchioles (Ball, Bindler, Cowen, & Shaw, 2017). While there are a variety of viruses that can cause bronchiolitis, respiratory syncytial virus (RSV) is the leading cause of bronchiolitis, and the leading cause of severe lower respiratory tract infections in young children (Walsh, 2017). Bronchiolitis occurs when a viral or bacterial infection invades the lower respiratory tract, causes inflammation and obstruction of the bronchioles (Ball et al., 2017). RSV attacks and kills the mucosal cells lining the small bronchi and bronchioles, obstructing the bronchioles and irritating the airway (Ball et al., 2017). This irritation leads to excessive mucus production, cough, wheezing, hyperexpansion of the lungs, hypoxia, and respiratory distress (Zhou et al., 2015). Current nursing care for infants and young children with RSV bronchiolitis focuses on supporting the child, maintaining respiratory function, and supporting fluid balance and rest.

Background

According to the Centers for Disease Control and Prevention (CDC), RSV infections lead to 57,527 hospitalizations and 2.1 million outpatient visits among children younger than 5 years old in the United States each year (CDC, 2016). In fact, RSV is the most important reason previously healthy infants are admitted to the hospital, predominantly due to an immature immune system and smaller dimensions of the airways of the lungs of infants and young children (Pickles & DeVincenzo, 2015). Infants who were born prematurely are at an even higher risk for a RSV infection causing hospitalization than infants born at term (Figueras-Aloy et al., 2016).

RSV is an extremely common infection, and by the age of 2 years, almost all children have been infected with RSV at least once (Figueras-Aloy et al., 2016). The transmission of RSV happens most effectively through contact of nasal secretions; RSV can survive for several hours on hard surfaces and hands, so the virus is transmitted via direct contact with objects that have been contaminated (Walsh, 2017). The season for RSV infections in the United States starts in October, peaks in December through February, and finishes in March or April (Bont et al., 2016).

Although all people contract RSV several times throughout their lifetimes, infants and young children are at the greatest risk for severe complications from the virus. The risk factors for an RSV infection progressing to severe bronchiolitis have been identified: less than 3 months at the time of infection, premature birth, and/or underlying immunodeficiency or cardiopulmonology disease

(Pickles & DiVincenzo, 2015). These risk factors are all important, but the age of infection seems to be the most significant risk factor. In fact, 80% of infants hospitalized with a RSV infection younger than the age of 2 months had no significant past medical history (Pickles & DiVincenzo, 2015). Additionally, studies have shown that the disease can impact a child long after the child's hospital discharge. In fact, children who were hospitalized as infants with RSV bronchiolitis have a higher prevalence of asthma when compared to matched control infants (Mejias & Ramillo, 2015).

RSV bronchiolitis should be considered in any infant presenting with acute symptoms of lower respiratory tract infections, especially during the winter months (Pickles & DiVincenzo, 2015). A conclusive diagnosis is made by taking a posterior nasopharyngeal wash or swab specimen and conducting an enzyme-linked immunoabsorbent assay (ELISA) or a immunofluorescent assay to identify the specific virus causing the symptoms (Ball et al., 2017). Additionally, a chest radiograph should be obtained. A child with bronchiolitis will have a chest x-ray showing hyperinflation, patchy atelectasis, and signs of inflammation (Ball et al., 2017). Clinical manifestations can also support a diagnosis of RSV. Children with an RSV infection will present with nasal congestion, cough, intermittent low-grade fever, wheezing, tachypnea, and poor feeding, with possible vomiting or diarrhea (Ball et al., 2017; Pickles & DiVincenzo, 2015). A child with a more significant infection will present with increased tachypnea, significant wheezing and coughing, poor fluid intake, and a distended abdomen, related to hyperexpansion in the lungs (Ball et al., 2017; Pickles & DiVincenzo, 2015).

Clinical Aspects

ASSESSMENT

The most important areas to assess in a young child presenting with RSV bronchiolitis are the child's airway and respiratory function. This can be done using good observation skills noting how quickly the infant is breathing and if retractions are noted, and by using pulse oximetry to determine oxygenation (Ball et al., 2017). Infants with RSV bronchiolitis can progress into severe disease quite easily, but identifying which patients will exhibit a progressively worse disease is difficult (Mejias & Ramillo, 2015), making the need for close observation of subtle changes in patients' status important. Parental and caregiver education also becomes very important, as many children with an RSV infection can be managed at home. The families need to help their child by encouraging rest, proper fluid intake and comfort, while being able to recognize when the patient's status may be declining (Potts & Mandleco, 2012). Children who are showing signs of respiratory distress and/or dehydration may require hospitalization. A hospitalized infant with RSV bronchiolitis may require humidified oxygen, nasal suctioning, intravenous (IV) fluids, input and output (I&O) monitoring, and daily weights (Ball et al., 2017).

As previously mentioned, treatments for RSV are mostly supportive therapies. At this time, there is no specific treatment for RSV, and medications are generally not prescribed for RSV infections (Ball et al., 2017). Palivizumab (Synagis) is a medication given to protects infants from RSV, but it is reserved for only high-risk infants who meet criteria outlined by the American Academy of Pediatrics (Walsh, 2017). This medication is given monthly, up to five times, during an infant's first winter, and it provides a passive immunity protection (Ball et al., 2017; Walsh, 2017).

NURSING INTERVENTIONS, MANAGEMENT, AND IMPLICATIONS

One of the most important nursing-related problems surrounding RSV of the hospitalized infant is being careful to not spread this contagious disease from one patient to another. Proper handwashing and isolation precautions for the RSV patient are crucial. These patients require contact precautions, which include gloves and gowns (Walsh, 2017). It is also important to continually promote adequate respiratory status, fluid balance, nutrition, rest, and comfort (Ball, Bindler, Cowen, & Shaw, 2017). Finally, nursing professionals must educate the parents and caregivers about the disease and its normal progression. Parents will need guidance in understanding bronchiolitis and respiratory distress, and recognizing signs and symptoms their infant's disease is getting more severe or improving. Additionally, parents and family may need emotional support due to the stress of the child's hospitalization and caring for a sick infant (Ball & Bindler, 2017).

OUTCOMES

The expected outcome of nursing care for an infant infected with RSV is complete recovery without further complications. Within 24 to 72 hours, the production of mucus will begin to decrease, aiding in improved respiratory function (Ball & Bindler, 2017). Once the virus runs its course, most infants and young children return to their pre-RSV health. Their breathing and feeding patterns should return to normal, and any weight lost because of poor feeding should be regained quickly. The incidence of reinfection can occur, but as the child grows, the severity of the disease will lessen. As noted before, there is a higher incidence of children who were severely infected with RSV and required hospitalization, acquiring asthma later in life (Meijias & Ramilo, 2015), making an RSV infection an important component of the patient's medical history.

Summary

A RSV infection in infants and young children can differ in its severity, making it vital for health care professionals to recognize subtle changes in the patients' status, especially related to respiratory function. Early recognition, supportive nursing interventions and thorough parent/caregiver teaching are crucial in managing patients infected with RSV.

Ball, J., Bindler, R., Cowen, K., & Shaw, M. (2017). *Principles of pediatric nursing: Caring for children* (7th ed.). New York, NY: Pearson.

Bont, L., Checchia, P., Fauroux, B., Figueras-Aloy, J., Manzoni, P., Paes, B., . . . Carbonell-Estrany, X. (2016). Defining the epidemiology and burden of severe respiratory syncytial virus infection among infants and children in Western countries. *Infectious Diseases and Therapy, 5*(3), 271–298. doi:10.1007/s40121-016-0123-0

Centers for Disease Control and Prevention. (2016). Respiratory syncytial virus infection (RSV). Retrieved from https://www.cdc.gov/rsv/research/us-surveillance.html

Figueras-Aloy, J., Manzoni, P., Paes, B., Simões, E., Bont, L., Checchia, P., . . . Carbonell-Estrany, X. (2016). Defining the risk and associated morbidity and mortality of severe respiratory syncytial virus infection among preterm infants without chronic lung disease or congenital heart disease. *Infectious Diseases and Therapy, 5*(4), 417–452. doi:10.1007/s40121-016-0130-1

Mejias, A., & Ramilo, O. (2015). New options in the treatment of respiratory syncytial virus disease. *Journal of Infection, 71*, S80–S87. doi:10.1016/j.jinf.2015.04.025

Pickles, R., & DeVincenzo, J. (2015). Respiratory syncytial virus (RSV) and its propensity for causing bronchiolitis. *The Journal of Pathology, 235*(2), 266–276. doi:10.1002/path.4462

Potts, N., & Mandleco, B. (2012). *Pediatric nursing: Caring for children and their families* (3rd ed.). Clifton Park, NY: Delmar.

Walsh, E. (2017). Respiratory syncytial virus infection: An illness for all ages. *Clinics in Chest Medicine, 38*(1), 29–36. doi:10.1016/j.ccm.2016.11.010

Zhou, L., Xiao, Q., Zhao, Y., Huang, A., Ren, L., & Liu, E. (2015). The impact of viral dynamics on the clinical severity of infants with respiratory syncytial virus bronchiolitis. *Journal of Medical Virology, 87*(8), 1276–1284. doi:10.1002/jmv.24111

■ BURNS: CLASSIFICATION AND SEVERITY

Melanie Gibbons Hallman
Lamon Norton

Overview

Burns result from thermal, electrical, chemical, mechanical, or radioactive injury to tissues. The extent of burn depth varies from superficial, involving the epidermis, to deeper structures, including muscle, bone, and organs, particularly the lungs (Stavrou et al., 2014). The cardiovascular and nervous systems are significantly impacted by electrical and lightning insults, potentially resulting in immediate cardiac or respiratory arrest (Moore, 2015b). Each year, more than 265,000 deaths occur worldwide related to burns, producing life-altering changes for victims and their families (Zuo, Medina, & Tredget, 2017). Serious burns result in a cascade of physiological responses that can influence morbidity and mortality for affected patients (Jewo & Fadeyibi, 2015).

Background

Annually, more than 500,000 people in the United States are evaluated in emergency departments for burns annually. Burns and fires are the fifth most common cause of accidental death in children and adults, and account for an estimated 3,500 adult and child deaths per year. Burn-risk is highest in children. Younger children are more likely to sustain scald burns, whereas children older than 6 years of age are more likely to experience burns from flames. Toddlers and children are more often burned by a scalding or flames and nearly 75% of all scalding burns in children are preventable. Most children ages 4 and younger who are hospitalized for burn-related injuries suffer from scald burns (65%) or contact burns (20%). Children with scald burns that have clear lines of demarcation and in a stocking or glove formation should be evaluated for child abuse (Hazinski, Mondozzi, & Baker 2014).

Hot tap water burns cause more deaths and hospitalizations than burns from any other hot liquids. The most common etiologies of burns are thermal (flame, steam, scalds), electrical (alternating current [AC] and direct current [DC], lightning) and chemical (alkaline and acid). The length of time that tissues are exposed to a burn source, the intensity of the source, and skin thickness determine the degree of burn (Rau, Spears, & Petruska, 2014). Burns impart injury by damaging skin surfaces, by impairing airways and lungs via inhalation burns, and by ingesting chemicals or objects capable of causing mucosal burns. Multiple organs, tissues, and body systems are susceptible to burns as primary or secondary injuries. Complications of burn shock, infection, respiratory compromise, and multisystem organ failure may result in death (Stavrou et al., 2014). Prevention or rapid correction of these complications is essential to achieving desirable outcomes for burn victims.

Thermal burns may directly affect only the epidermis and dermis, or may involve deeper structures of fat, muscle, and bone. The extent of injury caused by electrical burns is determined by the type of electrical current; either low voltage (less than a 1,000 volts) or high voltage (more than 1,000 volts). Severity is also determined by the length of time the victim is in contact with an electrical current. Lower voltage and less time exposed to the electrical source usually impart less severe injury (Moore, 2015b). Chemical burns require early identification and rapid decontamination and treatment. The concentration and acidity or alkalinity of a chemical, combined with the length of time the skin or mucosa is exposed to the agent, determine the significance of a chemical burn (Moore, 2015a).

Burn depth is categorized as first (superficial), second (partial thickness), and third degree (full thickness), with a deepest fourth-degree category being possible (Zuo et al., 2017). First-degree burns commonly are superficial and involve the epidermis only, requiring little or no treatment. Second-degree burns include both superficial and deep partial-thickness burns. Superficial partial-thickness burns include injuries to the epidermis and the outermost dermis. Redness, swelling, and discomfort or pain accompany these burns. Deep partial-thickness burns damage both the epidermal and dermal layers, causing necrosis and intercellular edema, resulting in blister formation. Second-degree burns are typically more painful than first-degree burns, with loss of skin integrity and subsequent fluid depletion. Full-thickness burns damage the epidermis, dermis, and subcutaneous tissue. Tissue necrosis evolves, producing eschar (leathery, sloughing, dead tissue) and leaving no protective barrier for remaining structures. Eschar increases the risk for bacterial infection in burns. Edema, inflammation, and vasodilation accompany this type of burn, and little or no sensation remains (Rau et al., 2014). Complications, including shock, infection, respiratory compromise, and multisystem organ failure are common in burn injuries and evolve during the acute phase of injury (Stavrou et al., 2014).

Clinical Aspects

Determining the percentage of total body surface area (TBSA) and depth of burns is an early step in burn resuscitation (Stavrou et al., 2014). Selection of appropriate resuscitation fluid and the correct amount to infuse over the first 24 hours following burn injury directly affect burn wound healing and chances for survival (Cancio, 2014). There are multiple tools available to calculate the approximate area of burns in the prehospital and acute phase settings. The rule of nines, modified Lund and Browder chart, and Parkland formula are among the most common measurement systems used for this purpose. More advanced methods for determining burn extent, such as laser Doppler imaging, may be initiated 2 to 5 days following preliminary burn resuscitation in order to avoid over-resuscitation with fluids, which poses an additional danger to patient outcomes (Martin, Lundy, & Rickard, 2014). The starting point for fluid resuscitation is typically between 2 and 4 mL/kg/TBSA/24 hr (Lundy et al., 2016).

ASSESSMENT

Evaluation and definitive management of airway, breathing, circulation, and fluid resuscitation are the most crucial elements of care for burn patients with life-threatening injuries. Early intubation is imperative for patients sustaining airway burns. A detailed history of injury, including time, mechanism, voltage if electrical source of injury, details of decontamination for chemical sources, a chemical safety data sheet if available, associated trauma, syncope, smoke exposure, abuse potential, and prehospital treatment should be obtained. Wet linens should be rapidly replaced with sterile dry linens. All jewelry and clothing should be removed, and careful evaluation of nonburn injuries should be done. Placement of urinary catheter and nasogastric tube should be accomplished during the reassessment phase of care (Cancio, 2014).

NURSING INTERVENTIONS, MANAGEMENT, AND IMPLICATIONS

Multiple factors must be considered following the acute phase of burn resuscitation. Hypothermia is an early complication of burns. The greater the surface area burned, the more vulnerable the patient is to development of hypothermia. It is important that the patient be kept warm and dry in order to conserve energy expended from the postburn hypermetabolic state. Persistent hypermetabolism and muscle wasting in extensive burns requires early nutritional reinforcement, but balancing calories and the composition of nutrients must be individualized to avoid overconsumption and increased risk for hyperglycemia (Rowan et al., 2015). Pruritus (itching) is an unfortunate and very common result of burns. It occurs in almost every pediatric burn patient, and in as much as 87% of affected adults. Itching may not respond favorably to anti-inflammatory drugs and other analgesics (Stavrou et al., 2014). Optimal management of pruritus should be addressed after patient stabilization during hospitalization, and in discharge planning.

Contractures manifest related to loss of skin elasticity, and pose great risk of loss of physical function. Mobilization of joints should begin as soon as possible during hospitalization. Essentially every body system and organ can be affected following a significant burn injury. Duodenal ulcers, anemia, hypermetabolic syndrome, insulin resistance, and liver dysfunction may develop in response to injury. In addition, other common sequelae, including central nervous system inflammation, cardiac dysfunction, and respiratory compromise, may develop. Compartment syndrome from circumferential burns may develop acutely, necessitating escharotomy or fasciotomy in any area of the body. Kidneys may be damaged by lactic acidosis and urine myoglobin production (Rau et al., 2014). Elevation in urine myoglobin levels is commonly associated with rhabdomyolysis, an associated complication of significant burn injuries (Moore, 2015b). Monitoring urine output is important in guiding titration of fluid resuscitation. It is important that IV fluids for burn resuscitation be initiated early, and that fluid intake and output be accurately measured, recorded, and reported. The urine output goal for adults is 30 to 50 mL/hr, and for children, weighing 30 kg or less, 1 mL/kg/hr (Lundy et al., 2016).

Deep vein thrombosis (DVT) prevention strategies should begin immediately in burn patients, since these injuries result in a hypercoagulable state (Zuo et al., 2017). Nurses should anticipate initiation of anticoagulant prophylaxis therapy. Burn severity impacts the degree of pain that patients experience. Long-term pain and sensory dysfunction accompany more extensive burns. Acutely burned patients may experience pain in the form of many abnormal sensations, including burning, dullness, itching, and dysesthesia (Rau et al., 2014). Frequent pain assessment and response to specific medications are important to determine the most effective pain treatment options for individual patients.

OUTCOMES

Prevention of infection in burn patients is crucial to survival. Burn sepsis typically presents within the first week postinjury. The most common causes of burn sepsis include pneumonia, central vascular access devices, and burn-injured skin. It is essential that health care workers maintain sterile technique and adhere to strict infection control practices while caring for burn patients. Antibiotic selection is carefully determined by specimen cultures to avoid pathogen resistance (Zuo et al., 2017). Significant burn wounds often require wound debridement and advanced wound care. Skin grafting is necessary for almost all full-thickness burns. Aesthetic changes related to deeper burns can have lasting effects on mental, emotional, and social well-being. Anxiety and depression are common especially within the first year after injury. Symptoms of posttraumatic stress disorder may emerge during the recovery process (Stavrou et al., 2014). Psychosocial support is essential in provision of holistic patient care, and to improve long-term outcomes.

Rapid communication with a regional burn center is advised by American Burn Association guidelines for patients with burn extent greater than 10% TBSA. Patients with inhalation injuries; burns associated with trauma; burns of the hands, feet, perineum, genitalia, or over major joints regardless of surface area burned; any third-degree burn; electrical, chemical, or lightning injuries; pediatric patients; and special needs patients, including those with social, emotional, or rehabilitation needs, require consultation with a burn center (Cancio, 2014).

Summary

Burn injuries pose significant challenges to children of all ages related to acute and long-term care. Children are much more vulnerable to changes in the temperature of the environment because they produce and lose heat faster than adults. Knowing what to do in case a burn or thermal injury occurs can help prevent a medical emergency. Nurses should remain current and knowledgeable regarding burn pathophysiology, assessment, and treatment significant to the pediatric population. Awareness of the most current evidence-based care available to burn patients assists nurses to provide them relative and efficient care.

Cancio, L. C. (2014). Initial assessment and fluid resuscitation of burn patients. *Surgical Clinics of North America, 94*(4), 741–754. doi:10.1016/j.suc.2014.05.003

Hazinski, M. F., Mondozzi, M. A., & Baker, R. A. U. (2014). Shock, multiple organ dysfunction syndrome, and burns in children. In K. L. McCance, S. E. Huether, V. L. Brashers, & N. S. Rote (Eds.), *Pathophysiology: The biologic basis for disease in adults and children* (7th ed., pp. 1699–1727). St. Louis, MO: Elsevier.

Jewo, P. I., & Fadeyibi, I. O. (2015). Progress in burns research: A review of advances in burn pathophysiology. *Annals of Burns and Fire Disasters, 28*(2), 105–115.

Lundy, J. B., Chung, K. K., Pamplin, J. C., Ainsworth, C. R., Jeng, J. C., & Friedman, B. C. (2016). Update on severe burn management for the intensivist. *Journal of Intensive Care Medicine, 31*(8), 499–510. doi:10.1177/0885066615592346

Martin, N. A. J., Lundy, J. B., & Rickard, R. F. (2014). Lack of precision of burn surface area calculation by UK Armed Forces medical personnel. *Burns, 40,* 246–250. doi:10.1016/j.burns.2013.05.009

Moore, K. (2015a). Hot topics: Chemical burns in the emergency department. *Journal of Emergency Nursing, 41*(4), 364–365. doi:10.1016/j.jen.2015.04.017

Moore, K. (2015b). Hot topics: Electrical injuries in the emergency department. *Journal of Emergency Nursing, 41*(5), 455–456. doi:10.1016/j.jen.2015.06.006

Rau, K. K., Spears, R. C., & Petruska, J. C. (2014). The prickly, stressful business of burn pain. *Experimental Neurology, 261,* 752–756. doi:10.1016/j.expneurol.2014.08.023

Rowan, M. P., Cancio, L. C., Elster, E. A., Burmeister, D. M., Rose, L. F., Natesan, S., . . . Chung, K. K. (2015). Burn wound healing and treatment: Review and advancements. *Critical Care, 19*(1), 243–255. doi:10.1186/s13054-015-0961-2

Stavrou, D., Weissman, O., Tessone, A., Zilinsky, I., Holloway, S., Boyd, J., & Haik, J. (2014). Health related quality of life in burn patients—A review of the literature. *Burns, 40*(5), 788–796. doi:10.1016/j.burns.2013.11.014

Zuo, K. J., Medina, A., & Tredget, E. E. (2017). Important developments in burn care. *Plastic and Reconstructive Surgery, 139*(1), 120e–138e. doi:10.1097/PRS.0000000000002908

■ CANCERS OF CHILDHOOD

Breanne M. Roche

Overview

Cancer develops when a single cell proliferates uncontrollably and the cell is independent of the laws governing the remainder of the body. The balance between cellular division and cellular loss is disrupted leading to uncontrolled cellular growth. According to the National Cancer Institute (NCI) in 2017, there was an estimated 10,270 new cases of cancer in children aged 0 to 14 years in the United States (NCI, 2017). Childhood cancer is a devastating diagnosis that can affect family dynamics. Nurses are at the forefront of care when it comes to caring for the child with an oncological disease.

Background

Fewer than 1% of all cancers are found in children (American Cancer Society, 2016). Out of more than 10,000 new cases annually, about 10% of these children die from their disease (NCI, 2017). Although survival rates continue to improve, and more than 80% of children with cancer survive 5 years or more, cancer remains the leading cause of death from disease among children (American Cancer Society, 2016). The types of cancer that develop in children are different from those in adults. The most common types of childhood cancers aged 0 to 14 years include acute lymphocytic leukemia (ALL), brain tumors, and neuroblastoma. The adolescent and young adult (AYA) aged 15 to 29 years population is a unique group of patients. The incidence of cancer in this age group represents 2% of all cancers. The most common types of cancers in the United States for patients aged 15 to 19 years old include lymphoma, germ cell tumors, brain tumors, malignant melanoma, and ALL (Kline, 2014).

The etiology of childhood cancer is unknown although it is likely that the interaction among many different factors both environmental and host contribute to its development (Kline, 2014). Only 5% of all childhood cancers are caused by an inherited mutation (NCI, 2017). With an inherited mutation, there are DNA changes in every cell in the body that may be linked to an increased risk to develop cancer, or these inherited mutations lead to syndromes that can predispose a child to cancer (American Cancer Society, 2016). For example, children with Down syndrome are at increased risk for the development of ALL and acute myelogenous leukemia (Fragkandrea, Nixon, & Panagopoulou, 2013). Most pediatric cancers are not caused by inherited DNA changes, but rather they develop as a result of an acquired mutation that occurs in one cell in the body during cellular division, and it has the potential to escape apoptosis and proliferate uncontrollably (American Cancer Society, 2016). Unlike adult cancers, lifestyle factors are not associated with the development of childhood cancer. There are a few environmental factors such as radiation exposure that may increase a child's risk for the development of cancer.

Cancer diagnosis in children is often delayed because the presenting symptoms are nonspecific and resemble benign conditions like a common viral illness (Fragkandrea et al., 2013). The diagnosis of pediatric cancer includes a thorough history and examination, labs, imaging, or tissue biopsy. There is oftentimes a lag time between presenting symptoms and diagnosis, which creates a great deal of uncertainty for the family. Treatment varies according to the type of malignancy and may include chemotherapy, radiation therapy, surgery, or bone marrow transplant.

Clinical Aspects

ASSESSMENT

Nursing assessment is a vital component in caring for the oncological child and may vary depending on the type of malignant process. Most signs and symptoms of childhood cancer are because of the following: (a) changes in blood cell production owing to bone marrow infiltration by tumor or an acute or chronic disease, (b) a mass resulting in compression of vital structures or organs, and (c) tumor by-products causing electrolyte disturbances or altered immunologic responses (Kline, 2014). Effective nursing care for pediatric oncology patients includes accurate records of history, physical examination, and lab values. The nurse must be able to recognize abnormal laboratory findings in association with physical examination findings to create and execute an effective nursing care plan.

Physical examination findings will be correlated with common chief complaints. Examination findings related to alterations in blood cell production include pallor (conjunctivae, oral mucosa, nail beds, and skin), petechiae or purpura, fever, infection, or fatigue (Kline, 2014). Dermatological findings are oftentimes associated with bone marrow function (Fragkandrea et al., 2013). A mediastinal mass may be present in a newly diagnosed patient with leukemia, lymphoma, neuroblastoma or other abdominal/pelvic tumors that can cause respiratory compromise. Examination may indicate signs of respiratory distress, including retractions, nasal flaring, grunting, and wheezing. An abdominal mass could be indicative of a tumor, hepatosplenomegaly, distended bladder, or retained stool (Kline, 2014). Symptoms associated with an abdominal mass may include gastrointestinal (nausea, vomiting, constipation or diarrhea), urinary (hematuria, retention), or respiratory (dyspnea related to increased abdominal pressure). Signs and symptoms of central nervous system (CNS) tumors vary according to the location of the tumor but may include loss of developmental milestones, irritability, early morning or post-nap headaches, cranial nerve palsies, diplopia, nystagmus, or ataxia (Kline, 2014).

Accurate record of vital signs is imperative in the oncological child. A fever is a medical emergency and not a symptom in these patients, but rather an indication of an underlying problem that has the potential to rapidly progress to life-threatening sepsis in an immunocompromised patient (Kline, 2014). Rectal temperatures are avoided in these patients because of potential injury of the rectal mucosa and a patient's risk of thrombocytopenia and neutropenia leading to unintentional bleeding or infection. Chills are a serious implication that a fever is brewing and could be one of the first signs of the showering of bacteria in the bloodstream. Tachycardia is a common sign that may be from anemia, anxiety, hypovolemia, shock, fever, or pain. Tachypnea may be a sign caused by anxiety, hypoxia, fever, pain, or respiratory compromise. Hypotension is a medical emergency and rapid fluid resuscitation is critical to prevent septic shock, hemorrhage, or dehydration.

Nursing assessment also includes monitoring for signs of toxicity related to therapy and oncological emergencies. Chemotherapy agents, radiation therapy, or biological response modifiers can all cause toxicity to the child with cancer (Kline, 2014). Understanding therapy-related side effects would help the nurse develop a safe nursing care plan. Oncological emergencies are life-threatening events that can occur during the treatment course of the child with cancer (Kline, 2014). They include hyperleukocytosis, tumor lysis syndrome, septic shock, typhlitis, spinal cord compression, and the inappropriate antidiuretic hormone secretion syndrome (Kline, 2014). Thorough nursing assessment can lead to early recognition of oncologic emergencies and rapid intervention preventing complications.

Proper assessment of the child with cancer is ongoing from diagnosis through survivorship. Children who have survived cancer are at risk for late effects of cancer treatment, and therefore meticulous assessment of late effects is imperative. Late effects of cancer treatment depend on the type of therapy used, which may affect every organ of the body.

NURSING INTERVENTIONS, MANAGEMENT, AND IMPLICATIONS

Every organ system in the body could be compromised with an oncological process. Nursing care of the child with cancer should focus on the prevention of infection, education and anticipatory guidance to the patient and caregivers regarding diagnosis, treatment, and medications. Some of the more common nursing-related problems include bone marrow suppression, impairment of the immune system leading to an increased risk of infection, altered electrolytes as a result of malignancy or therapy, nausea and vomiting associated with chemotherapy agents, and altered family dynamics related to a cancer diagnosis.

Nursing management for the child with cancer is comprehensive and family-centered. It is focused on managing the treatment side effects while providing ongoing education to the patient and family. With chemotherapy, bone marrow suppression is an expected side effect, and therefore, nurses must be comfortable educating families regarding blood counts and routine administration of blood products. Nursing interventions also include assessing for evidence of infection, and understanding a fever is a medical emergency. With a fever, nurses should anticipate clinician orders such as obtaining blood cultures from each lumen of a central line and antibiotic administration. Nursing care also includes providing emotional support to the patient and family during this vulnerable time period. Supportive care measures must be part of the nursing care plan and include managing post-op pain from surgical resection, a new central line placement, or advanced disease and nausea, vomiting, constipation, fatigue, and mucositis.

OUTCOMES

Outcomes when caring for the child with cancer include safe chemotherapy administration, improved treatment delivery, and proper education for the patient and family regarding the diagnosis and treatment, minimizing side effects from therapy, improving the quality of life for the child, and monitoring for late effects of cancer treatment in the pediatric cancer survivor. Palliative care plays a crucial role for these children and families. If a child reaches the end-of-life spectrum, outcomes include a safe transition to the end-of-life continuum, respecting and honoring the patient and family, and effective symptom management control.

Summary

Childhood cancer is rare, but the nurse caring for these children and families has a pivotal role from diagnosis throughout treatment and survivorship. Accurate physical examinations, assessment of vital signs and potential complications, and recognizing anticipated side effects of therapy are crucial components for the oncology nurse.

American Cancer Society. (2016). Key statistics for childhood cancers. Retrieved from http://www.cancer.org/cancer/cancerinchildren/detailedguide/cancer-in-children-key-statistics

Fragkandrea, J., Nixon, J. A., & Panagopoulou, P. (2013). Signs and symptoms of childhood cancer: A guide for early recognition. *American Family Physician, 88*(3), 185–192. Retrieved from https://www.aafp.org/afp/2013/0801/p185.html

Kline, N. (Ed). (2014). *Essentials of pediatric hematology/oncology nursing* (4th ed.). Chicago, IL: Association of Pediatric Hematology/Oncology Nurses.

National Cancer Institute. (2017). Childhood cancers. Retrieved from https://www.cancer.gov/types/childhood-cancers

■ CEREBRAL PALSY

Rachael Weigand

Overview

Cerebral palsy (CP) is defined as "a group of disorders of the development of movement and posture, causing activity limitation that are attributed to nonprogressive disturbances that occurred in the developing fetal or infant brain. The motor disorders of CP are often accompanied by disturbances of sensation, cognition, communication, perception, or behavior, and may be accompanied by a seizure disorder" (Jackson Allen, Vessey, & Schapiro, 2010, p. 326). The damage to the brain is nonprogressive; however, the effects of CP can worsen with time, growth, and maturity.

CP occurs in approximately two out of every 1,000 births and is the most common physical disability in childhood (Kirby et al., 2011). The incidence, prevalence, and most common causes of cerebral palsy vary over time because of continuing changes in prenatal and pediatric care. CP is a chronic disorder affecting multiple different body systems. Many different elements must be dealt with to manage children diagnosed with this disorder, including motor disability.

Background

The classification of CP is based on the type and distribution of the motor disruption. The damage has occurred in the motor cortex and pyramidal tracts in the brain. The severity and distribution of the neurological impairments vary significantly among children. There are four types of movement disorders seen in children with CP. These types are spastic, dystonia, athetosis, and ataxia. Children can fall under a "mixed" category, but only if there is a clear description of each type of movement disorder present (Jackson Allen et al., 2010).

Spasticity is characterized by increased muscle tone and is the most common motor difficulty (Hasnat & Rice, 2015). The signs of spastic CP include persistent primitive reflexes, such as an ongoing Moro reflex, rooting reflex, palmar reflex, exaggerated stretch reflexes, positive Babinski reflex, ankle clonus, and development of contractures as the child grows (Jackson Allen et al., 2010). Spastic CP affects 70% to 80% of children with CP (Delgado et al., 2010). Spasticity can be further broken down based on limb distribution, diplegia, hemiplegia, or quadriplegia.

Diplegia refers to the dysfunction of all extremities with the lower extremities more affected than the upper extremities. Children with spastic diplegia may have relatively intact hand function (Glader & Barkoudah, 2017). Hemiplegia is dysfunction of one side of the body, with the upper extremity more affected than the lower extremity. Quadriplegia refers to all extremities affected by increased muscle tone. These quadriplegic children are often severely handicapped with deficits of intellectual disability, communication, vision, epilepsy, feeding difficulties, and possible pulmonary disease (Glader & Barkoudah, 2017).

Dystonia is defined as slow and twisting, abnormal movements of the trunk or extremities that may involve abnormal posturing and can remain in that position. Dystonia can occur in dyskinetic CP, but is also commonly present in spastic CP. Dyskinesia is described as abnormal involuntary movements after initiation of voluntary movements. Children experience manifestations of rigid muscle tone when awake, although experiencing decreased tone when asleep or idle. In athetosis, the basal ganglia are damaged that is illustrated by slow, writhing movements. Choreoathetoisis is a form of athetosis that includes erratic, rapid, and random movements (Jackson Allen et al., 2010).

Many risk factors are associated with the development of CP. Risks can occur during the prenatal period, birth, perinatal, childhood, or an unknown period. Prematurity and low birth weight represents the largest risk factors. In addition, risk factors that could be prevented include teratogens and infections during pregnancy. CP is multifactorial, and many risk factors can contribute to its development (Jackson Allen et al., 2010). Lastly, for babies who are born at full term, risks for CP development include placental abnormalities, birth defects, low birth weight, meconium aspiration, instrumental/emergency Caesarean delivery, birth asphyxia, neonatal seizures, respiratory distress syndrome, hypoglycemia, and neonatal infection (McIntyre et al., 2012).

There are many associated problems related to CP, which include disabilities with motor function, cognitive function, feeding and nutrition, bowel and gastrostomy-tube dependence, bladder, dental, osteoporosis, pulmonary, skin, pain, behavioral, and emotional and intellectual disability (Jackson Allen et al., 2010). Epilepsy occurs in about 25% to 45% of patients with CP, and seizures are most commonly seen in spastic quadriplegia and hemiplegia (Glader & Barkoudah, 2017). Children with CP can get tired or frustrated faster than other children without the disorder. Owing to the prolonged reflexes, children can overreact to stimulation much more frequently. They also can become more demanding or uncooperative (Jackson Allen et al., 2010).

Clinical Aspects

ASSESSMENT

The evaluation of children who are suspected of CP begins with a thorough history and physical examination. It is diagnosed based on physical, functional, and developmental abilities. There is no specific test confirming the diagnosis. Clinical manifestations noted are delayed gross motor development, abnormal cognitive performance, alterations of muscle tone, abnormal postures, reflex abnormalities, and other associated disabilities such as learning disability, seizures, and sensory impairment (Jackson Allen et al., 2010).

Specific clinical signs that warrant suspicion of CP include poor head control and clinched hands at 3 months, no side protective reflexes at 5 months, extended Moro and atonic neck reflexes past 6 months, no parachute reflex after 10 months, crossing of the midline to reach objects before 12 months, and hand preference before 18 months (Jackson Allen et al., 2010). Behavioral manifestations during infancy such as irritability, weak cry, poor extraction, excessive sleep patterns, and little interest in surroundings may indicate CP. A diagnosis is not given till the child is 18 to 24 months old because of development and the rapid changes that can occur. Research shows that it is difficult to diagnose a specific CP syndrome till around age 5 because many of the developmental milestones have not been reached to see the true delays caused by CP (Glader & Barkoudah, 2017).

NURSING INTERVENTIONS, MANAGEMENT, AND IMPLICATIONS

Children diagnosed with CP may experience impaired physical mobility related to decreased muscle strength and control, sensory/perceptual alteration related to cerebral damage, altered nutrition—less than body requirements related to difficulty in chewing, swallowing, high metabolic needs, and seizure activity. Children may experience ineffective management of therapeutic regimens related to excessive demands made on the family. The children have complex care needs. They may experience diversional activity deficit related to poor social skills, altered learning, language development, and reasoning (Sparks & Taylor, 2011).

The first objective is the early identification of CP and then to accelerate the process of referrals to the proper community resources (Liptak & Murphy 2011). Positive signs of CP that nurses may observe are ongoing primitive reflexes and absent or delayed developmental milestones. Nurses need to be aware of the basic red flags that indicate CP.

Basic management of children with CP requires a patient and family-centered medical home, physiotherapy, physical therapy, speech therapy, occupational therapy, and orthotics. Treatment goals are aimed at promoting social and emotional development, communication, education, nutrition, mobility, and maximal independence in activities of daily living (Glader & Barkoudah, 2017). After proper assessment of the child and his or her needs, interventions should be implemented beginning with the least invasive method. Studies show that effective treatments include medications; functional therapies, including physiotherapy, occupational therapy, speech therapy, and constraint-induced movement therapy; orthoses, casting and splinting; weight-bearing exercises; and multilevel orthopedic surgery (Jackson Allen et al., 2010).

A primary goal of management is to increase the child's function. Nurses should promote optimal growth and development, maximize the joint range of motion, optimize muscle control and balance, provide means of communication, means of locomotion, and promote childhood independence (Jackson Allen et al., 2010). Research has also shown that the combination of interventions from all areas of management can improve a child's function, self-care, and activities of daily living.

OUTCOMES

Children with CP often struggle with dysphagia and therefore may not meet nutritional requirements (Liptak & Murphy 2011). A child's ability to feed himself or herself can range based on the severity of the child's condition. The degree of oral motor function, however, may require tube feeding. Gastroesophageal reflux disease (GERD) is also common in children with this condition, and nurses should assess risk for aspiration. Educating families on this issue as well as appropriate posturing when eating is a key intervention. Drooling can be excessive and persistent in children with CP. Psychosocially, the excessive drooling can be embarrassing. Working with the children to help them swallow, remind them how to swallow, and assessment of posture (i.e., head control, positioning, and mouth closure) can help maintain the secretions.

Evidence shows that high-quality health care for children with CP depends on collaborations among parents, health care providers, including dentists, and community agencies (i.e., educational services, recreational programs, and parent groups) with ongoing monitoring of the child's health and function (Liptak & Murphy, 2011, p. e1324). Optimizing health and well-being for children with CP and their families involves family-centered care provided in the medical home (Liptak & Murphy 2011). If an infant or child is hospitalized, the nurse should maintain the at-home regimen as much as possible.

There are a variety of notable responsibilities that a parent must take on when raising and caring for a child with CP. The first aspect addressed is the psychological effect on siblings and parents. There is a direct impact on the quality of life that affects the family members of the child who is suffering from CP. The family often requires psychological help and support. The nurse should help guide children and their families in the right direction to help find a strong support system, including parent support and advocacy groups, respite programs, and community programs for recreational and adaptive sports (Liptak & Murphy 2011).

Summary

CP is the most common motor disability condition in children and adolescents. It represents a distressing and difficult condition that is experienced by a multitude of families throughout the world. However, with proper treatment and care, this disease can be combatted to preserve a high level of function and a suitable quality of life. Providers and families affected by this disease must work together to treat diagnosed children with the utmost personal, financial, and medical responsibility.

Delgado, M. R., Hirtz, D., Aisen, M., Ashwal, S., Fehlings, D. L., McLaughlin, J., . . . Vargus-Adams, J. (2010). Practice parameter: Pharmacologic treatment of spasticity in children and adolescents with cerebral palsy (an evidence-based review): Report of the Quality Standards Subcommittee of the American Academy of Neurology and the Practice Committee of the Child Neurology Society. Neurology, 74, 336–343. doi:10.1212/WNL.0b013e3181cbcd2f

Glader, L., & Barkoudah, E. (2017). Clinical features and classification of cerebral palsy. In C. A. Armsby, UpToDate. Retrieved from https://www.uptodate.com/contents/clinical-features-and-classification-of-cerebral-palsy

Hasnat, M. J., & Rice, J. E. (2015). Intrathecal baclofen for treating spasticity in children with cerebral palsy. *Cochrane Database of Systematic Reviews, 2015*(11). doi:10.1002/14651858.CD004552.pub2

Jackson Allen, P., Vessey J. A., & Schapiro, N. (2010). *Primary care of the child with a chronic condition* (5th ed.). St. Louis, MO: Mosby.

Kirby, R. S., Wingate, M. S., Van Naarden Braun, K., Doernberg, N. S., Arneson, C. L., Benedict, R. E., ... Yeargin-Allsopp, M.(2011). Prevalence and functioning of children with cerebral palsy in four areas of the United States in 2006: A report from the Autism and Developmental Disabilities Monitoring Network. *Research in Developmental Disabilities, 32*, 462–469. doi:10.1016/j.ridd.2010.12.042

Liptak, G. S., Murphy, N. A., & the Council on Children With Disabilities. (2011) Providing a primary care medical home for children and youth with cerebral palsy. *American Academy of Pediatrics, 128*, e1321–e1329. doi:10.1542/peds.2011-1468

Mcintyre, S., Taitz, D., Keogh, J., Goldsmith, S., Badawi, N., & Blair, E. (2012). A systematic review of risk factors for cerebral palsy in children born at term in developed countries. *Developmental Medicine & Child Neurology, 55*, 499–508. doi:10.1111/dmcn.12017

Sparks, S. & Taylor, C. M. (2011). *Nursing diagnosis pocket guide*. Philadelphia, PA: Lippincott Williams & Wilkins.

■ CHILD ABUSE AND NEGLECT

Patricia M. Speck
Pamela Harris Bryant
Tedra S. Smith
Sherita K. Etheridge
Steadman McPeters

Overview

For a majority of states (46 out of 50), child abuse and neglect are serious public health problems. Among states contributing to a report published in 2016, there were 6.6 million children in 3.6 million reports of child abuse and neglect nationwide; authorities validated 2.2 million or 61%, with an incidence rate of 29 per 1,000 children (U.S. Department of Health and Human Services [HHS], 2016, p. ix). Professionals who have contact with children as part of their job are mandatory reporters responsible for more than 45% of the reported cases (p. ix). Of the children evaluated, the majority had one report (83%), and some had two or more reports (16%; p. x). The children with validated experiences were neglected (75%) and physically abused (17%), but if the child experienced both, only one category counted toward maltreatment (p. x). Other types of maltreatment constitute the remaining percentage of validated reports. The mortality rate was 2.13 deaths per 100,000, or 1,546 fatalities (p. x). Boys had a higher fatality rate than girls (2.48 vs. 1.82 per 100,000), and Caucasians died more frequently (43%), followed by different minority populations of children (African American—30.3%; Hispanic—15.1%; p. x). The financial impact of abuse and neglect of children in 2008 was $124 billion (Fang, Brown, Florence, & Mercy, 2012). Perpetrators of child abuse and neglect were mostly women (54.1%), White (48.8%), mistreating two or more children (HHS, 2016, p. x).

Background

The Child Abuse Prevention and Treatment Act (CAPTA), with reauthorization, defined behaviors as acts of child abuse and neglect as:

> Any recent act or failure to act on the part of a parent or caretaker which results in death, serious physical or emotional harm, sexual abuse or exploitation; or an act or failure to act, which presents an imminent risk of serious harm. (HHS, 2016, p. viii)

Maltreatment includes psychological maltreatment (emotional abuse), neglect (including endangerment), physical and sexual abuse (HHS, 2016, p. viii). The Justice for Victims of Trafficking Act of 2015 (JVTA) requires states to report the number of identified sex trafficked children younger than 18 years, allowing states to provide services and report identified victims up to 24 years (Civic Impulse, 2017). Of the adults aged 18 years rescued, overwhelmingly introduction to the industry began between the ages of 12 and 14 years. These legislative mandates at the national and state levels are helpful to the registered nurse responsible for evaluating injury in pediatric populations and reporting suspicions of abuse or neglect.

The changes in the federal reporting system, specifically how child abuse and neglect cases are reported and understanding the nuances of abuse, lowered the prevalence and incidence of child maltreatment in the past 20 years. In 2014, four to five children lost their lives every day to child abuse or neglect (HHS, 2016, p. x). The deceased children are younger than 2 years (70%), unable to escape the danger, dependent on the parent caregiver, and include another smaller group between 2 and 5 years (10%; HHS, 2016, p. x). Another group with falling victimization rates is the adolescent group ranging between 12 and 20 years. In the 1990s, violent crime was at an all-time high, where adolescents experienced violent victimizations including physical assaults, robberies, and sexual crimes (Child Trends, 2015). Although falling, there are persistent patterns, including increasing age, which exposes teens to increasing vulnerability (independence) and therefore, violent crimes, such as physical and sexual assaults (52 per 1,000, compared with 35 per 1,000 among adolescents ages 15 to 17 years, and 34 per 1,000 among adolescents ages 18 to 20 years; Child Trends, 2015, para 5). Additionally, females versus males, aged 18 to 20 years, were six times more likely to be victims of rape (6:1 per 1,000; Child Trends, 2015, para 7). White teens were more likely to be victimized than the African- or Hispanic-descent teens (Child Trends, 2015, para 8).

The children most at risk for child abuse and neglect are in chaotic or traumatized families, many experiencing social and personal environments not conducive to development or emotional health. Disparities and social determinants as risk factors diminish attainment of health outcomes. Social determinants include the environment and attitudes, exposure to crime and violence, disease and diminished access to health care, personal and support systems (HHS, Office of Disease Prevention and Health Promotion, 2017). Chronic stress in environments, whether from the individual's disease, the family, the community or the system, increase hormonal dysregulation predisposing the child to an increased risk of violence and disease (McEwen, 1998).

Building on the stress and adaptation theories of the 1990s, emerging science focuses on the epigenetic transference of cellular environments that predispose offspring to poor health outcomes (Whitman & Kondis, 2016). In fact, physically and sexually victimized children display at least one mental health disorder by the age of 18 years (Silverman, Reinherz, & Giaconia, 1996), which, when passed to their children, are predictive of future victim experiences (Child Trends, 2017).

A tool to measure adverse childhood experiences (ACE) validated that there is a connection between ACE and health outcomes, including early death (Felitti et al., 1998). The research continues. Diseases once thought to be a result of genetics may be a result of physical changes following significant ACEs; in fact, the impact of ACEs affects all human body systems where earlier stress results in high-risk behaviors, chronic disease, and early death (Anda et al., 2009; Brown et al., 2009).

Pregnant women and their developing fetus(es), newborns, infants, and children exposed to violence experience elevated stress hormones and begin a quest to escape or calm the "fear" response. The neuroendocrine system creates the brain stem irritation response (fear) to a threat and the hormonal sequelae of several hormonal pathways, including the hypothalamic–pituitary–adrenal axis (HPA axis; Nestler, Hyman, & Malenka, 2009). The resulting "fight-or-flight" response causes an elevation in stress hormones cascading and triggering other hormones in the stressed environment of the body. The hormones in the stress response originate from the primitive emotional midbrain, stimulated by the brain stem in response to fear, resulting in a constellation of symptoms, called "general adaptation syndrome" (GAS; Selye, 1974). *The victim is responding normally to abnormal stresses.* However, the stress hormones change end-organ function. Today, research documents change in response to chronic stress, for example, digestion, immune system, mood, anxiety, energy storage (fat), and other deleterious alterations, specifically in a child's brain architecture, affecting learning, behavior, and long-term health (Child Welfare, 2015). The child is handicapped socially and developmentally by the exposure, usually without sensitive identification and intervention to mitigate the normal response to serious stresses in the family. The negative health outcomes include behavioral aberrations, hypertension, obesity, autoimmune diseases, poor school performance, adoption of risk behaviors (with subsequent disease or injury), and others. Understanding the underlying physiology of stress and trauma in childhood prepares the registered nurse to address obvious symptoms that lead to future poor health choices and outcomes for the child.

Clinical Aspects

An important fact for the practicing registered nurse is the recognition that child abuse or neglect occurs by a parent (HHS, 2016). Each state defines child abuse differently, but all states follow federal legislation (p. viii), so the practicing registered nurse must be familiar with his or her state legislation related to reporting child maltreatment. If there is a suspicion of child abuse, the registered nurse (caring for a pediatric patient) is a mandatory reporter in every state and all U.S. territories (HHS, 2016; Parrish, 2016).

In the interim, the registered nurse receives *education* about abuse and neglect to successfully screen and document developmental milestones at all ages and developmental stages. The first requirement is to understand elements of abuse and neglect, which include emotional abuse, such as words belittling the child to outright screaming obscenities at the child, physical abuse, such as pinching, pushing, slapping, shoving the child at any developmental age or chronologic age, and outcomes from the abuse, which include depression, self-injurious behavior, suicide, or homicide (HHS, 2016).

ASSESSMENT

Screening for stresses and developmental milestones identifies at-risk children and gives the registered nurse an opportunity to provide anticipatory guidance and intervention (Larkin, Shields, & Anda, 2012), which may include reporting the event(s) to the state's child services agency. The registered nurse caring for pediatric populations needs a strong institutional policy and procedure for the management of abused and neglected pediatric patients, as well as the skills to identify, mitigate, and prevent early relational stresses between the child and the child's primary parent or caretaker. The ACE questions, when asked at every visit, provide the opportunity to intervene on multiple levels, and is an important vital sign to monitor to prevent child abuse and neglect. The assessment domains for pediatric registered nurse providers include the areas of "language, literacy, and math," and also "interpersonal interaction, and opportunities for self-expression" (Snow & Van Hemel, 2008, p. 22). Guidelines and validated tools for assessment at each developmental stage prepare the registered nurse provider to assist non-offending parents with a comprehensive plan for intervention to mitigate the impact of abuse and neglect (p. 7). Functional approaches for the registered nurse require special training in the assessment of all children, including those with challenges and deficits in abilities (p. 22). Parents from a variety of cultures, including minority and immigrant families (p. 22), also positively respond to the anticipatory guidance provided by the registered nurse.

NURSING INTERVENTIONS, MANAGEMENT, AND IMPLICATIONS

Using the totality of nursing education, the registered nurse, as an expert in growth and development of children, incorporates Maslow's hierarchy of needs to include trusting one's environment at all developmental stages. When the closest caregiver (usually a parent) is unable or unwilling to provide the nurture, recognition is the first step to plan the necessary interventions to protect the safety of the child. Recommending prevention and parenting programs for at-risk families is a good first step, including home visitation, or more frequent visits, or phone calls to check on the well-being of the mother and child. This is particularly important for the teen mother, who may be surviving a chaotic upbringing, experiencing the predictable high-risk behaviors and teen pregnancy.

All child assessments should be head to toe and include all mucous membrane areas (eye, ear, nose, throat [EENT], and anogenital). The expectation with each visit is that the child evaluation includes behavior and skin injuries, asking about the manner and cause of the injury detected, and if serious or inconsistent, reasons for the delay. The registered nurse assessment for child abuse or neglect is descriptive only, documenting objective information, and monitoring activity between mother or caregiver and infant/child. If the registered nurse is the first to suspect abuse or neglect, he or she is a mandated reporter, regardless of other professionals' opinions.

OUTCOMES

Not all injury or neglect is intentional, so the institutions designated to complete the comprehensive evaluation of the child, family, and social situation, is mandated to exercise legal authority over the child's safety. Throughout the process, the registered nurse role is therapeutic and helpful, explaining the process of reporting and providing clarity to the process of the investigation. The registered nurse works with the institutional team to provide nursing care, assessment, and documentation, important for the safety of and planning for the pediatric patient. In the event of child removal, the registered nurse's role is to comfort the nonoffending parent, provide community resources, and explain (to his or her ability) processes through anticipatory guidance.

Summary

Children depend on safe and secure environments created by their parent(s) or caregiver, specifically to provide the love and support for all developmental stages and ages. Child abuse and neglect represent an inability of the responsible adult to nurture the child. During pregnancy, the stress of the mother transfers to the fetus and can result in spontaneous abortion. After delivery, lack of maternal nurture arrests the infant's development and changes the brain architecture, so the child is unable to navigate a learning environment. Stress creates anxiety in older children, which leads to the overproduction of stress hormones, crippling the capacity of the child to move through Maslow's basic hierarchical steps toward adulthood and independence.

Domestic violence, poverty, trafficking of human families, war, drug use (covered in other chapters), neglect, and abuse by parent/caregiver create additional stress responses in the infant and child that doom the child to adopt risky behaviors beginning as young as 6 or 8 years of age. Registered nurses are in the position to recognize the child subjected to violence and the subsequent stress. The developmental milestones provide clues for the pediatric registered nurse to begin the inquiry into ACEs, scales measuring depression and anxiety, and other validated methods for assessing mother and child. Recognition of the health signs of hypertension, obesity, risk behavior, mental health diagnoses, neglect, and other signs of fear in an infant or child provide the opportunity for all registered nurses to intervene, report, and participate in interprofessional team collaboration to create safe and secure environments for all children.

Anda, R. F., Dong, M., Brown, D. W., Felitti, V. J., Giles, W. H., Perry, G. S., . . . Dube, S. R. (2009). The relationship of adverse childhood experiences to a history of premature death of family members. *BMC Public Health, 9*, 106. doi:10.1186/1471-2458-9-106

Brown, D. W., Anda, R. F., Tiemeier, H., Felitti, V. J., Edwards, V. J., Croft, J. B., & Giles, W. H. (2009). Adverse childhood experiences and the risk of premature mortality. *American Journal of Preventive Medicine, 37*(5), 389–396. doi:10.1016/j.amepre.2009.06.021

Child Trends. (2015). Violent crime victimization. Retrieved from http://www.childtrends.org/?indicators=violent-crime-victimization

Child Welfare Information Gateway. (2015, April). *Understanding the effects of maltreatment on brain development.* Washington, DC: U.S. Department of Health and Human Services, Children's Bureau. Retrieved from https://www.childwelfare.gov/pubPDFs/brain_development.pdf

Civic Impulse. (2017). H.R. 181—114th Congress: Justice for victims of trafficking act of 2015. Retrieved from https://www.govtrack.us/congress/bills/114/hr181

Fang, X., Brown, D. S., Florence, C. S., & Mercy, J. A. (2012). The economic burden of child maltreatment in the United States and implications for prevention. *Child Abuse & Neglect, 36*(2),156–165. doi:10.1016/j.chiabu.2011.10.006

Felitti, V. J., Anda, R. F., Nordenberg, D., Williamson, D. F., Spitz, A. M., Edwards, V., . . . Marks, J. S. (1998). Relationship of childhood abuse and household dysfunction to many of the leading causes of death in adults: The adverse childhood experiences (ACE) study. *American Journal of Preventive Medicine, 14,* 245–258. doi:10.1016/S0749-3797(98)00017-8

Larkin, H., Shields, J. J., & Anda, R. F. (2012). The health and social consequences of adverse childhood experiences (ACEs) across the lifespan: An introduction to prevention and intervention in the community. *Journal of Prevention and Intervention in the Community, 40*(4), 263–270. doi:10.1080/10852352.2012.707439

McEwen, B. S. (1998). Stress, adaptation, and disease: Allostasis and allostatic load. *Annals of the New York Academy of Sciences, 840,* 33–44. doi:10.1111/j.1749-6632.1998.tb09546.x

Nestler, E. J., Hyman, S. E., & Malenka, R. C. (2009). *Molecular neuropharmacology: A foundation for clinical neuroscience* (2nd ed.). New York, NY: McGraw-Hill Medical.

Parrish, R. (2016). Legal system intervention in cases of child maltreatment. In A. P. Giardino, L. Shaw, P. M. Speck, & E. R. Giardino (Eds.), *Recognition of child abuse for the mandated reporter* (pp. 321–356). St. Louis, MO: STM Learning.

Selye, H. (1974). *Stress without distress.* Philadelphia, PA: Lippincott.

Silverman, A. B., Reinherz, H. Z., & Giaconia, R. M. (1996). The long-term sequelae of child and adolescent abuse: A longitudinal community study. *Child Abuse & Neglect, 20*(8), 709–723. doi:10.1016/0145-2134(96)00059-2

Snow, C. E., & Van Hemel, S. B. (Eds.). (2008). *Early childhood assessment: Why, what, and how.* Washington, DC: National Research Council of the National Academies. doi:10.17226/12446

U.S. Department of Health and Human Services, Administration for Children and Families, Administration on Children, Youth and Families, Children's Bureau. (2016). Child maltreatment 2014. Retrieved from http://www.acf.hhs.gov/programs/cb/research-data-technology/statistics-research/child-maltreatment

U.S. Department of Health and Human Services, Office of Disease Prevention and Health Promotion. (2017, January 13). Determinants of health. Retrieved from https://www.healthypeople.gov/2020/about/foundation-health-measures/determinants-of-health

Whitman, B. V., & Kondis, J. (2016). Understanding the short-term and long-term effects of child abuse. In A. P. Giardino, L. Shaw, P. M. Speck, & E. R. Giardino (Eds.). *Recognition of child abuse for the mandated reporter* (pp. 165–178). St. Louis, MO: STM Learning.

■ CYSTIC FIBROSIS

Karen Vosper

Overview

Cystic fibrosis (CF) is a complex and multisystem disease, characterized by thickened tenacious secretions in the respiratory tract, sweat glands, gastrointestinal tract, pancreas, and other exocrine tissue. It is the most common life-shortening autosomal recessive disorder of the exocrine glands. Typical respiratory manifestations of CF include persistent, productive cough, difficulty clearing secretions, and frequent respiratory infections. Typical gastrointestinal manifestations include large bulky malodorous stools; impaired absorption of fat, protein, and carbohydrates resulting in poor weight gain and growth and malnutrition; as well as excess losses of sodium and chloride in sweat (National Heart, Lung, and Blood Institute, 2016).

Background

In the United States, CF occurs in approximately 1:3,000 Whites, predominately of European descent; 1:9,200 Hispanics; 1:10,900 Native Americans; 1:15,000 African Americans; and 1:100,000 Asian Americans (Lahiri et al., 2016). Gender is not a factor in the disease incidence. Median predicted survival for CF patients in the United States in 2015 was 41.6 years (95% confidence interval: 38.5–44.0 years), and the median age at death was 29.1 years. Overall, 5% of deaths occur in individuals younger than 13 years (CFF Registry Report, 2015). Although CF is a multisystem disease, lung involvement is the major cause of morbidity and more than 90% of mortality.

The gene that causes CF was discovered in 1989 and is located on the long arm of chromosome 7, known as the *CF transmembrane regulator* (CFTR) gene (Stern, 2006). People with CF either have too few CFTR proteins at the cell surface, CFTR proteins that do not work properly, or both. The defective CFTR proteins result in the poor flow of salt and water in and out of the cells. As a result, abnormally thick and sticky mucus forms and obstructs the epithelial tissues throughout the body, such as the lungs, sinuses, pancreas, intestine, reproductive system, and sweat glands. Thick and sticky airway secretions, a combination of mucus and pus, build up in the lungs causing chronic lung infections and progressive lung damage. In the gastrointestinal tract, there is a reduced ability to absorb nutrients, and digestive enzymes from the pancreas that are critical to the breakdown and absorption of fats, calories, and nutrients do not reach the small intestine, resulting in malabsorption, steatorrhea, and malnutrition (Davis, 2006).

The sweat test is considered the gold standard for diagnosing CF. It can be done on an individual of any age. It has three technical parts: localized sweat stimulation induced by iontophoresis of pilocarpine, collection, and analysis. The preferred site for sweat collection is the flexor surface of the forearm. The chance of urticaria or burn to the skin after iontophoresis is possible. For all patients, sweat chloride values greater than or equal to 60 mmol/L is considered positive for CF. A positive result on the sweat chloride test indicates that CF is nearly certain (Collie, Massie, Jones, LeGrys, & Greaves, 2014).

Currently, all 50 states and the District of Columbia screen newborns for CF, but the method for screening may differ from state to state. All screening algorithms in current use in the United States rely on testing for immunoreactive trypsinogen (IRT) as the primary screen for CF. The presence of high levels of IRT, typically elevated in CF-affected infants, indicates the need for a second tier of testing, which determines the positive or negative outcome of the screen. The second tier testing relies on IRT again or DNA testing. All babies with a positive newborn screen (NBS) will be required to have a confirmatory sweat test. As a characteristic of all NBSs, most infants with a positive CF NBS result will not have CF (Farrell et al., 2008).

Clinical Aspects

ASSESSMENT

Assessment of the child with CF focuses on respiratory and gastrointestinal function. Typical respiratory manifestations of CF include a persistent cough, cough with sputum production, and pulmonary function tests consistent with obstructive airway disease. The onset of clinical symptoms varies widely, because of differences in CFTR genotype and other individual factors, but pulmonary function abnormalities often are detectable even in the absence of symptoms. As the disease progresses, chronic bronchitis and progressive bronchiectasis develop and are accompanied by acute exacerbations, characterized by increased cough, tachypnea, increased sputum production, malaise, anorexia, and weight loss. Digital clubbing is often seen in patients with moderate to advanced lung disease. Clinicians need to inquire about the frequency and character of the patient's cough, as well as quality and quantity of sputum production. Auscultation of the chest for breath sounds, crackles, and wheezes accompanies assessment of respiratory rate, work of breathing, use of accessory muscles, position of comfort, and any cyanosis or clubbing of the extremities.

NURSING INTERVENTIONS, MANAGEMENT, AND IMPLICATIONS

Management of CF focuses on minimizing pulmonary complications, promoting growth and development, and facilitating coping and adjustment of the child and family. Early intervention and monitoring for respiratory and gastrointestinal disease in children with CF are vital to improve outcomes. Evidence-based nutrition goals and pulmonary and nutritional care guidelines for children with CF have been published by the CF Foundation. More than 85% of patients are pancreatic insufficient at birth and others often gradually lose function over time. If the patient is taking pancreatic enzymes, evaluating response to enzymes should be a routine part of the nutritional assessment. Inquire about pancreatic enzyme dose and amount, appetite, weight loss, stool history, steatorrhea, flatus, abdominal bloating, constipation, and abdominal pain.

For infants and children with CF, airway clearance at least twice daily is a critical intervention that is increased during illness. Airway clearance for infants involves manual percussion, vibration, and postural drainage. For older infants and children, a high-frequency chest compression vest may be used. Inhaled hypertonic saline may be used to assist with mobilization of secretions. Inhaled recombinant human DNase (Pulmozyme) is given daily to decrease sputum viscosity and help clear secretions. Inhaled bronchodilators and anti-inflammatory agents are prescribed for some children. Aerosolized antibiotics are often prescribed and may be given in the home as well as in the hospital. *Pseudomonas aeruginosin* has been long recognized as a significant pathogen in the disease progression. Other pathogens can lead to worsening symptoms and can speed the decline in lung function (Lahiri et al., 2016).

Pancreatic enzymes must be administered with all meals and snacks to promote adequate digestion and absorption of nutrients. In the infant and young child, the enzymes capsule can be opened and mixed with a small amount of applesauce. Supplemental fat-soluble vitamins are prescribed to promote adequate digestion and absorption of nutrients and optimize nutritional status. Increased-calorie, high-protein diets are recommended, and sometimes supplemental high-calorie formula, either oral or via tube feeling. It can be difficult to maintain a schedule that requires hours of treatments daily as well as close attention to high-calorie diet, enzyme supplementation, vitamins, and oral and aerosolized antibiotics (Schindler, Michel, & Wilson, 2015).

Nurses in the outpatient, inpatient, home care, and school settings need to help others understand the increased calorie and salt requirements of those with CF and support the plan of care. Maintaining infection control practices in the primary care provider's office, schools, and hospital setting is key to minimizing the risk for acquisition and spread of pathogens. The nurse is in a position to help people with CF and their families fit the complex medical care into their daily routine. Promoting health, quality of life, and education about the signs and symptoms of potential problems is a primary focus of a nurse.

OUTCOMES

The expected outcomes for CF respiratory management are aimed at slowing the progression of the lung disease, minimizing pulmonary complications, maximizing lung function, and preventing infection. The expected outcomes of evidence-based nutritional goals are centered on maintaining 50th percentile weight/length from birth to 24 months and body mass index (BMI) at the 50th percentile for 2 to 20 years of age (Schindler et al., 2015).

Summary

Advances in science have led to increased survival among patients with CF such that, currently, nearly half of the CF population in the United States is older than 18 years, which far exceeds survival rates of previous decades. The disease demands significant adaptations by children and their families, many of which can be challenging and stressful. Families commonly face a set of significant obstacles accessing CF care. Obtaining and maintaining adequate health insurance, cost of prescription medications, disease-related out-of-pocket expenses, lost work days, as well as travel to specialists and CF care centers can tax family resources. Delays in or denial of coverage for medications and treatment can be extremely difficult.

Children face their challenges associated with medication and nutrition regimens, pulmonary therapy, missed school days owing to illness, difficulty engaging in extracurricular activities with peers, often resulting in the sense of social isolation. Effective partnerships among children, families, clinicians, and community agencies are critical to the quality of life and sustained health. The nurse plays an essential, and long-lasting role throughout the life of a person with CF contributing direct care, advocacy, and education to help each achieve his or her best health and quality of life.

Collie, J. T. B., Massie, R. J., Jones, O. A. H., LeGrys, V. A., & Greaves, R. F. (2014). Sixty-five years since the New York heat wave: Advances in sweat testing for cystic fibrosis. *Pediatric Pulmonology, 2014* (49), 106–117. doi:10.1002/ppul.22945

Cystic Fibrosis Foundation. (2015). *Patient registry annual data report.* Retrieved from https://www.cff.org/Our-Research/CF-Patient-Registry/2015-Patient-Registry -Annual-Data-Report.pdf

Davis, P. B. (2006). Cystic fibrosis since 1938. *American Journal of Respiratory and Critical Care Medicine, 173*(5), 475–482. doi:10.1164/rccm.200505-840OE

Farrell, P. M., Rosenstein, B. J., White, T. B., Accurso, F. J., Castellani, C., Cutting, G. R., . . . Campbell, P. W., III. (2008). Guidelines for diagnosis of cystic fibrosis in newborns through older adults: Cystic Fibrosis Foundation consensus report. *Journal of Pediatrics, 153*(2), S4–S14. doi:10.1016/j.jpeds.2008.05.005

Lahiri, T., Hempstead, S. E., Brady, C., Cannon, C. L., Clark, K., Condren, M. E., . . . Davis, S. D. (2016). Clinical practice guidelines from the Cystic Fibrosis Foundation for preschoolers with cystic fibrosis. *Pediatrics, 3*(22). Retrieved from https://pediatrics .aappublications.org/content/early/2016/03/22/peds.2015-1784

National Heart, Lung, and Blood Institute. (2016). What are the signs and symptoms of cystic fibrosis? Retrieved from https://www.nhlbi.nih.gov/health/health-topics/topics/ cf/signs

Schindler, T., Michel, S., & Wilson, A. (2015). Nutrition management of cystic fibrosis in the 21st century. *Nutrition in Clinical Practice, 30*(4), 488–500. doi:10.1177/088 4533615591604

Stern, R. (2006). The diagnosis of cystic fibrosis. *The New England Journal of Medicine, 336*(7), 487–491.

■ DEVELOPMENTALLY APPROPRIATE COMMUNICATION

Nanci M. Berman

Overview

Developmentally appropriate communication applies skills of communication that are aligned with the developmental stage of the patient as defined by the theoretical frameworks of Piaget, Erikson, and Freud (Ball, Bindler, & Cowen, 2013, 2014). Effective, developmentally appropriate communication can affect the emotional well-being, medical compliance, and preparation of patients to care for themselves into adulthood (Bell & Condren, 2016; Brand, Fasciano, & Mack, 2016). Developmentally appropriate communication in nursing keeps the patient at the center of triadic communication between nurse, parent, and child, which is a unique factor in the pediatric population (Brand et al., 2016).

Background

Communication is a process where the sender encodes a message that is sent to the receiver who decodes the message and responds, providing feedback to the original sender for decoding (D'Amico & Barbarito, 2015). Communication can have positive and negative effects on behavior. In pediatric nursing, the way in which the message is encoded and sent can make a significant difference in the behavior and emotion that results during decoding. The patient's developmental age and previous experience contribute to his or her ability to decode information (Bell & Condren, 2016). Nurses who identify the patient's developmental age and exhibit appropriate approaches to interactions and communication gain a greater trust from the parent/caregiver and have a greater effect on the future nurse-to-patient encounters (Salmani, Abbaszadeh, & Rassouli, 2014). These encounters provide an opportunity to build and sustain a relationship that provides mutual respect between the patient, parent, and nurse, each in their significant role promoting well-being and providing care (Salmani et al., 2014).

Communication can be verbal, nonverbal, or abstract. Verbal communication includes pace, intonation, simplicity, clarity, timing, and adaptability that accompany the spoken words (Ball et al., 2013; Pearson Education, 2015). Nonverbal communication, posture, gait, facial expression, and gestures can be interpreted during the process of communication to be supportive or contradictory to verbal communication (Ball et al., 2013; Pearson Education, 2015). Verbal and nonverbal messages should be consistent and congruent for the nurse to gain trust and credibility. Children who play with dolls or cars as they see others do or teenagers who dress to make a statement are exhibiting abstract communication (Ball et al., 2013).

Therapeutic communication is the process of interacting and sharing information in a professional–patient relationship. For the purpose of this discussion, the focus is on the relationship between nurse and child or nurse and family. This relationship is founded on mutual respect and trust between the patient/parent and nurse (Pearson Education, 2015). Therapeutic communication includes verbal and nonverbal communication that is meaningful and adjusted to the situation. Techniques include the use of broad, open-ended statements, active listening, physical presence, and clarification (Pearson Education, 2015).

Clinical Aspects

ASSESSMENT

Developmentally appropriate communication is specific to the patient's developmental and cognitive age, which may differ from one's chronological age. Humans communicate from birth, initially with cries, followed by pointing and grunting, and proceeding eventually to putting words together to create meaningful sentences. Communication aids in alleviating fears, building trusting relationships, and developing confidence to sustain treatment plans. Erik Erikson's *theory of psychosocial development* and Jean Piaget's *theory of cognitive development* are most often used as frameworks for nursing care of the pediatric patient. Erikson (1979) categorizes the stages of psychosocial development as birth to 1 year of age: trust versus mistrust; ages 1 to 3 years: autonomy versus shame and doubt; ages 3 to 6 years: initiative versus guilt; ages 6 to 12 years: industry versus inferiority; and ages 12 to 18 years: identity versus role confusion. Piaget (1976) provides four stages of cognitive development age: birth to 2 years: sensory motor; ages 2 to 7 years: preoperational; ages 7 to 11 years: concrete operational; and 12 years of age and older: formal operational.

To organize the following presentation of developmentally appropriate approach and communication, Erikson and Piaget's stages are combined. Examples are presented for the newborn, infant, toddler and preschooler, school-age, and adolescent. Newborns communicate with cries to get their basic needs such as feeding, clean clothes, and comfort met (Ball et al., 2013). Human voice and touch, kangaroo care, gain a greater importance for this stage, especially for those born prematurely (Ball et al., 2013). Infants continue to need comforting touch and predominately communicate nonverbally, making it important for the nurses caring for this patient to use voice inflection and facial expression to engage (Ball et al., 2013). Toddlers and preschoolers need time to process their thoughts without interruptions and are gaining their independence, requiring time commitments from the nurse (Ball et al., 2013). Nurses who provide simple responses, simple directions, and choices that result in the decision of the child to be acceptable while carving out time for responses allow for the greatest exchange with this age group. School-age children are exploring the world around them, initiating activities, and engaging in groups (Ball et al., 2013). Patients at this stage like to take part in decisions that affect them. Nurses should clarify the extent of patient involvement in decision making before initiating conversations (Brand et al., 2016). Communicating at the same physical level of the patient and including the patient in the conversation allows the patient the ability to answer the question, allowing the parent/caregiver to answer after the patient for any required clarification (Ball et al., 2013). Adolescents are seeking their position into adulthood (Ball et al., 2013). Nurses should build a rapport with this age group by active listening and presenting a nonjudgmental attitude.

NURSING INTERVENTIONS, MANAGEMENT, AND IMPLICATIONS

Adjustments to the approach and techniques for communication may vary based on the physiological, psychological, and emotional state of the patient. For example, patients diagnosed with autism spectrum disorder, attention deficit disorder, mental retardation, or developmental delay, adjusting the approach may require combining skills from more than one stage to produce meaningful communication, trust, and respect. As another example, children with chronic conditions may regress to an earlier stage or mature to a higher cognitive or developmental stage that requires tailoring to individual needs.

OUTCOMES

Outcomes of developmentally appropriate communication are increasingly reported.

Relationship-based care provides an example of an approach to improving patient safety, satisfaction, and motivation, which are grounded in trusting relationships with a foundation in developmentally appropriate, highly individualized communication (Bell & Condren, 2016). Research has established that patients are more likely to take appropriate doses of medication, at the correct intervals, for the prescribed amount of time when their education is presented in ways that are appropriate for their stage of cognition and development (Bell & Condren, 2016).

Summary

Nurses play an integral role in the relationship, satisfaction, and adherence to medical treatment, and are more effective when they apply developmentally appropriate communication and approaches with the patients. As children mature and seek input into their medical care, shared decision-making frameworks should be considered as a means to maintain the therapeutic relationship, promote satisfaction, and achieve adherence to treatment plans.

Ball, J. W., Bindler, R. C., & Cowen, K. J. (2013). *Child health nursing: Partnering with children and families* (3rd ed.). Upper Saddle River, NJ: Pearson.

Ball , J. W., Bindler, R. C., & Cowen, K. J. (2014). *Principles of pediatric nursing: Caring for children* (6th ed.). Upper Saddle River, NJ: Pearson.

Bell, J., & Condren, M. (2016). Communication strategies for empowering and protecting children. *The Journal of Pediatric Pharmacology and Therapeutics, 21*(2), 176–184. doi:10.5863/1551-6776-21.2.176

Brand, S. R., Fasciano, K., & Mack, J. W. (2016, October 10). Communication preferences of pediatric cancer patients: Talking about prognosis and their future life. *Support Care in Cancer, 10*, 769–774. doi:10.1007/s00520-016-3458-x

D'Amico, D. T., & Barbarito, C. (2015). *Health and physical assessment in nursing* (3rd ed). Hoboken, NJ: Pearson.

Erikson, E. (1979). *Childhood and society* (2nd ed.). New York, NY: W. W. Norton.

Pearson Education. (2015). *Nursing a concept-based approach to learning* (2nd ed.). Hoboken, NJ: Pearson.

Piaget, J. (1976). *The child and reality: Problems of genetic psychology.* A. Rosin (Trans.). New York, NY: Grossman.

Salmani, N., Abbaszadeh, A., & Rassouli, M. (2014, December). Factors creating trust in hospitalized children's mothers towards nurses. *Iranian Journal of Pediatrics, 24*(6), 729–738. Retrieved from https://www.ncbi.nlm.nih.gov/pmc/articles/PMC4442835/pdf/IJP-24–729.pdf

■ DIABETES

Julia E. Blanchette

Overview

Diabetes mellitus (DM) is a chronic metabolic disorder in which the body does not metabolize carbohydrates, fats, and proteins because of progressive loss or function of pancreatic beta cells resulting in hyperglycemia (American Diabetes Association [ADA], 2017). The majority of pediatric patients with diabetes have type 1 diabetes (T1D) although some have type 2 diabetes (T2D) or other forms (ADA, 2017). Despite medical advances, a majority of children with T1D do not obtain optimal glycemic control resulting in higher mortality rates, shortened average life spans, and risk of long-term complications (ADA, 2017; Juvenile Diabetes Research Foundation [JDRF], 2016). Nurses focus on the prevention of decline in health status and future complications. Care delivery is focused on family-centered self-management care to maintain optimal and safe glycemic control for children with DM (ADA, 2017).

Background

There are more than 200,000 Americans younger than 20 years living with T1D (JDRF, 2016). Since the past decade, there has been a 21% increase in the prevalence of childhood T1D (Centers for Disease Control and Prevention [CDC], 2014; JDRF, 2016). The annual increase in the prevalence of childhood T2D is expected to quadruple in the coming 40 years (CDC, 2014). Both types of DM are polygenic and have many disease progression factors (ADA, 2017). Common environmental factors associated with the development of T1D and T2D include dietary factors, endocrine disruption, environmental toxins, gut microbiome composition, and infection (ADA, 2017). Children who are at risk for T1D are those who have a family member with T1D or autoimmune diseases such as celiac disease or Hashimoto's thyroiditis (ADA, 2017). A majority are Whites who have inherited complex risk factors from both parents, although there may be no previous family history of DM (ADA, 2017). Children at risk for T2D include those who have a body mass index (BMI) greater than the 85% for sex and age, weight greater than the 120% for ideal height, a family history of T2D in first- and second-degree relatives, and are Native American, African American, Hispanic, or Asian/South Pacific Islander ethnicity (ADA, 2017).

The onset of T1D occurs suddenly and most frequently in children younger than 4 years of age and during adolescence (ADA, 2017). It is a multifactorial disease caused by autoimmune destruction of insulin-producing pancreatic beta cells in those who are predisposed (ADA, 2016). Hyperglycemia or increased blood glucose occurs because of a decreased secretion of insulin (ADA, 2017). Fat is then used as an energy source when glucose is unavailable to the cells for metabolism-causing diabetes ketoacidosis (DKA), an acute life-threatening form of metabolic acidosis, which presents in at least one third of T1D onset (ADA, 2017). The onset of T2D is less common than T1D in childhood and occurs because of insulin resistance and the relative decrease in insulin secretion, resulting in elevated glucose levels (ADA, 2017). Insulin resistance is when the body is less able to use insulin resulting in reduced absorption of glucose into the cells for fuel (ADA, 2017). Insulin resistance causes excess production of glucose from the liver and dysfunction or total loss of function of the pancreatic beta cells (ADA, 2017).

Diabetes management for optimal glycemic control includes insulin administration, blood glucose monitoring, carbohydrate counting, treatment of hyperglycemia, treatment of hypoglycemia, exercise, nutrition therapy, family counseling, stress management, and self-monitoring of trends in insulin requirement and glucose levels (ADA, 2017). In the hospital, diabetes management includes a monitored initiation of insulin therapy via hospital protocol, fluid replacement, and family-centered diabetes education (ADA, 2017). Basal and bolus insulin administration occur through an intravenous (IV), insulin pumps, insulin syringe, or insulin pen. Basal insulin is a continuous insulin in small doses over a 24-hour period (ADA, 2017). Basal administration occurs via infusion of rapid-acting or one daily dose of long-acting insulin analogs (ADA, 2017). Bolus insulin is for hyperglycemia and carbohydrate corrections and is determined based on the patient's weight and blood sugar targets; a sliding scale regimen is strongly discouraged for inpatient settings (ADA, 2017). However, those with T2D may not be insulin dependent and may have tailored pharmacological treatment such as Metformin and increased physical activity (ADA, 2017).

Despite knowledge of risk factors, medical advances, and technology advances in diabetes care, children with DM still have higher mortality rates owing to complications than the rest of the population, especially during pubertal years because of the increased insulin sensitivity (ADA, 2017). Of the children living with DM, less than one third obtain the recommended glycemic control targets placing them at high risk for DKA and complications (JDRF, 2015).

Clinical Aspects

ASSESSMENT

The child's history, key physical assessment findings, and laboratory data are vital components of nursing care for children with DM. Children with both types of DM often present with polydipsia, polyphagia, blurred vision, and polyuria (ADA, 2017). Many children present with weight loss and flu-like symptoms, which have been present for several weeks (ADA, 2017). Diagnosis of DM in children occurs when symptoms manifest, and A1C is greater than or equal to 6.5%, a casual plasma glucose level is greater than or equal to 200 mg/dl, or a fasting plasma glucose level is greater than or equal to 126 mg/dl (ADA, 2017). Although DM diagnosis occurs under the same glycemic criteria, classification of the type of diabetes is important in determining therapy. Children with T2D may have conditions or signs associated with insulin resistance such as acanthosis nigricans (dark velvety patches) on the skin folds, hypertension, dyslipidemia, polycystic ovarian syndrome, history of small for gestational age at birth, or maternal history of gestational diabetes mellitus (ADA, 2017). Children at risk should be screened every 3 years after the age of 10 years or at the onset of puberty if it occurs earlier (ADA, 2017). Those with T2D do not typically present with DKA (ADA, 2017).

Physical assessment for a hospitalized child with DM should focus on detecting and preventing DKA. Children with T1D often present with DKA at diagnosis through infection, insulin pump failure, expired insulin, the omission of insulin and inadequate insulin, mental health issues, lack of family or social support; after trauma or after surgery can also cause DKA (ADA, 2017). Assessment should focus on the changes in the cardiovascular system (hypotension, arrhythmias, widening pulse rate), respiratory system (Kussmaul respirations, respiratory rate, acid–base disturbance), neurologic system (pupillary changes, altered level of consciousness), and integumentary system (dry mucous membranes, sunken eyes, decreased skin turgor; ADA, 2017). A child in DKA may also complain of abdominal pain, nausea, vomiting, and have fruity breath (ADA, 2017). Diagnosis of DKA occurs when plasma glucose is greater than 250 mg/dL, arterial pH is greater than 7.3, serum bicarbonate is greater than 15 mEq/L and moderate, or greater ketonuria is present (ADA, 2017). Management of DKA includes isotonic IV fluids, electrolyte replacement, regular IV insulin (0.1 unit/kg/hr), potassium supplementation, and phosphate supplementation (ADA, 2017). If cerebral edema occurs, it must be treated with mannitol (ADA, 2017).

Blood glucose is monitored at least every hour and is managed based on hospital protocols to prevent hyperglycemia and hypoglycemia (ADA, 2017). Young children may not be able to communicate hypoglycemia symptoms efficiently. In addition, children with complications may have hypoglycemia unawareness (ADA, 2017). Children who are not new to diabetes may have continuous blood glucose monitors to prevent hypoglycemia unawareness. The child is not required to take off a continuous monitor, although you should still monitor the child's blood glucose via the hospital's policy.

A plan for preventing and treating hypoglycemia (blood glucose below 70 mg/dL) is established for each patient and episodes are documented (ADA, 2017). Signs of hypoglycemia include sudden heart palpitations, fatigue, pallor, shakiness, anxiety, diaphoresis, hunger, and irritability (ADA, 2017). Hypoglycemia occurs from a sudden reduction of corticosteroids, reduced oral intake, extra insulin, and increased physical activity (ADA, 2017). It typically requires treatment of 15 g of fast-acting carbohydrates and when the blood sugar rises, a complex carbohydrate (ADA, 2017). If a patient is unresponsive with severe hypoglycemia (less than 40 mg/dL), glucagon or IV dextrose may be administered.

NURSING INTERVENTIONS, MANAGEMENT, AND IMPLICATIONS

Nursing care of the hospitalized child with DM should focus on the prevention of DKA and severe hypoglycemia. Priority nursing-related problems include imbalanced nutrition less than body's requirements, fluid volume deficit, the risk of injury (for hypoglycemia), the risk of infection, fatigue, and knowledge deficit related to new diabetes diagnosis or self-management skills.

Evidence-based practice supports interventions to improve glycemic control. According to evidence-based practice, diabetes self-management education includes medical nutrition therapy, psychosocial support at diagnosis and regularly after that in a developmentally appropriate manner. These interventions result in a less frequent decline in health status and improved glycemic control (ADA, 2017). The use of a team-based approach and shared decision making between the youth and family members results in improved diabetes self-efficacy, protocol adherence, and positive metabolic outcomes (ADA, 2017). Moreover, evidence-based practice suggests that the child should have periodic assessments to determine the need for self-care skills education. Premature transfer of diabetes care from the parent to the child can result in nonadherence and deterioration in glycemic control (ADA, 2017). Psychosocial and family issues should also be assessed to ensure that adherence to diabetes self-management is not impacted; early detection of depression, anxiety, and eating disorders can minimize adverse effects on diabetes management and improve glycemic control (ADA, 2017).

OUTCOMES

The results of evidence-based nursing care are to incorporate family-centered self-management to reach optimal glycemic control, to prevent DKA and severe hypoglycemia. Monitoring for changes in physical assessment and blood glucose changes can provide evidence for intervening with blood glucose levels. It is vital to monitor children's blood glucose levels frequently and to pay attention to signs and symptoms of decline in health status.

Summary

Treatment plans for optimal glycemic outcomes incorporate family dynamics, mental health, developmental readiness, and physiological changes. Hospitalized children with DM can rapidly progress into DKA or severe hypoglycemia if not monitored and managed appropriately. Changes in glucose and insulin patterns can be related to physical growth, puberty, insulin pump failure, a decline in mental health, and children beginning to provide their self-care. Educating families to recognize these developmental changes and the signs and symptoms of DKA, hyperglycemia, and hypoglycemia is vital in the prevention of poor health outcomes.

American Diabetes Association. (2017). Standards of medical care in diabetes—2017: Summary of revisions. *Diabetes Care, 40*(Suppl. 1), S4–S5. doi:10.2337/dc17-S003

Centers for Disease Control and Prevention. (2014). *National diabetes statistics report, 2014.* Retrieved from https://www.cdc.gov/diabetes/pdfs/data/2014-report-estimates-of-diabetes-and-its-burden-in-the-united-states.pdf

Juvenile Diabetes Research Foundation. (2015). JDRF 2015 annual report. Retrieved from http://www.jdrf.org/annualreport/2015

Juvenile Diabetes Research Foundation. (2016). JDRF 2016 annual report. Retrieved from http://www.jdrf.org/annualreport/2016/html5/index.html?page=1&noflash

■ FAILURE TO THRIVE

Mary Alice Dombrowski

Overview

Failure to thrive (FTT) describes the occurrence of insufficient weight gain over a period. Although there are varying definitions, commonly used criteria for FTT include a consistent weight gain less than 3% to 5% and/or crossing over two major percentiles with consecutive measurement over a period (Jaffe, 2011; Keane, 2015). Although FTT could occur in any age group, FTT in pediatrics is typically reserved to describe poor weight gain during the first 2 to 3 years of life. Untreated FTT is associated with poor linear growth (height), disease, behavioral challenges, and cognitive delay (McLean & Price, 2015). All children, regardless of socioeconomic status or race, should be monitored for FTT. Careful nursing assessment, application of appropriate nursing intervention, and comprehensive parental education are essential components of nursing care. Successful and early interventions have lifelong implications for improved mental and physical health (Cole & Lanham, 2011; Motil & Duryea, 2015).

Background

In the United States, FTT occurs in approximately 5% to 10% of children in primary care settings and 3% to 5% of those in the hospital setting (Cole & Lanham, 2011; Kirkland et al., 2015). Eighty percent of children present with FTT before the first 18 months of life (Cole & Lanham, 2011). Poor linear growth, a natural consequence of early FTT, is estimated to be much higher throughout the world especially in developing countries given the poor access to adequate nutrition and medical care (Karra, Subramanian, & Fink, 2016). Gender is affected equally (Habibzadeh, Jafarizadeh, & Didarloo, 2015). During this period of critical brain growth, untreated FTT can lead to significant developmental delay (Jaffe, 2011; McLean & Price, 2015). FTT may occur secondary to underlying biological, psychosocial, and environmental circumstances, or a combination of these circumstances (Jaffe, 2011, Kirkland et al., 2015). Regardless of its contributing factors, FTT occurs when there are too little calories ingested to meet energy demands of the body (Jaffe, 2011).

Biological risk factors may begin prenatally. Intrauterine growth retardation and exposure to a harmful substance in utero puts an infant at risk for developing FTT. Children born with chromosomal disorders or birth defects, such as cleft lip, can have early challenges with feeding mechanics. Others may have medical conditions with high-energy demands (i.e., heart disease, chronic infection, or endocrine disorders) or poor intestinal absorption (i.e., cystic fibrosis, or short bowel syndrome) necessitating high-calorie diets (Jaffe, 2011; McLean & Price, 2015).

Many psychosocial conditions contribute to the development of failure to thrive. Children raised in poverty with little food or poor living conditions may find it difficult to obtain food (Habibzadeh et al., 2015). Parents with mental illness, addiction, poor education, or little social support are at increased risk of having children with FTT (Habibzadeh et al., 2015). Lack of parental guidance and role modeling may encourage children to develop disordered eating patterns (Jaffe, 2011; McLean & Price, 2015) or choose foods with little nutritional value. Often, parents have unrealistic expectations regarding food. Some very young children develop phobias associated with eating (Kirkland et al., 2015).

Many children with FTT are not identified or go untreated. Poor access to medical care, no or limited insurance, inaccurate measurements, or dismissal of growth concerns by primary care providers prevent children from receiving nutritional intervention. Untreated FTT may cause growth stunting, immune disorders, medical complications, developmental delay, and lower cognitive function throughout the life span (Jaffe, 2011). There is even some evidence that early FTT increases the likelihood of hostility as an adult (Jaffe, 2011). Interventions include aggressive nutritional supplementation, family education (Jaffe, 2011; McLean & Price, 2015), and sometimes medications like cyproheptadine to stimulate appetite (Sant'Anna et al., 2014).

ASSESSMENT

Assessment of FTT is multifaceted and includes careful consideration of the child, family, and environment. Medical history including complications of pregnancy and labor, gestational age, birth weight, birth length, and birth head circumference should be obtained as well as newborn screening results. Feeding method, food intolerances, feeding difficulties, vomiting, diarrhea, sleep difficulties, history of illness, and achievement of developmental milestones should be recorded. Caregiver cultural beliefs and feeding practice should be discussed. Parental ability to make formula or food, feeding routine, and family living conditions, as well as other child care providers, are important factors to consider in FTT (McLean & Price, 2015; Wilson, 2015). The most important aspect of the physical examination includes appropriate measurement of weight, length, and head circumference. Infants and toddlers should be undressed and in dry diapers before measurement. Measurements need to be plotted on the appropriate pediatric growth chart; the World Health Organization (WHO) growth chart is used for children 2 years of age and younger, while the Centers for Disease Control and Prevention (CDC) growth chart is used for children older than 2 years of age (Keane, 2015). Medical conditions associated with unique growth patterns, including prematurity, Down syndrome, or Turner syndrome, have their charts that should be used (Jaffe, 2011). Physical examination findings common in FTT include small head size and prominent forehead (Keane, 2015), thin appearance, decreased activity, thin hair, and rash. Bruising, burns, or scarring may be signs of physical abuse. The child may appear to have a syndrome face suggesting an underlying genetic condition. Mouth mucous membranes may appear dry, teeth discolored, and breath smells atypical. Abdomens may look distended, and bowel sounds may be more or less active. Genitals should be examined for trauma. Infant muscle tone, ability to suck and swallow, and quality of movement must be documented. Behaviors of concern include the inability to meet eyes and poor responsiveness to visual, verbal, or tactile stimuli (McLean & Price, 2015; Wilson, 2015). There is very little evidence to support the use of laboratory testing in FTT. However, it may be used to screen for other associated conditions of poor nutrition including anemia and celiac disease (McLean & Price, 2015). The practitioner may want to consider reviewing a complete blood count, comprehensive metabolic panel, and stool studies for fats and reducing substances (Jaffe, 2011; McLean & Price, 2015). The primary nursing problem is ensuring that the child's nutritional needs are being met. Nursing interventions should focus on identifying contributing factors to pediatric FTT, correcting the child's nutrition deficit, and addressing parental educational and social needs. Nursing interventions include parental education regarding growth and development, assisting health care providers in developing a plan of care, implementing the plan of care, and encouraging parental participation in feeding goals. In many cases, this involves parental education and setting realistic short- and long-term goals for weight gain. Implementing a plan of care may include demonstrating proper mixing and administration of infant or toddler formula, placement and assessment of nasogastric tube placement, assessment of gastrostomy tube sites, management of enteral feeding, and administration of medications used to stimulate appetite (Ralph & Taylor, 2014; Wilson, 2015). Depending on the contributing factors and circumstances of FTT, nursing diagnoses may include insufficient breast milk, ineffective breastfeeding, ineffective infant feeding pattern, imbalanced nutrition—less than body requirements—impaired swallowing, risk for electrolyte imbalance, feeding self-care deficit, impaired parenting, risk for disproportionate growth, and risk for delayed development (Ralph & Taylor, 2014).

OUTCOMES

Weight gain is the primary expected outcome for pediatric FTT. In addition, parents should be able to describe weight goals and interventions to achieve those goals. Nursing interventions include ensuring that the child receives adequate nutrition and/or is working with a team of providers to correct underlying obstacles to obtain adequate nutrition. This may include intensive parental nutrition and feeding skills education, working with the medical team to treat underlying medical conditions, addressing social factors, providing home nursing visits, and in some cases, assisting with the removal of the child from his or her home (McLean & Price, 2015).

Summary

Pediatric failure to thrive occurs when there is insufficient caloric intake, and its effects may lead to poor cognitive and physical health outcomes for the child. Its etiology is often multifaceted and stems from underlying biological, psychosocial circumstances. Primary nursing goals include correction of nutritional deficiency and family education. Successful interventions and corrected nutritional deficiencies have lifelong implications for improved mental and physical health.

Cole, S. Z., & Lanham, J. S. (2011). Failure to thrive: An update. *American Family Physician, 83*(7), 829–834. Retrieved from https://www.aafp.org/afp/2011/0401/p829.html

Habibzadeh, H., Jafarizadeh, H., & Didarloo, A. (2015). Determinants of failure to thrive (FTT) among infants aged 6–24 months: A case-control study. *Journal of Preventive Medicine and Hygiene, 56*, E180–E186. Retrieved from http://www.jpmh.org/index.php/jpmh/article/view/451

Jaffe, A. (2011). Failure to thrive: Current clinical concepts. *Pediatrics in Review, 32*, 100–108. doi:10.1542/pir.32-3-100

Karra, M., Subramanian, S. V., & Fink, G. (2016). Height in healthy children in low- and middle-income countries: An assessment. *American Journal of Clinical Nutrition, 105*, 121–126.

Keane, V. (2015). Assessment of growth. In R. M. Kliegman, B. F. Stanton, J. W. St. Germe III, & N. F. Schor (Eds.), *Nelson textbook of pediatrics* (20th ed., pp. 84–89) Philadelphia, PA: Elsevier.

McLean, H. S., & Price, D. T. (2015). Failure to thrive. In R. M. Kliegman, B. F. Stanton, J. W. St. Germe III, & N. F. Schor (Eds.), *Nelson textbook of pediatrics* (20th ed., pp. 249–251). Philadelphia, PA: Elsevier.

Motil, K. J., & Duryea, T. K. (2017). Failure to thrive (undernutrition) in children younger than two years: Etiology and evaluation. In J. E. Drutz, C. Jensen, & C., Bridgemohan (Eds.), *UpToDate*. Retrieved from https://www.uptodate.com/contents/failure-to-thrive-undernutrition-in-children-younger-than-two-years-etiology-and-evaluation

Ralph, S. S., & Taylor, C. M. (2014). *Spark's & Taylor's nursing diagnosis reference manual* (9th ed.). Philadelphia, PA: Wolters Kluwer Health/Lippincott Williams & Wilkins.

Sant'Anna, A. M. G. A., Hammes, P. S., Porporino, M., Martel, C., Zygmuntowicz, C., & Ramsay, M. (2014). Use of cyproheptadine in young children with feeding difficulties and poor growth in a pediatric feeding program. *Journal of Pediatric Gastroenterology and Nutrition, 59*(5), 674–678. doi:10.1097/MPG.0000000000000467

Wilson, D. (2015). Health problems of the infant. In M. J. Hockenberry & D. Wilson (Eds.), *Wong's nursing care of infants and children* (10th ed., pp. 452–784). St. Louis, MO: Mosby/Elsevier.

■ FLUID AND ELECTROLYTE IMBALANCES

Michael D. Gooch
Celeste M. Alfes

Overview

Fluid and electrolyte balance is essential for homeostasis and assures adequate cellular perfusion and function, and is the key to maintaining electrolyte balance as well. Sodium (Na^+), potassium (K^+), calcium (Ca^{2+}), and magnesium (Mg^{2+}) play key roles in maintaining cell membrane stability, muscle contractions, cardiac and neuronal conduction, and bone health. This balance may be altered by numerous processes including numerous medications, diseases, alterations in the pH, and nutrition. A thorough history including medication review, physical examination, and analysis of laboratory data is often needed to identify an imbalance, assess for complications, and formulate a plan of care. Nurses should be able to recognize the diagnostics needed to properly identify an imbalance, the associated clinical manifestations, and initial management of these derangements.

Background

Water makes up 50% to 60% of our total body weight, although this varies by age, sex, and muscle and fat composition (Hall, 2016; Harring, Deal, & Kuo, 2014; Kamel & Halperin, 2017). Water is contained in various compartments and can be shifted around if needed by the body. The intracellular space accounts for two thirds of our total body water. The remainder is extracellular and includes intravascular (plasma) and interstitial spaces. Water balance is regulated by the hypothalamic–neurohypophyseal–renal axis; during acute illness this axis is often altered leading to imbalances in many hospitalized patients (Knepper, Kwon, & Nielsen, 2015). By releasing vasopressin or antidiuretic hormone (ADH), altering the thirst response, and altering renal water excretion, this axis works to maintain a serum osmolality of 280 to 295 mmol/kg; as with any lab the accepted values vary. Osmolality is a measure of the concentration of solutes in a solution (Hall, 2016; Harring et al., 2014; Kamel & Halperin, 2017). The higher the osmolality, the higher the concentration of solutes. Osmolality must be balanced between intracellular and extracellular compartments to maintain equilibrium and cell membrane integrity (Kamel & Halperin, 2017; Sterns, 2015). Sodium is the primary extracellular solute and directly influences osmolality, as well as how fluids shift among the body's compartments. Fluid movement is also influenced by plasma proteins, glucose, and other electrolytes.

Sodium is the most abundant extracellular cation, with an accepted normal range of 135 to 145 mEq/L. Hyponatremia is considered the most common electrolyte imbalance encountered in the hospitalized patient (Cho, 2017). It is estimated that 15% of admitted adults have hyponatremia with an overall mortality rate of 3% to 29% (Harring et al., 2014). The degree of hyponatremia is often assessed based on the serum and urine Na^+ concentrations and osmolality. Isotonic hyponatremia (osmolality 280–295 mmol/kg) is characterized by a normal serum osmolality and may result from elevated serum lipids or proteins. Hypertonic hyponatremia (osmolality greater than 295 mmol/kg) may be caused by hyperglycemia or osmotic diuretics (Cho, 2017; Craig, 2015; Harring et al., 2014; Kamel & Halperin, 2017).

The most common fluid and electrolyte imbalance is hypotonic hyponatremia (osmolality less than 280 mmol/kg). Children are at particular risk of developing hyponatraemia encephalopathy (Lamont & Crean, 2014). Hypotonic patients can further be categorized as hypovolemic, euvolemic, and hypervolemic. Hypovolemia occurs when there is a loss of both water and Na^+ from the body, for example, excessive gastrointestinal (GI) or genitourinary (GU) losses. The Na^+ loss usually exceeds the water loss, and these patients often appear dehydrated. Euvolemia occurs when excess free water is gained most often related to ADH release or function, and there is no excess of serum Na^+. This may include hypothyroidism, cortisol insufficiency, syndrome of inappropriate antidiuretic hormone (SIADH), exogenous free water intake, and use of certain drugs including thiazide diuretics and 3,4-methylenedioxymethamphetamine (MDMA, ecstasy). As the free water is gained, the serum Na^+ is lowered, but there is usually no loss of Na^+. However, the patient does not appear dehydrated or volume overloaded. Hypervolemia occurs when there is an increased retention of both body water and Na^+ often because of renal disease, heart failure, or cirrhosis. Water is retained more than Na^+, leading to a decrease in the serum Na^+. These patients usually appear volume overloaded (Cho, 2017; Craig, 2015; Harring et al., 2014; Kamel & Halperin, 2017; Sterns, 2015).

Hypernatremia is most often associated with a decrease in free water intake which leads to cellular dehydration and an increased osmolality. This can be seen in patients with a decreased thirst reflex and those without easy access to water, for example, limited mobility, extremes of age, and comatose states. It is also associated with diabetes insipidus (DI); because of the lack of ADH, the kidneys cannot adequately regulate water balance. Excess loss of water worsens hypernatremia, but unless the thirst reflex is altered or there is limited access to water, insufficient free water intake is the primary cause of hypernatremia (Cho, 2017; Craig, 2015; Harring et al., 2014; Kamel & Halperin, 2017).

Potassium is the most abundant intracellular cation with an accepted serum range of 3.5 to 5.0 mEq/L. Potassium plays a key role in maintaining the resting membrane potential of cardiac and muscle cells. Hypokalemia may be related to increased loss from the GI or GU tract, cellular shifts from alkalosis and beta-2 stimulation, or inadequate dietary intake. Hypomagnesemia can also lead to hypokalemia. Hyperkalemia may result from medications that increase K^+ levels, inadequate excretion as seen in renal failure, cellular shifts seen with acidosis and significant tissue trauma, or maybe a measurement error because of cell hemolysis from the lab draw, often referred to as *pseudohyperkalemia* (Combs & Buckley, 2015; Gooch, 2015; Hall, 2016; Kamel & Halperin, 2017; Medford-Davis & Rafique, 2014).

Calcium plays an essential role in the neuromuscular function and bone health. A normal Ca^{2+} level is often considered to be 8.5 to 10.5 mg/dL or an ionized level of 4.6 to 5.3 mg/dL. About half of the serum Ca^{2+} is bound to proteins; the remainder is free or ionized. Almost all (99%) of the body's Ca^{2+} is stored in the bones. Hypocalcemia most often results from inadequate intake or gastrointestinal (GI) absorption, a chronic kidney disease that results in vitamin D deficiency, hypoparathyroidism, or from massive blood transfusions. In the setting of hypoalbuminemia, hypocalcemia may be noted and is often considered a pseudohypocalcemia. Evaluating the ionized Ca^{2+} level can help determine if a true imbalance exists. Hypercalcemia most often develops from hyperparathyroidism or, in cases of higher levels, malignancy is a prime cause. It is estimated that 20% to 30% of cancer patients experience hypercalcemia (Chang, Radin, & McCurdy, 2014; Cho, 2017; Gooch, 2015; Hall, 2016; Love & Buckley, 2015).

Magnesium is the second most common intracellular cation and plays a similar role as Ca^{2+} in regards to the nervous system. When outside the normal range of 1.8 to 2.5 mg/dL it may influence K^+ and Ca^{2+} levels. Hypomagnesemia is more common and often results from altered dietary intake or absorption or increased urinary excretion. Hypermagnesemia is rare and often associated with renal failure but could be related to medications that increase magnesium levels (Chang et al., 2014; Cho, 2017; Love & Buckley, 2015).

Clinical Aspects

ASSESSMENT

It is common for acutely ill patients to have one or more imbalances. The nurse should be observant for risk factors and signs or symptoms of these imbalances. Both Na^+ imbalances may present similarly, and lab data is needed to properly identify and manage the patient. The patient may have altered mental status, weakness, headache, or seizures. Management is guided by the lab values, clinical findings, and rapidity in which symptoms started. Hypovolemia should be corrected as the patient condition allows. In the stable hyponatremic patient, free water restrictions may be all that is required to stabilize the patient. In the unstable seizing patient, a bolus of hypertonic (3%) saline may be required. In most patients, increasing the serum Na^+ by 4 mEq/L is all that is needed to reduce cerebral edema and resolve the seizures. In patients with SIADH or hypervolemic hyponatremia, a vasopressin antagonist may be administered to block ADH receptors in the kidneys and limit the reabsorption of water (Cho, 2017; Craig, 2015; Gooch, 2015).

NURSING INTERVENTIONS, MANAGEMENT, AND IMPLICATIONS

Fluid administration to the pediatric patient is an integral part of the medical management of hospitalized children (Lamont & Crean, 2014). Intravenous (IV) fluids are frequently administered to hospitalized children to provide sufficient water, electrolytes, and glucose to maintain homeostasis during recovery from illness (Lamont & Crean, 2014). Variations in age, size, underlying physiology, and disease processes should be considered and in general younger children require more fluid per kilogram than older children owing to a higher metabolic rate, higher body surface area to volume ratio, and a reduction in renal concentrating ability (Lamont & Crean, 2014). Total body water percentages vary with age, most likely seen as a higher percentage of body water in the very young compared to the older pediatric patient (Lamont & Crean, 2014).

Hypernatremia may be managed with isotonic IV fluids initially to restore perfusion. Loop diuretics may be used in volume-overloaded patients to increase the excretion of water and Na^+. In the setting of DI, desmopressin (DDAVP) may be given. An important caveat to the management of Na^+ imbalances is that the level should not be rapidly changed. If the serum Na^+ is increased too quickly, osmotic demyelination or central pontine myelinolysis may occur. If the serum Na^+ is reduced too rapidly, cerebral edema often develops. A guideline to prevent complications is to correct the level by no more than 1 to 2 mEq/L/hr and no more than 10 mEq/d (Cho, 2017; Craig, 2015; Gooch, 2015; Sterns, 2015). The more chronic the condition, the slower the correction.

Any patient suspected of having a K^+ imbalance should have his or her EKG quickly assessed. Patients may experience muscle cramps or weakness, which could progress to respiratory failure. Flattened or inverted T waves, the appearance of U waves, and ST depression are often seen with hypokalemia. Hypokalemic management is also based on the severity and may require oral or IV K^+ replacement. In the setting of hypomagnesemia, the Mg^{2+} imbalance will have to be corrected first (Cho, 2017; Combs & Buckley, 2015; Gooch, 2015; Medford-Davis & Rafique, 2014).

Of the electrolyte imbalances, hyperkalemia is the most lethal. If there is a concern for hyperkalemia, the ECG should quickly be assessed for the presence of peaked T waves, a prolonged PR interval, or a widened QRS. If these ECG changes are present, IV Ca^{2+} should be administered to stabilize the resting membrane potential of the cardiac cells and prevent life-threatening arrhythmias. Treatment should not be delayed while awaiting lab values. Hyperkalemia is managed two ways. First, high dose albuterol, insulin with glucose, or sodium bicarbonate may be given to shift the K+ back in the cells temporarily. Subsequently, the excessive K^+ should be eliminated. This is most effectively accomplished through hemodialysis, but loop diuretics or cation exchange resins may also be used with caution (Cho, 2017; Combs & Buckley, 2015; Gooch, 2015; Medford-Davis & Rafique, 2014).

Hypocalcemia cause neuromuscular excitability including muscle spasms, paresthesias, hyperactive deep tendon reflexes (DTRs), and eventually seizures. The ECG should also be assessed for a prolonged QT interval and bradycardia. Symptomatic patients may be managed with oral or IV Ca^{2+} replacement. Patients with hypercalcemia may have lethargy, muscle weakness, hypoactive DTRs, and at higher levels a shortened QT and widened QRS may be noted on the ECG. Patients may develop atrioventricular blocks which can progress to cardiac arrest in levels more than 15 mg/dL. Initially, IV fluids should be given to restore renal perfusion. Depending on the severity of the patient, hemodialysis may be used to remove the excess Ca^{2+}. In less severe cases, the patient may be given a loop diuretic, a bisphosphonate, a glucocorticoid, or calcitonin (Chang et al., 2014; Cho, 2017; Gooch, 2015; Love & Buckley, 2015).

Lastly, patients with low serum Mg^{2+} levels present similarly to those with hypokalemia and hypocalcemia and have weakness and muscle cramps. This can progress to neuromuscular and cardiac irritability. Treatment is focused on replacement with oral or IV Mg^{2+} depending on the patient's condition. Hypermagnesemia is similar to hypercalcemia, and patients experience blunted neuromuscular effects including lethargy, paralysis, decreased DTRs, and eventually hypotension, cardiac and respiratory compromise. Calcium may be administered to antagonize the Mg^{2+} and reverse neuromuscular weakness. If needed, dialysis is effective at removing the excess electrolyte in severe cases (Chang et al., 2014; Cho, 2017; Love & Buckley, 2015).

OUTCOMES

The fluid prescription for each pediatric patient should be individualized according to the clinical situation. Many hospitalized children are at risk of developing hyponatremia while receiving IV fluids, which may necessitate fluid restriction (Lamont & Crean, 2014). The nurse should include frequent monitoring and observation of the child to ensure the fluid orders are still appropriate. Often a urea and electrolyte profile should be checked at least every 24 hours in pediatric patients receiving IV fluids and more frequently if there are known electrolyte abnormalities (Lamont & Crean, 2014). Asymptomatic electrolyte abnormalities are common and will be detectable only by blood sampling; only fluids with a sodium content above 131 mmol/L should be used for an IV fluid bolus (Lamont & Crean, 2014).

Summary

Fluid and electrolyte balance is critical to maintaining all body functions. Sodium and water have an important relationship and imbalances are common in pediatric patients with acute problems. Patients with Na^+ imbalances often present with neurological changes and the imbalance cannot be aggressively corrected. Potassium is crucial for cardiac and muscle function; it can be life threatening and often requires rapid identification and correction to prevent complications. Calcium and Mg^{2+} both play an important role in neuromuscular function and can affect cardiac function as well. Nurses should evaluate for these imbalances in the acutely ill pediatric patient, recalling the patient may have more than one. Labs are often helpful, but history and physical examination findings are also important to identify the imbalance and manage the derangement.

Chang, W.-T. W., Radin, B., & McCurdy, M. T. (2014). Calcium, magnesium, and phosphate abnormalities in the emergency department. *Emergency Medicine Clinics of North America, 32*(2), 349–366. doi:10.1016/j.emc.2013.12.006

Cho, K. C. (2017). Electrolyte and acid-base disorders. In M. A. Papadakis, S. J. McPhee, & M. W. Rabow (Eds.), *Current medical diagnosis and treatment 2017* (56th ed., pp. 884–912). New York, NY: McGraw-Hill.

Combs, D. J., & Buckley, R. G. (2015). Disorders of potassium metabolism. In A. B. Wolfson, R. L. Cloutier, G. W. Hendey, L. J. Ling, C. L. Rosen, & J. J. Schaider (Eds.), *Harwood-Nuss' clinical practice of emergency medicine* (6th ed., pp. 1047–1052). Philadelphia, PA: Wolters Kluwer.

Craig, S. A. (2015). Disorders of sodium and water metabolism. In A. B. Wolfson, R. L. Cloutier, G. W. Hendey, L. J. Ling, C. L. Rosen, & J. J. Schaider (Eds.), *Harwood-Nuss' clinical practice of emergency medicine* (6th ed., pp. 1041–1047). Philadelphia, PA: Wolters Kluwer.

Gooch, M. D. (2015). Identifying acid-base and electrolyte imbalances. *The Nurse Practitioner, 40*(8), 37–42. doi:10.1097/01.NPR.0000469255.98119.82

Hall, J. E. (2016). *Guyton and Hall textbook of medical physiology* (13th ed.). Philadelphia, PA: Elsevier.

Harring, T. R., Deal, N. S., & Kuo, D. C. (2014). Disorders of sodium and water balance. *Emergency Medicine Clinics of North America, 32*(2), 379–401. doi:10.1016/j.emc.2014.01.001

Kamel, K. S., & Halperin, M. L. (2017). *Fluid, electrolyte, and acid-base physiology: A problem-based approach* (5th ed.). Philadelphia, PA: Elsevier.

Knepper, M. A., Kwon, T.-H., & Nielsen, S. (2015). Molecular physiology of water balance. *The New England Journal of Medicine, 372*(14), 1349–1358. doi:10.1056/NEJMra1404726

Lamont, S., & Crean, P. (2014). Fluid and electrolyte balance in children. *Paediatrics and Child Health, 24*(7), 273–277. doi:10.1016/j.paed.2013.11.001

Love, J. W., & Buckley, R. G. (2015). Disorders of calcium, phosphate, and magnesium metabolism. In A. B. Wolfson, R. L. Cloutier, G. W. Hendey, L. J. Ling, C. L. Rosen, & J. J. Schaider (Eds.), *Harwood-Nuss' clinical practice of emergency medicine* (6th ed., pp. 1052–1058). Philadelphia, PA: Wolters Kluwer.

Medford-Davis, L., & Rafique, Z. (2014). Derangements of potassium. *Emergency Medicine Clinics of North America, 32*(2), 329–347. doi:10.1016/j.emc.2013.12.005

Sterns, R. H. (2015). Disorders of plasma sodium. *The New England Journal of Medicine, 372*(13), 1267–1269. doi:10.1056/NEJMc1501342

■ INFLAMMATORY BOWEL DISEASE

Sharon Perry

Overview

Inflammatory bowel disease (IBD) is a chronic inflammatory disorder of the gastrointestinal tract that includes Crohn's disease, ulcerative colitis (UC), and inflammatory bowel disease unclassified (IBD-U). The location and degree of inflammation, as well as histological findings, determine the diagnosis. The incidence of IBD is increasing in children, and up-to-date investigation, diagnosis, and management are essential (Kammermeier et al., 2015). The role of the nurse in IBD is to educate patients and their families so that they are successful in the management of their disease.

Background

Around 25% of patients are diagnosed with IBD in the first two decades of life, with the most common time between 13 and 18 years, with the incidence increasing in the early second decade of life (Ye, Pang, Chen, Ju, & Zhou, 2015). The incidence of pediatric IBD is increasing worldwide; the highest rise occurring in developing countries is thought to be because of the influence of Western culture (Ye et al., 2015). In the United States, IBD in children and adolescents accounts for 30% of all patients diagnosed; in Canada, the incidence of pediatric IBD increased from 9.5/100,000 in 1994 to 11.4/100,000 in 2005 (Ye et al., 2015).

The exact etiology of IBD is unknown. The current concept is IBD has a multifactorial etiology, consistency of an overlap between genetics, environment, dysregulation of the immune system, and the microbiome. It has been linked to several genes, including *NOD2/CARD15* gene. Although the link between genetics and environment is unknown, previous research suggests that nonpathogenic intestinal bacteria trigger and perpetuate an uncontrolled inflammatory response. Microorganisms, including *Mycobacterium avium* paratuberculosis (MAP) and *Escherichia coli* adherent-invasive, have also been linked to IBD.

Crohn's disease and UC share many features, but do have some distinct differences. Clinical presentation, radiologic findings, and histological patterns can allow for differentiation of the two, but there can still exist clinical ambiguity among them in a single patient. In pediatric patients, IBD demonstrates unique characteristics in phenotype and severity. In Crohn's disease, the terminal ileum is most often involved and the disease progression in the first decade of diagnosis is well documented, along with more extensive disease than adults with Crohn's disease. In UC, pancolitis is the most common finding at diagnosis and is more likely to progress in the first decade.

Diagnosis is made by history, physical examination, laboratory results, and endoscopic findings. Once the diagnosis is made, there are several treatment options for patients, including steroids, exclusive enteral nutrition, immunomodulator medications, and biologic agents to induce and maintain remission. The role of the nurse is to provide support throughout their journey.

Clinical Aspects

ASSESSMENT

Diarrhea, rectal bleeding, abdominal pain, weight loss, and growth failure are common presenting symptoms of IBD. Patients may also present with extraintestinal manifestations, including aphthous ulcers, fever, anemia, joint pain, or skin rashes. Lab work is done to identify anemia, hypoalbuminemia, and elevated inflammatory markers. Stool studies to rule out an infectious process, including *Clostridium difficile* and bacterial infections, are part of the routine workup. Esophagogastroduodenoscopy (EGD) and colonoscopy remain the gold standard of IBD and can determine disease location and extent. Small-bowel imaging, such as magnetic resonance enterography, is obtained to rule out abscess, strictures, or fistulas in the portion of the small bowel out of reach from standard endoscopes. Video-capsule endoscopy can also be obtained to survey the mucosal lining of the small bowel. In most cases, this workup is done in the outpatient setting.

For IBD in the outpatient setting, the nurse is seen as a "first point of contact" for patients and their families. The nurse is responsible for recognizing a change in symptoms and early intervention during acute exacerbations, which may reduce admissions and emergency room visits (Leach et al., 2014). The nurse also coordinates medical management, future endoscopic procedures, and development of self-management strategies.

In the inpatient setting, effective nursing care is based on physical examination, interpretation of labs, recognition of medication reactions, and education. A change in the abdominal examination (increased pain, abdominal tenderness, or abdominal distention), increase in stool pattern, and/or onset of hematochezia are concerns related to an exacerbation or worsening disease. In addition, changes in albumin, hemoglobin, and inflammatory markers may indicate changes in disease status.

NURSING INTERVENTIONS, MANAGEMENT, AND IMPLICATIONS

Nursing care of the pediatric patient with IBD in the inpatient setting is focused on education allowing the patient to be discharged home with a basic knowledge of the disease. The focus of the outpatient nurse is disease management, medication adherence, and promotion of self-care, with the ultimate goal of successful transition to adult care at the appropriate time.

OUTCOMES

Research has shown that IBD nurse specialists have a positive impact on outcomes of patients with IBD. As valuable and cost-effective members of the health care team, nurses excel in providing educational materials on lifestyle, health maintenance, medications, and diagnostic testing, which help to improve patient education, satisfaction, and disease management. Hospital stays were also shown to decrease by 38%, and length of admissions decreased by 19% when an IBD specialist was involved in the patient's care (Stretton, Currie, & Chauhan, 2014).

Summary

Adolescents and children with IBD can thrive when it is detected early in the disease process and managed with the most effective medications. Diagnosis is multifactorial, and treatment options are continually expanding. The nurse plays a crucial role in providing the education necessary for IBD patients to achieve and sustain remission.

Kammermeier, J., Morris, M.-A., Garrick, V., Furman, M., Rodrigues, A., & Russell, R. (2015). Management of Crohn's disease. *Archives of Disease in Childhood, 101*(5), 475–480. doi:10.1136/archdischild-2014-307217

Leach, P., De Silva, M., Mountifield, R., Edwards, S., Chitti, L., Fraser, R., & Bampton, P. (2014). The effect of an inflammatory bowel disease nurse position on service delivery. *Journal of Crohn's and Colitis, 8*, 370–374. doi:10.1016/j.crohns.2013.09.018

Stretton, J., Currie, B., & Chauhan, U. (2014). Inflammatory bowel disease nurses in Canada: An examination of Canadian gastroenterology nurses and their role in inflammatory bowel disease care. *Canadian Journal of Gastroenterology and Hepatology, 28*(2), 89–93. doi:10.1155/2014/179309

Ye, Y., Pang, Z., Chen, W., Ju, S., & Zhou, C. (2015). The epidemiology and risk factors of inflammatory bowel disease. *International Journal of Clinical and Experimental Medicine, 8*(12), 22529–22542. Retrieved from https://www.ncbi.nlm.nih.gov/pmc/articles/PMC4730025

■ OBESITY

Rosanna P. Watowicz

Overview

Pediatric obesity is a major concern in the United States, affecting approximately 17% of children between 2 and 19 years of age. Defined as a body mass index (BMI) at the 95th percentile or above, obesity has been linked to several serious comorbidities, both physiological and psychological. Nurses play an important role in educating families around specific guidelines that have been developed for children with obesity.

Background

In children, obesity is defined as having a BMI at or above the gender-specific 95th percentile according to the Centers for Disease Control and Prevention (CDC) BMI-for-age growth charts. Most recent estimates indicate that 17% of the U.S. population between the ages of 2 and 19 years have obesity. The prevalence of obesity is higher for non-Hispanic Black children (19.5%) and Hispanic children (21.9%), compared to non-Hispanic White children (14.7%). The overall prevalence is also higher for 6- to 11-year-old children (17.5%) and 12- to 19-year-old children (20.5%).

Obesity comorbidities may include hypertension, sleep apnea, type 2 diabetes, hyperinsulinemia, nonalcoholic fatty liver disease, dyslipidemia, polycystic ovarian syndrome and other menstrual irregularities, and orthopedic conditions such as Blount's disease and slipped capital femoral epiphysis. Psychosocial comorbidities, including bullying or isolation from peers, decreased the quality of life, and anxiety or depression are also common (Barlow & Expert Committee, 2007).

In 2013, the American Heart Association brought attention to the additional health risks for children and adolescents with severe obesity. Consequently, a standardized definition of severe obesity was recommended (Kelly et al., 2013). Based on this recommendation, the most widely accepted definition of severe obesity is now 120% of the 95th percentiles of gender-specific BMI-for-age (i.e., 1.2 times the absolute BMI at the 95th percentile for the child's gender and age). Estimates indicate that 5.8% of the U.S. population aged 2 to 19 years have severe obesity (Ogden et al., 2016). Mirroring the trends for obesity overall, prevalence is higher for non-Hispanic Black and Hispanic children compared to non-Hispanic White children, and also for older children compared to younger children.

The etiology of obesity is extremely complex and most likely involves both environmental and genetic factors (Kumar & Kelly, 2017). Collectively referred to as "lifestyle behaviors," diet and physical activity play a large role in the development of obesity. High caloric consumption from sugar-sweetened beverages, fast foods or restaurant foods, and large portion sizes can contribute to energy imbalance. In addition, reduced physical activity and increased screen time contribute to decreased energy expenditure. Several additional environmental factors that are further outside of individual control, such as parental feeding styles, perinatal factors (i.e., maternal weight gain during pregnancy), breast feeding status, antibiotic use, gut microbiota, and adverse life experiences have also been implicated as causes of obesity. However, multiple gene sites related to appetite, satiety, and fat distribution have been identified as being associated with obesity, clearly indicating heritability (Barlow & Expert Committee, 2007). Certain medications, particularly antipsychotics, are known to contribute to weight gain, and for a small percentage of children, obesity may be related to a genetic syndrome such as Prader–Willi syndrome (Kumar & Kelly, 2017).

Clinical Aspects

ASSESSMENT

Nurses and other health care professionals should use BMI percentile to identify obesity in children aged 2 years and older. Weight and height should be measured at least annually, and BMI percentile should be calculated at each measurement. Many electronic health record systems can be configured to automatically calculate and display BMI percentile for children, which removes the burden of calculating BMI percentile from the medical staff. If BMI percentile is not available in the electronic health record, gender-specific BMI-for-age, CDC growth charts, or the CDC's (n.d.) online BMI percentile calculator should be used. The American Academy of Pediatrics does not recommend screening children for obesity before the age of 2 years.

Severe obesity is more difficult to assess as growth charts defining 120% of the 95th percentile are not readily available, nor are they easily configured into electronic health records. Clinicians may use an absolute BMI of 35 kg/m^2 or greater as a proxy for severe obesity in children. However, young children with severe obesity may not approach this BMI cutoff. For clinicians to whom it is important to know whether a child has obesity versus severe obesity, a manual calculation of 120% of the BMI at the 95th percentile for that child may be necessary (Kelly et al., 2013).

If a child is found to have obesity, the nurse may look for physical signs of the comorbidities related to obesity, such as elevated blood pressure, acanthosis nigricans (a darkening of the skin around the neck, which can be indicative of hyperinsulinemia), or problems with gait. The nurse may also ask about snoring, which may be a sign of obstructive sleep apnea. Common laboratory assessments for children with obesity include fasting blood glucose and/or hemoglobin A1c (HbA1c), fasting lipid panel, alanine transaminase (ALT), and aspartate aminotransferase (AST). Elevated values for any of these studies may indicate an obesity-related comorbidity (Kumar & Kelly, 2017).

Health care professionals should also assess diet and physical activity behaviors for children with obesity. Nutrition-related assessment may include sugar-sweetened beverage consumption, the frequency of dining out, fruit and vegetable consumption, and typical composition and portion size of meals and snacks. Physical activity behaviors may include the amount of daily or weekly active play or vigorous activity as well as the amount of daily screen time. Owing to the psychosocial comorbidities that are common among children with obesity, the quality of life is often assessed as well. Several validated tools exist to assess the quality of life in children, including the Pediatric Quality of Life Inventory (Peds-QL) and the Impact of Weight on Quality of Life-Kids (IWQOL-Kids; Bryant et al., 2014). The nurse may also ask the child about teasing or bullying experiences.

NURSING INTERVENTIONS, MANAGEMENT, AND IMPLICATIONS

Nursing-related problems for the child with obesity may include a knowledge deficit and/or imbalanced nutrition. To address these problems, nurses and other health care professionals should provide education around eight specific guidelines for families and children with obesity: (a) consume five or more servings of fruits and vegetables per day, (b) minimize sugar-sweetened beverages, (c) limit screen time to 2 hours per day or fewer (d) participate in 1 hour or more of physical activity per day, (e) eat breakfast daily, (f) limit meals outside the home, (g) eat family meals at least five or six times per week, and (h) allow the child to self-regulate his or her meals and avoid overly restrictive behaviors (Spear et al., 2007). In addition, children with obesity should be referred to a primary care provider or registered dietitian with additional training in pediatric weight management and behavioral counseling. Older children, or those with more severe obesity, may benefit from a referral directly to a multidisciplinary pediatric weight management clinic or tertiary care center where more aggressive options such as pharmacological treatment or weight loss surgery can be discussed.

OUTCOMES

In the early stages of obesity treatment, the goal is for the child to maintain his or her weight while age and height increase, thereby decreasing his or her BMI and BMI percentile. If a child loses weight, weight loss should be limited to an average of 2 pounds per week, with lesser weight loss suggested for younger children (Spear et al., 2007).

Summary

Pediatric obesity is a common yet complex disease with a variety of potential causes. Nurses play an important role in ensuring that BMI percentile is assessed and that the recommended education is provided. Children with obesity should also be referred to health care professionals with training in pediatric obesity management. The high prevalence of obesity has led to the existence of multidisciplinary weight management centers where nurses specialized in obesity are part of the treatment team. The goal for children with obesity should be weight maintenance or a weight loss of no more than 2 pounds per week

Barlow, S. E., & Expert Committee. (2007). Expert committee recommendations regarding the prevention, assessment, and treatment of child and adolescent overweight and obesity: Summary report. *Pediatrics, 120*(Suppl. 4), S164–S192. doi:10.1542/peds.2007-2329C

Bryant, M., Ashton, L., Brown, J., Jebb, S., Wright, J., Roberts, K., & Nixon, J. (2014). Systematic review to identify and appraise outcome measures used to evaluate childhood obesity treatment interventions (CoOR): Evidence of purpose, application, validity, reliability, and sensitivity. *Health Technology Assessment, 18*(51), 1–380. doi:10.3310/hta18510

Centers for Disease Control and Prevention. (2016). BMI percentile calculator for child and teen. Retrieved from https://nccd.cdc.gov/dnpabmi/calculator.aspx

Kelly, A. S., Barlow, S. E., Rao, G., Inge, T. H., Hayman, L. L., Steinberger, J., ... Daniels, S. R. (2013). Severe obesity in children and adolescents: Identification, associated health risks, and treatment approaches: A scientific statement from the American Heart Association. *Circulation, 128*(15), 1689–1712. doi:10.1161/CIR.0b013e3182a5cfb3

Kumar, S., & Kelly, A. S. (2017). Review of childhood obesity: From epidemiology, etiology, and comorbidities to clinical assessment and treatment. *Mayo Clinic Proceedings, 92*(2), 251–265. doi:10.1016/j.mayocp.2016.09.017

Ogden, C. L., Carroll, M. D., Lawman, H. G., Fryar, C. D., Kruszon-Moran, D., Kit, B. K., & Flegal, K. M. (2016). Trends in obesity prevalence among children and adolescents in the United States, 1988–1994 through 2013–2014. *Journal of the American Medical Association, 315*(21), 2292–2299. doi:10.1001/jama.2016.6361

Spear, B. A., Barlow, S. E., Ervin, C., Ludwig, D. S., Saelens, B. E., Schetzina, K. E., & Taveras, E. M. (2007). Recommendations for treatment of child and adolescent overweight and obesity. *Pediatrics, 120*(Suppl. 4), S254–S288. doi:10.1542/peds.2007-2329F

■ ORAL HEALTH

Marguerite DiMarco

Overview

Tooth decay or dental caries is one of the most prevalent chronic diseases in children, five times more common than asthma. Dental caries is an infectious disease that can be transmitted from mother or primary care taker to infant. Many health care professionals do not know about the pathology behind dental caries, or how serious oral disease can affect systemic health. In fact, the surgeon general called dental caries the "silent epidemic" especially affecting poor children. Many Americans lack a dental home and children are 2.5 times more likely not to have dental coverage. Dentists are declining, and many do not accept Medicaid, making it difficult for poor families to access dental care. Therefore, health professionals, including dentists/hygienists, physicians, physician assistants, nurse practitioners, nurses, and dieticians, need to work together to meet the oral health needs of infants, children, and adolescents (Office of Disease Prevention and Health Promotion, 2014).

Background

The primary cause of tooth decay is the bacterium *Streptococcus mutans*, which is the main contributor to tooth decay. Adults may have higher amounts of *S. mutans* in their mouths and can transmit it to their infant or child through the exchange of saliva. Frequent sugary snacking and drinking interacts with *S. mutans*, producing acids that can cause mineral loss from the teeth increasing the risk for tooth decay. Dental caries affects more children in the United States than any other chronic infectious disease. Tooth decay and other oral diseases that can affect children are preventable. Fluoride varnish can reduce cavities in preschool children by 30% to 40%. The American Dental Association (ADA) currently recommends 2.26% fluoride varnish for prevention of dental caries in children aged 6 years and younger. School-age children in second and sixth grades can have dental sealants placed on healthy molars, which has reduced the amount of caries in school-age and adolescent children. Unfortunately, the rates of caries continue to rise in the preschool-age group. Tooth decay in baby teeth contributes to an increased amount of decay in the permanent teeth (DiMarco et al., 2016).

Tooth decay of the front top teeth is referred to as *early childhood caries* (ECC), formerly called *baby bottle tooth decay*. The causes of ECC include poor oral hygiene, not enough fluoride, sleeping with a bottle or sippy cup, frequent snacking, bottle/sippy cup feedings containing beverages high in sugar, milk, or formula during the day or night, coating pacifiers with sweeteners like sugar or honey, and having a mother/caregiver or sibling who has had active tooth decay in the past 12 months. ECC and tooth decay in general are a multifactorial disease, and a child could have a few of these factors and not have decay, although other children may have only one factor and have decay. In addition, some foods called *cariogenic foods* such as cookies, juice or sweet drinks, chips, fruit roll-ups, and chewy candy cause tooth decay more than others. ECC develops in young children who use sippy cups or baby bottles constantly, and have poor nutrition with a history of eating frequently or eating the wrong foods (DiMarco et al., 2016).

The process of decay is influenced mostly by sugars that can be fermented by the bacteria in the mouth, causing a lower pH or acidic environment. This environment works on deteriorating the enamel of the tooth. This demineralization incites a cavity. Caries, in the primary dentition, leads to the same in permanent teeth. Another source of caries, aside from poor nutrition choices, is an infection. Mothers who pick up their child's pacifier and put the pacifier in their mouth to clean it off may inadvertently pass on the bacteria, *Mutans streptococci*, which causes dental caries. Along with passing the infection by saliva and mouth kissing the baby, the frequency of eating significantly increases the presence of *Mutans streptococci*. The constant change of the acidity of the mouth's saliva causes a wearing down of the protective enamel setting up the possibility of decay. A human's saliva can cause remineralization of the tooth's enamel. Eating foods that keep the acidity of saliva high continues to cause demineralization and the potential for dental caries. The more the teeth are bathed in anything other than water or healthy saliva, the greater the chance of demineralization. Despite our understanding of the risk factors associated with caries in early childhood, it remains one of the largest untreated conditions in preschool children (Griffin et al., 2014).

Oral health has been linked to physical health, social acceptance, and well-being. During these early years of physical growth, appropriate nutrition is essential. If chewing is painful, children refuse to eat crunchy fresh fruit or vegetables because they cause too much discomfort. Socially, children are sensitive to being different from others. If teeth are decayed or eroded, it sets them up for social bullying, even at a young age. The normal eruption of teeth permits children successful language development. Proper speech, sturdy teeth, and attractive smiles permit children greater access to their social worlds and help them achieve not only physical health but social acceptance as well. Lack of access to care and untreated dental conditions in children contribute to emergency room visits, expensive treatments, dysfunctional speech, compromised nutrition and growth, and an estimated 52 million missed hours of school per year, 189 million hours of lost work, not to mention the pain and suffering. Untreated caries can lead to infection, and infections in the mouth can spread to the blood causing infections in the brain, mouth abscesses, sinus infections, cellulitis, endocarditis, and sepsis to mention a few. Unborn babies are affected if their mothers have dental disease and periodontal disease; the infant could be born having a low birth weight, be premature or even still born (Norris, DiMarco, & Thacker, 2013).

Clinical Aspects

The American Academy of Pediatric Dentistry (AAPD) and the American Academy of Pediatricians (AAP) recommend that primary care providers and other health professionals include the following oral health prevention strategies: (a) perform periodic risk assessments to determine the child's relative risk of developing dental caries; (b) provide anticipatory guidance to parents about oral hygiene, diet, and fluoride exposure; (c) apply appropriate preventive therapies, such as fluoride varnish; and (d) help parents establish a dental home for their children by 12 months of age (Griffin et al., 2014).

ASSESSMENT

Nurses can perform an oral-screening assessment of the lips, tongue, teeth, gums, inside the cheeks, and the roof of the mouth to assess for dental caries or other oral conditions such as abscesses or trauma. An oral health screening takes about 2 minutes; no diagnosis is made that requires a dentist, and the nurse can guide management. The nurse can do a knee-to-knee examination with the parent facing him or her and the child lying down on the nurse's and parent's knees facing the parent. With a gloved hand, the nurse lifts the lip, views the soft tissue, the teeth, and the entire mouth. Any light such as a flashlight can be used for screening. A tongue blade or tooth brush can be used to move the tongue and view the teeth (Norris et al., 2013).

NURSING INTERVENTIONS, MANAGEMENT, AND IMPLICATIONS

Anticipatory guidance to parents and the child should be given not only during well-child examinations but also in the hospital when doing an oral examination and/or brushing the child's teeth. Children who are at high risk are special-needs children, children with cancer, and/or children on ventilators. Nurses should follow special hospital procedures to prevent ventilator-associated pneumonia (VAP) with children on ventilators. Oral care with chlorhexidine has been studied, and meta-analyses suggest that oral care with chlorhexidine can reduce VAP rates in this population by 10% to 30%. The American Dental Association recommends beginning oral hygiene a few days after birth. Wipe the gums with a gauze pad after each feeding to remove plaque and residual formula that could harm erupting teeth. When teeth erupt, brush them gently twice a day with a child-size toothbrush and water. Fluoride toothpaste is recommended for children older than 2 years. After oral hygiene, rinse and suction the mouth. Keep the oral mucosa and lips clean, moist, and intact using sponge-tipped applicators dipped in nonalcohol nonperoxide mouth rinse (Klompas et al., 2014). Here are some tips for well or stable children:

1. Have your very own toothbrush that no one else uses.
2. Brush at least 2 minutes twice a day (after breakfast and before bed) with an adult brushing the child's teeth before bedtime until age 7 years.
3. Use a smear of fluoride toothpaste on a soft toothbrush until child spits well.
4. Once able to spit well and not swallow, increase fluoride paste to a small pea size or the size of the child's smallest fingernail.
5. Drink water after eating sweets to rinse off the teeth.
6. If a toddler carries a sippy cup around while playing, fill with water only.
7. If going to bed, fill bottles or sippy cups with water only.
8. Be cautious, if nursing your baby, that you take the baby off the breast once asleep.

9. Limit fruit juice to 4 ounces daily, 3 cups of milk, and otherwise, DRINK WATER.
10. Encourage fresh vegetables and protein-rich foods as snacks, and limit candy (Norris, DiMarco, & Thacker, 2013).

OUTCOMES

Dental problems can have deadly outcomes if not treated. Help parents establish a dental home. If a dental problem is assessed that needs immediate attention of a dentist, be aware of the resources available in your hospital or community. Some hospitals have a dentist on call or a dental clinic affiliated with the hospital. Dental schools, safety net clinics, and health departments are other sources. If these are not available in your community, make a list of private dentists and what insurances they accept.

Summary

Dental caries and oral health problems are common with children. These problems can have deadly outcomes if not treated. It is often difficult for poor families to access a dentist. Interprofessional collaboration is needed to help address the oral health problem. Nurses working in every area can help with the oral health problem. Nurses have initiated Smiles for Life: A National Oral Health Curriculum. This program presents oral health education to nurses and other health professionals in web-based modules. This article touched on some of the problems of oral health with children. A free curriculum, Smiles for Life, is available online with more detail than discussed in this article (http://smilesforlifeoralhealth.org/buildcontent.aspx?tut=555&pagekey=62948&cbreceipt=0).

DiMarco, M. A., Fitzgerald, K., Taylor, E., Marino, D., Huff, M., Biordl, D., & Mundy, E. (2016). Improving oral health of young children: An interprofessional demonstration project. *Pediatric Dental Care, 1,* 113. doi:10.4172/pdc.1000113

Griffin, S., Barker, L., Wei, L., Li, C.-H., Albuquerque, M., & Gooch, B. (2014). Use of dental care and effective preventive services in preventing tooth decay among U.S. children and adolescents—Medical Expenditure Panel Survey, United States, 2003–2009 and National Health and Nutrition Examination Survey, United States, 2005–2010. *Morbidity and Mortality Weekly Report, 63*(Suppl. 2), 54–60. Retrieved from https://www.cdc.gov/mmwr/pdf/other/su6302.pdf

Klompas, M., Branson, R., Eichenwald, E. C., Greene, L. R., Howell, M. D., Lee, G., . . . Berenholtz, S. M. (2014). Strategies to prevent ventilator-associated pneumonia in acute care hospitals: 2014 update. *Infection Control and Hospital Epidemiology, 35*(8), 915–936. doi:10.1086/677144

Norris, M., DiMarco, M. A., & Thacker, S. A. (2013). Open wide: Tips for performing oral health screening on young children during fluoride varnish application. *Nurse Practitioner, 38*(9), 14–21.

Office of Disease Prevention and Health Promotion. (2014). *Healthy people 2010: Progress reviews area 21: Oral health presentations.* Washington, DC: U.S. Department of Health and Human Services. Retrieved from https://www.cdc.gov/nchs/healthy_people/hp2010/focus_areas/fa21_oral2.htm

■ ORTHOPEDICS

Michelle Calabretta
Emily Canitia
Michelle A. Janas

Overview

Pediatric orthopedic nursing encompasses care of both the trauma and the surgical patient. Patients of all ages are affected by orthopedic issues, from the infant with a congenital club foot to the teenager with a femur fracture from a motor vehicle accident. Surgeries can range from correction of a spinal deformity to acute treatment of a fracture. The predominant focus of the pediatric orthopedic specialty is on fracture care. An increase in physical activity, such as sports and recreational activities, places the pediatric population at high risk for orthopedic injury, specifically upper extremity fractures (Shah, Buzas, & Zinberg, 2014). Many of these patients require surgical nursing care in an inpatient hospital setting. Specialized pediatric orthopedic nursing care and knowledge are essential for the successful treatment and recovery course of these patients.

Background

Fractures in children are an important public health issue and a frequent cause of emergency room visits and inpatient hospital stays. According to the National Electronic Injury Surveillance System (NEISS), nearly one in every five children experiences a fracture sometime during childhood or adolescence (Naranje, Erali, Warner, Sawyer, & Kelly, 2016). The annual incidence of fractures increases with age, with children between 10 and 14 years of age having the highest incidence of fractures. There is no gender difference in younger age groups; however, for older age groups, fractures are more prevalent in males. Children in urban areas or with lower socioeconomic status are also at an increased risk (Shah et al., 2014).

Fractures of the upper extremity in children are much more common than those of the lower extremity. The most common anatomic area for fracture is the distal radius, followed by the elbow and fingers. For lower extremities, the tibia is more commonly fractured than the femur. Supracondylar humerus fractures are the most common in children aged 7 years and younger. Fractures of the femur are most prevalent for ages 0 to 3 years. Falls from playground equipment, trampolines, bicycles, and sports account for a majority of fractures, and there is a higher incidence of these injuries during summer and school holidays (Shah et al., 2014).

Fracture diagnosis is usually made with a plain radiograph. Although a majority of pediatric fractures can be treated nonoperatively, some fractures that are open, displaced, or unstable may require surgical treatment. Surgical treatment depends on the severity of the fracture and ranges from closed reduction to open reduction and internal fixation with hardware. Most orthopedic injuries require a period of immobilization by casting.

Although most pediatric patients recover completely and return to full function after treatment for a fracture, all fractures are associated with a significant potential for complications. Some serious complications can include vascular injury, peripheral nerve injury, pain, and compartment syndrome. Fortunately, most neuropraxia resolve spontaneously over time with adequate fracture reduction. Compartment syndrome can occur with the initial injury if the swelling is greater than the compartment of the muscle and tissues, or postoperatively if the cast material becomes too tight (Nguyen, McDowell, & Schlechter, 2016). Any of these complications can lead to premature disability and a decreased quality of life. Nursing assessment and clinical knowledge in the care of pediatric fractures can contribute to timely and safe treatment for the patient.

Clinical Aspects

ASSESSMENT

Key elements of the nursing assessment of the pediatric orthopedic patient include a thorough pain assessment and neurovascular checks. Pain management can pose a particular challenge during the acute stage of care. Children and parents are often fearful following an injury, which can make pain assessment challenging. Ineffective pain management can play a major role in patient recovery time, cost of the stay, and overall patient satisfaction. Consistent communication and collaboration with the patient and caregiver(s) are crucial in maintaining pain control (Schroeder et al., 2016).

The use of pain scales such as the Face, Legs, Activity, Cry, Consolability (FLACC), Wong's faces, or a 1 to 10 numerical scales are key elements in assessing patient pain. The use of these pain scales requires a detailed assessment of physiological, behavioral, and patient/caregiver verbal reports. Behavioral assessment is often helpful in measuring pain in the young child, especially after a surgical procedure when measuring sharp procedural pain (Wilson, Curry, & Hockenberry, 2009). Older children are usually able to describe the presence and nature of their pain.

Neurovascular monitoring is a fundamental part of the postoperative assessment and recognition of neurovascular deterioration is crucial. Early recognition of neurovascular compromise prevents detrimental damage such as functional loss, contractures, amputation, infection, and renal failure (Large, Agel, Holtzman, Benirschke, & Krieg, 2015). It is important to know that neurovascular deterioration can occur late after trauma, surgery, or cast application. Neurovascular checks include frequent assessment of the six Ps of acute compartment syndrome: pain, pressure, pallor, paresthesia, pulselessness, and poikilothermia (Howard-Hill, 2014). Postoperative pain is to be expected. However, pain that is not consistent with the surgery or is not relieved by pain medication should raise concern. The feeling of pins and needles is concerning and should not be dismissed. Pulses should be monitored closely as should color and temperature; a pale, cool limb should be examined thoroughly.

Neurovascular checks in the pediatric patient can prove to be most difficult because of lack of language skills and the patient's inability to articulate signs and symptoms of discomfort. Therefore, a meticulous assessment of the limb is vital. Visually assess the limb, checking for color and swelling. Check for temperature with superficial touch. The limb should be warm to the touch and pink in color. Capillary refill should be less than 3 seconds. Pulses should be palpated thoroughly, and strength of pulses should be documented.

NURSING INTERVENTIONS, MANAGEMENT, AND IMPLICATIONS

Immobilization of a fracture is achieved with a type of cast applied to the extremity or area of the fracture. Most often a two-sided plaster splint with a mold on the posterior and anterior aspects of the extremity is used. With only two solid sides of a cast, this allows for swelling of the extremity. The fracture causes a significant amount of swelling in the first 24 to 48 hours. If the cast were solid circumferentially during this time, a tourniquet effect of the limb in the event of excessive swelling could be created. A hard cast is applied later for better protection. Although casting provides stability required to facilitate musculoskeletal healing, there are certain risks associated with immobilization by casting. Excessive internal swelling remains a potential risk once a hard cast is applied. The fascia compartments of the limb or the hard cast may not be able to accommodate a large amount of swelling. Frequent assessment is needed by the nurse to provide early diagnosis and intervention is required with casting complications. It is imperative that the nurse be able to accurately identify and intervene if complications arise. It is important first to calm the family and the child to improve the accuracy of the initial evaluation. This includes identifying and assessing the pain of the child (Wilson et al., 2009).

If there is a change in the neurovascular assessment of the patient and acute compartment syndrome is suspected, call the patient's medical team for an urgent review. If the limb has a bandage or plaster cast, completely split the cast and cut the dressing to skin level. Elevate the limb to the height of the heart, and continue to assess neurovascular status as your facility deems necessary, but usually every 15 to 30 minutes. If there is a circumferential cast in place, the cast can be valved. Valving a cast is a noninvasive procedure, which can be done quickly at the bedside. The cast is cut on one or two sides as well as the bottom layer and slightly opened to allow for increased room for swelling and circulation. High-energy fractures carry a higher risk for significant swelling to the extremity than an injury caused by a low energy force (Nguyen et al., 2016). It is important to understand the etiology of the injury to anticipate the potential complications and interventions.

OUTCOMES

Orthopedic injuries are often painful and traumatic for both the patient and the family. The nurse plays a vital role in the care of these patients. If the complications of an orthopedic injury are caught early, proper interventions can be initiated, and damage to the patient can be limited. Without early identification of a complication, the patient may require further surgical intervention and can have lasting physical consequences.

Summary

Nursing care of the pediatric orthopedic patient requires a specialized knowledge of not only the population but also of the orthopedic condition. The developmental level of the patient must be taken into consideration when caring for these patients. Orthopedic injuries and conditions are often painful. The nurse must know how to appropriately assess and treat the pain associated with either an orthopedic surgical intervention or injury. This includes the use of the correct pain scale corresponding to the developmental level of the patient, attention to the external environment contributing to the pain or stress of the patient, and appropriate use and dosage of medications. Care of the pediatric orthopedic patient requires patience and vigilance by the nurse. With appropriate observation, assessment, and intervention, these patients can recover well following an orthopedic surgery or injury.

Howard-Hill, A. (2014). Acute compartment syndrome. *Dissector, 42*(3), 20–22.

Large, T. M., Agel, J., Holtzman, D. J., Benirschke, S. K., & Krieg, J. C. (2015). Interobserver variability in the measurement of lower leg compartment pressures. *Journal of Orthopaedic Trauma, 29*(7), 316–321. doi:10.1097/BOT.0000000000000317

Naranje, S. M., Erali, R. A., Warner, W. C., Jr., Sawyer, J. R., & Kelly, D. M. (2016). Epidemiology of pediatric fractures presenting to emergency departments in the United States. *Journal of Pediatric Orthopaedics, 36*(4), e45–e48. doi:10.1097/BPO.0000000000000595

Nguyen, S., McDowell, M., & Schlechter, J. (2016). Casting: Pearls and pitfalls learned while caring for children's fractures. *World Journal of Orthopedics, 7*(9), 539–545. doi:10.5312/wjo.v7.i9.539

Schroeder, D. L., Hoffman, L. A., Fioravanti, M., Medley, D. P., Zullo, T. G., & Tuite, P. K. (2016). Enhancing nurses' pain assessment to improve patient satisfaction. *Orthopaedic Nursing, 35*(2), 108–117. doi:10.1097/NOR.0000000000000226

Shah, N. S., Buzas, D., & Zinberg, E. M. (2014). Epidemiologic dynamics contributing to pediatric wrist fractures in the United States. *Hand, 10*(2), 266–271. doi:10.1007/s11552-014-9710-2

Wilson, D., Curry, M., & Hockenberry, M. (2009). The child with musculoskeletal or articular dysfunction. *Wong's essentials of pediatric nursing* (8th ed.). St. Louis, MO: Mosby/Elsevier.

■ OSTEOMYELITIS

Mary Variath
Jane F. Marek
Celeste M. Alfes

Overview

Osteomyelitis (OM), or inflammation of the bone, is usually caused by bacterial infection. Bone infections in children are primarily hematogenous, although incidents secondary to surgery, penetrating trauma, or infection in a contiguous site are reported (Kalyoussef, Windle, Domachowske, Steele, & Noel, 2016). OM is inflammation of the bone caused by a variety of infectious organisms (i.e., bacteria, fungi, or viruses) that results in tissue destruction of the affected bone. OM is a complex disease in its pathophysiology, clinical presentation, and management, making accurate diagnosis and treatment a challenging process. The symptoms of OM include the history of local inflammation, erythema, and/or swelling. In addition, patients with OM may present with a low-grade fever, malaise, and fatigue, along with nonspecific chronic pain at the site of infection (Malhotra, Schulz, & Kallail, 2015). OM may affect any bone, resulting in the progressive bone destruction leading to the formation of sequestra. OM can be acquired through contiguous spread from adjacent soft tissue, joint, and blood infections, or direct inoculation of microorganisms into the bone as a result of trauma or surgery (Malhotra et al., 2015). Other risk factors include diabetes, vascular insufficiency, dialysis treatment, intravenous drug use, and immunosuppression. If untreated, OM can become a life-threatening illness because of bacteremia and sepsis. Therefore, early diagnosis, identification of the causative organism, and prompt treatment can prevent recurrent infection, chronic disease, and complications.

Background

Approximately 50% of OM in children occurs in preschool-age children (Kalyoussef, 2016). Young children experience acute hematogenous osteomyelitis because of the rich vascular supply seen in developing bones. Circulating organisms tend to infect in the metaphyseal ends of the long bones because of the slower circulation in the loops of the metaphyseal capillary loops (Kalyoussef, 2016).

OM is an ancient disease and is one of the most difficult infectious diseases to diagnose and treat (Malhotra et al., 2015). OM can affect people of all ages, and in children, preponderance in males is observed in all age groups (Kalyoussef, 2016). Increased incidence in males may be related to increased trauma owing to risk-taking behavior or other physical activities that predispose to bone injury (Kalyoussef, 2016).

Major causative bacterial organisms include *Pseudomonas aeruginosa*, *Staphylococcus aureus*, *Streptococcus pyogenes*, and *Streptococcus pneumoniae*. Infection with drug-resistant organisms is of particular concern. For unknown reasons, *Haemophilus influenza* type B is shown to affect joints rather than bones alone. In addition, fungal or mixed bacteria are associated with skull, vertebrae, and/or long-bone OM. In fact, about 75% to 95% skull OM are reported to be of fungal origin (Johnson & Batra, 2014; Peltola & Pääkkönen, 2014).

Bacteria can reach the bone through direct inoculation from traumatic wounds, open fractures, implanted hardware, by spreading from adjacent tissue affected by various infections, such as cellulitis, septic arthritis, or by hematogenous spread following bacteremia. OM resulting from hematogenous spread is more common in children; boys are more commonly affected than girls. In developed countries approximately eight in 100,000 children are affected with OM annually; in developing countries, the incidence is higher, especially in resource-poor places where patients present with advanced disease and survivors experience serious and long-lasting complications (Peltola & Pääkkönen, 2014). Salmonella species are reported to be a common cause of OM in developing countries as well as in patients with sickle cell disease. OM usually results from adjacent tissue inflammation and infection, as in the case of osteomyelitis of the skull as a result of contiguous spread from an infected sinus or penetrating trauma (Malhotra et al., 2015). Skull base osteomyelitis, although rare, is associated with 10% to 20% mortality rate and affects primarily patients with diabetes and/or immunocompromised men in their 60s (Conde-Díaz et al., 2017).

Treatment depends on the etiology of the infection. Debridement of the affected bone was once considered the primary method of treatment; however, long-term systemic antimicrobial therapy has replaced debridement as the first-line therapy (Conde-Díaz et al., 2017; Johnson & Batra, 2014). In severe cases, antimicrobial therapy needs to be continued for several weeks to avoid recurrent or chronic infection.

Surgical intervention is indicated if the patient does not respond to antimicrobial treatment or has persistent soft tissue infection, joint infection, or bone abscess. Goals of surgical management are debridement of necrotic bone and tissue, management of dead space, restoration of vascular supply, and adequate wound closure. Surgical techniques include bone debridement and resection, stabilization using an external fixator (including the Ilizarov technique), revascularization procedures, and as for last resort, amputation. Infection following fracture fixation and prosthetic joint infection may result in removal of the hardware, systemic antibiotic therapy, and fracture fixation or joint revision after resolution of infection. Local antibiotic therapy with antibiotic-impregnated beads (antibiotic bead pouch) and spacers may be considered with joint infections and open fractures complicated with OM. In persons with extensive soft tissue involvement, hyperbaric oxygen treatment, vacuum-assisted wound closure (VAC), and skin grafting may be indicated.

Clinical Aspects

ASSESSMENT

Long-bone osteomyelitis is classified by the Cierny–Mader system, which is used to guide treatment. Symptoms of osteomyelitis may include pain, persistent sinus tract or wound drainage, poor wound healing, and presence of fever. Bony necrosis may not occur for 6 weeks after the onset of infection (Spencer, 2015). A thorough history and physical assessment are critical to determine the initial injury, infection, or precipitating event.

NURSING INTERVENTIONS, MANAGEMENT, AND IMPLICATIONS

OM can be classified as acute if the duration of the illness has been less than 2 weeks, subacute for a duration of 2 weeks to 3 months, and chronic for longer than 3 months in duration. Classic clinical manifestations in children include the inability to walk, fever and focal tenderness, visible redness and swelling around the affected bone. Symptoms are dependent on the affected bone. For example, spinal OM in adults is characteristically manifested as back pain, whereas pain on a digital rectal examination suggests sacral OM.

Diagnosis is determined by the patient's history, clinical presentation, and diagnostic testing. Laboratory testing is nonspecific to osteomyelitis and includes complete blood count and differential, C-reactive protein, and erythrocyte sedimentation rate. Bone biopsy and wound and blood cultures are performed to identify the causative organism and develop the antibiogram (Peltola & Pääkkönen, 2014). Selection of imaging techniques is based on clinical findings. In some cases, plain radiographs may be sufficient for diagnosis. If plain films are normal or inconclusive, MRI is the most sensitive for OM; CT or scintigraphy can also be used, especially if a long bone is affected or if symptoms are not localized.

OUTCOMES

Nursing interventions include managing pain, monitoring the neurovascular status of the affected extremity, administering antibiotic therapy, preventing further infection, supporting and immobilizing the affected area, preventing further injury, teaching the patient and family about medications, antibiotic therapy, treatments, prognosis, and rehabilitation therapy. Nurses can take an active role in infection control education that helps to control OM development and prevent complications (Spencer, 2015).

Summary

OM usually involves long-term treatment and recurrence rates are high. Prompt identification of the offending organism and appropriate antibiotic therapy are key in optimizing patient outcomes. Owing to the complexity of the illness, a multidisciplinary team approach is necessary. Physical and occupational therapy referrals are often indicated, and the patient may require help with activities of daily living and the use of assistive devices until weight bearing is permitted. As a result of the length of treatment, psychosocial support of the patient and family are important interventions. Treatment goals include limb preservation and prevention of complications including pathologic fracture and further injury, flexion contractures, muscle atrophy, and systemic complications. Identification of persons at risk for and prevention of infection are important nursing considerations.

Conde-Díaz, C., Llenas-García, J., Parra Grande, M., Terol Esclapez, G., Masiá, M., & Gutiérrez, F. (2017). Severe skull base osteomyelitis caused by *Pseudomonas aeruginosa* with successful outcome after prolonged outpatient therapy with continuous infusion of ceftazidime and oral ciprofloxacin: A case report. *Journal of Medical Case Reports, 11*(1), 48. doi:10.1186/s13256-017-1221-7

Johnson, A. K., & Batra, P. S. (2014). Central skull base osteomyelitis: An emerging clinical entity. *The Laryngoscope, 124*(5), 1083–1087. doi:10.1002/lary.24440

Kalyoussef, S. (2016). Pediatric osteomyelitis. In R. Steele (Ed.), *Medscape*. Retrieved from http://emedicine.medscape.com/article/967095-overview

Malhotra, B., Schulz, T., & Kallail, K. J. (2015). When anemia, atypical plasma cells, and a lytic bone lesion are not myeloma: An unusual presentation of osteomyelitis. *Kansas Journal of Medicine, 8*(4), 151–152.

Peltola, H., & Pääkkönen, M. (2014). Acute osteomyelitis in children. *The New England Journal of Medicine, 370*(4), 352–360. doi:10.1056/NEJMra1213956

Spencer, D. (2015). Implications of underlying pathophysiology of osteomyelitis in diabetics for nursing care. MSN Student Scholarship. Paper 68. Retrieved from http://digitalcommons.otterbein.edu/stu_msn/68

■ PEDIATRIC EMERGENCIES

Rachel Tkaczyk

Overview

In 2010, the Centers for Disease Control and Prevention (CDC) database reported a total of 129.8 million emergency department visits in the United States. Of those visits, 25.5 million visits consisted of patients younger than 15 years, and an additional 20.7 million visits were patients between 15 and 24 years (Centers for Disease Control and Prevention, 2012). When it comes to the emergency room setting, there is no one universal definition as to what constitutes a "pediatric emergency." Subsequently, levels of care and the associated acuity in the emergency setting often differ among various institutions. Despite varying definitions and management techniques, the approach to identifying, assessing, and treating a pediatric emergent situation must be systematic. To achieve successful outcomes, the medical staff must be equipped with the knowledge to appropriately recognize and treat all pediatric emergency scenarios.

Background

Pediatric patients, who accounted for 17.4% of the emergency room visits in 2010 in the United States, present unique challenges that can ultimately hinder an emergency room's ability to provide the best possible care (Macias, 2013). Obtaining a complete history and performing a thorough assessment in the pediatric population can be accompanied by many unique challenges. Particularly in the emergency setting, the time constraint alone can elicit a sense of urgency that affects the overall quality of the patient intake and triage. This section explores several challenges that may be encountered during the evaluation and treatment of pediatric emergencies.

One identified difficulty when attempting to obtain an accurate history is the lack of an established rapport with the patient and his or her family. This can contribute to an incomplete, and often inadequate, extraction of critical information. Often the history taking is not given enough devoted time, and a therapeutic relationship is not established. This is problematic as the health history typically provides 85% of the information that is needed for the medical team to make a diagnosis (Reuter-Rice & Bolick, 2012). As stated earlier, another barrier is the element of time, and possibly the lack thereof. In the trauma scenario, resuscitation takes precedence over the acquisition of a health history. However, it is important to realize that this does not negate the significance of the health history. Rather it is necessary to recognize the limitation and employ strategies to overcome it (Reuter-Rice & Bolick, 2012).

There are several key elements of the pediatric emergent intake. Although obtaining a history is significant, another key element is the pediatric assessment and physical examination (Scott et al., 2014). Both components are used to answer the critical questions: Is there an immediate life threat? Regarding severity, where does the patient fall? Will the patient need admission? What evidence supports the providers' differential diagnoses? In summary, the goal of assessing the pediatric patient in the emergent setting is to determine the severity of the situation and whether treatment is indicated. Often, this requires the initial assessment but also reassessment. When it comes to the overall treatment of a seriously ill or injured child, the goal is to provide a systematic approach that is consistent across all institutions. The recommended model for all pediatric life support courses consists of the general assessment, secondary assessment, and tertiary assessment (American Heart Association, 2015).

For example, in the case of a pediatric patient who presents with concern for sepsis, four physical examination signs are recommended for early detection of pediatric septic shock, before hypotension occurs. They include alteration in mental status, decreased capillary refill, cold extremities, and peripheral pulse quality (Scott et al., 2014). These changes can be subtle, particularly with the provider who does not have an established baseline for a patient as a primary care provider may have had (Reuter-Rice & Bolick, 2012). Research has shown that several barriers to this practice of frequent reassessment exist and include a lack of time, increased workload, and at times a lack of nursing knowledge specific to the situation (Pretorius, Searle, & Marshall, 2015). This again reinforces the need to provide a systematic and standardized approach to the assessment of the pediatric patient. With those skills, the medical team is equipped with the tools to recognize signs of impending respiratory distress, failure, and shock. Without the ability to assess and intervene quickly, pediatric patients are at greater risk and can progress to cardiopulmonary failure, which can lead to an arrest (AHA, 2015).

Clinical Aspects

ASSESSMENT

To meet the need for high-quality care in this population, several health care systems have integrated quality improvement methods to improve access, safety, and ultimately better the care delivered to this patient population (Macias, 2013). As discussed, one of the barriers to obtaining a thorough history from the beginning of the medical course is the lack of a developed therapeutic relationship with the patient and family. The American Academy of Pediatrics (AAP) and the American College of Emergency Physicians (ACEP) continually recognize the patient and family as significant decision makers in the patient's overall care. Patient- and family-centered care is a method of health care that recognizes the essential role of the patient and family. The goal is to focus and implement collaboration among the patient, family, and medical professionals (AAP Committee on Pediatric Emergency Medicine & ACE Physicians Pediatric Emergency Medicine Committee, 2006).

NURSING INTERVENTIONS, MANAGEMENT, AND IMPLICATIONS

The AAP and ACEP have issued several recommendations to improve the patient and medical team therapeutic relationship, which comes with its emergency room specific challenges. They continue to reinforce the necessity to validate a family and patient's concerns. Family members should be given the option to be present for all aspects of their child's care while in the emergency room. It is also essential that information is provided to the family during all interventions, regardless of the family's decision to be present or not (AAP Committee on Pediatric Emergency Medicine & ACE Physicians Pediatric Emergency Medicine Committee, 2006).

OUTCOMES

In addition to information gathering, one of the key elements to improved outcomes in the pediatric emergency setting is early recognition and intervention. As stated previously, the sense of urgency and time constraint, increased work load, and inadequate knowledge can contribute to poor outcomes. The objective observation was recently studied to assess strengths and weaknesses during a pediatric resuscitation. The overall goal was to assess how well the medical providers in a pediatric emergency room adhered to cardiopulmonary resuscitation (CPR) guidelines during a resuscitation. During this study, 33 children received CPR under video recording. The results demonstrated appropriate compression rate, duration of pauses, and compression depth. It did show that there tended to be hyperventilation as well as the inability to coordinate the compression–ventilation ratio during the resuscitation. The overall recommendations included various training modalities for CPR among staff and evaluation of its effectiveness (Donoghue et al., 2015). This particular study is only one example of how a pediatric institution implemented a quality initiative to assess potential limitations and areas that required additional education. It demonstrates an overall approach to identify barriers to care, assess any shortcomings, and ultimately provide education to correct and improve certain practices.

Summary

The pediatric population is unique in many aspects when compared to the adult population, particularly in the emergency care setting. There are several challenges that the medical team faces, beginning from the moment the patient enters into their care and extends throughout treatment. Several strategies can be used to overcome those challenges and provide optimal care. It is of paramount importance that the medical team identifies any barriers to obtaining a thorough history and performing an in-depth assessment. Continued focus on ever evolving education is also essential. With a consistent and systematic approach to pediatric emergency care, outcomes continue to improve.

American Academy of Pediatrics, Committee on Pediatric Emergency Medicine & American College of Emergency Physicians, Pediatric Emergency Medicine Committee. (2006). Patient- and family-centered care and the role of the emergency physician providing care to a child in the emergency department. *Pediatrics, 118*(5), 2242–2244.

American Heart Association. (2015). *Pediatric advanced life support.* Elk Grove, IL: American Academy of Pediatrics.

Centers for Disease Control and Prevention. (2012). Reasons for emergency room use among U.S. children: National Health Interview Survey, 2012. Retrieved from https://www.cdc.gov/nchs/products/databriefs/db160.htm

Donoghue, A., Hsieh, T.-C., Myers, S., Mak, A., Sutton, R., & Nadkarni, V. (2015). Videographic assessment of cardiopulmonary resuscitation quality in the pediatric emergency department. *Resuscitation, 91,* 19–25. doi:10.1016/j.resuscitation.2015.03.007

Macias, C. (2013). Quality improvement in pediatric emergency medicine. *Academic Pediatrics, 13*(6 Suppl.), S61–S68. doi:10.1016/j.acap.2013.06.007

Pretorius, A., Searle, J., & Marshall, B. (2015). Barriers and enablers to emergency department nurses' management of patients' pain. *Pain Management Nursing, 16*(3), 372–379. doi:10.1016/j.pmn.2014.08.015

Reuter-Rice, K., & Bolick, B. (2012). *Pediatric acute care: A guide for interprofessional practice* (1st ed.). Burlington, MA: Jones & Bartlett.

Scott, H. F., Donoghue, A. J., Gaieski, D. F., Marchese, R. F., & Mistry, R. D. (2014). Effectiveness of physical exam signs for early detection of critical illness in pediatric systemic inflammatory response syndrome. *BMC Emergency Medicine, 14,* 24. doi:10.1186/1471-227X-14-24

■ SEIZURE DISORDER

Kathleen Maxwell

Overview

The majority of seizures are idiopathic. Seizures can present at any age and clinically can be described as convulsions, staring spells, muscle spasms, and odd sensations. Seizure types include febrile seizures, benign familial neonatal seizures, focal seizures, and generalized seizures, including absence epilepsy and juvenile myoclonic epilepsy (JME). Epilepsy has been defined by the International League Against Epilepsy (ILAE) as at least two unprovoked seizures occurring more than 24 hours apart, one unprovoked seizure, and the probability of further seizures similar to the general recurrence risk (at least 60%) after two unprovoked seizures occurring over the following 10 years and a diagnosis of an epilepsy syndrome (Fisher et al., 2014). Seizures that are provoked by changes in electrolytes, high fevers, or alcohol or drug withdrawal are not classified as epilepsy. Individuals can have a combination of provoked and unprovoked seizures. In children, brain malformations, intracranial lesions, or trauma can provoke seizures.

Background

Seizure disorders can be a chronic condition for many individuals, and chronic seizures can cause problems that impact social development and feelings that they are not like everyone else. This perceived feeling of social difference could also impact their psychological development. Furthermore, cognitive development can be impacted as a consequence of seizure frequency and medication side effects.

Clinical Aspects

ASSESSMENT

The evaluation of a patient with a seizure disorder consists of getting a detailed history of the event. This description includes what the child looked like before the event (if it was witnessed from the start), details of the event itself, whether the child lost consciousness and continence, how long the event lasted, and how long it took the individual to return to baseline. A thorough medical and developmental history is obtained. Labs, including a complete blood count (CBC), toxicology screen, and comprehensive metabolic panel (CMP), may be ordered depending on the circumstances surrounding the seizure. Neuroimaging studies, a head MRI, and an EEG are indicated.

Seizure disorders can be broken down into two main groups: focal and generalized. Generalized seizures involve both sides of the brain. They are associated with a loss of consciousness but not necessarily with shaking or convulsions. Generalized seizures are further delineated as absence (brief staring that may have associated automatisms) or tonic (stiffening), atonic (loss of tone), myoclonic (sudden, quick jerks), or clonic (jerking). The definition of status epilepticus has been revised to include seizure length as well as the time point that the seizure is now considered continuous seizure activity and the time after which there is a risk of long-term consequences (Trinka et al., 2015).

There are certain childhood epilepsies that are considered benign. These entities remit and require shortened or no medical intervention. Benign familial neonatal seizures affect otherwise healthy neonates. In general, seizures are brief and are associated with a period of apnea, causing cyanosis, and generalized tonic–clonic or focal–clonic movements (Park, Shahid, & Jammoul, 2015). The majority of infants with this seizure type have their seizures abate spontaneously. The infants can be started on phenobarbital with about 75% of infants responding to this treatment and continued for several weeks before weaning. Parents need to be aware of the increased risk of seizure recurrence later in life (Kaddurah, 2017).

Febrile seizures are a common occurrence in childhood affecting 2% to 5% of the pediatric population that is between 6 and 60 months of age. Febrile seizures occur in the presence of a fever not concomitant with an intracranial infection, a metabolic disorder, or in children who have a history of afebrile seizures (Shinnar & Shinnar, n.d.). Daily anticonvulsant therapy is not recommended for children with simple febrile seizures. Treatment options include the use of a benzodiazepine such as clonazepam orally disintegrating tablets, rectal diazepam gel, or buccal midazolam. These treatments can shorten the duration of the febrile seizure and are tolerated with less potential side effects than a daily anticonvulsant.

Sudden unexplained death in epilepsy (SUDEP) is defined as an unexpected, witnessed or unwitnessed, death in patients with epilepsy, with or without evidence of a seizure, an excluding documentation of status epilepticus, drowning, or trauma, with no toxicological or anatomic cause of death found on postmortem (Keddie et al., 2016). Individuals with epilepsy have a 24- to 28-fold increase of dying unexpectedly compared to the general population. Risk factors to SUDEP include poor seizure control, especially generalized tonic–clonic seizures, nighttime seizures, decreased supervision, polytherapy with antiepileptic medications, comorbid psychiatric conditions, and increased incidence of medication noncompliance (Tomson, Surges, Delamont, Haywood, & Hesdorffer, 2016).

Focal seizures arise from the temporal lobe and can be termed "temporal lobe epilepsy." Children can demonstrate automatisms and motor manifestations as part of their seizure pattern. These motor behaviors can change depending on the age of the child. In the 0- to 3-year-old age group, the child's motor manifestations may be difficult to differentiate from generalized seizures as the behaviors seen may be bilateral and symmetric, appearing more consistent with seizures arising from the frontal lobe. Children in the 3- to 6-year age range may have automatisms that are easier to disseminate, such as dystonic posturing, eye/mouth or head deviation, as well as having an awareness of an aura. Children older than 6 years and into adolescence may report similar automatisms and auras as adults. Auras may include a confusion state before seizure onset, a feeling of déjà vu, an olfactory aura, lip smacking, dystonic posturing of an extremity, or aimless movements (Nickels, Wong-Kisiel, Moseley, & Wirrell, 2012).

Treatment options for focal seizures include, but are not limited to, the following medications: carbamazepine, oxcarbazepine, phenytoin, levetiracetam, zonisamide, and perampanel. Multiple factors influence medication choice. Children often require a medication that either comes in a liquid preparation or one that can easily be chewed or crushed. In general, medications that are administered daily or twice a day (BID) have a greater likelihood of compliance compared to three times a day (TID) or four times a day (QID) regimens. Any seizure medication has the potential to cause lethargy, so it is often advantageous to start with a bedtime dose and titrate up slowly to improve tolerability.

Childhood absence epilepsy is the most common of all childhood epilepsies with females having a higher rate of occurrence than males. Absence seizures are brief staring spells that may or may not have associated automatisms. The associated automatisms may include a repetitive eye blink, lip movement, finger picking/rubbing, trunk arching, or eyelid twitching (Park et al., 2015). This type of seizure manifests between 4 and 10 years of age with the highest prevalence between 5 and 6 years of age (Park et al., 2015). The prognosis for this type of seizure is good as the majority of children with just absence seizures have their seizures abate after 6 to 7 years (Vrielynck, 2013). Studies have shown about 40% of individuals with absence seizures develop a generalized tonic–clonic seizure. It may initially be thought to be inattentiveness or attention deficit hypertensive disorder (ADHD) with the child. Parents need to monitor the child for accidental injuries, such as falling when they experience a seizure, as well as comorbid conditions including ADHD, anxiety, self-esteem issues, and depression (Tenney & Glauser, 2013). Treatment options include ethosuximide, valproate, and lamotrigine. Ethosuximide is often the first choice as it has a high rate of treatment success with minimal side effects. When ethosuximide has tolerability issues, it is usually with the gastrointestinal (GI) system. Most often, dosing BID or TID and taking with food can minimize GI upset. A valproate is an option especially if the individual has also had a generalized convulsion.

JME consists of bilateral myoclonic jerks, usually most prevalent in the early morning after waking, generalized convulsions, and absence seizures. JME syndrome occurs most frequently in individuals aged 13 to 15 years (Park et al., 2015). Long-term seizure control by medication has been seen in as many as 75% to 90% of patients with a diagnosis of JME (Rossi, 2013). Individuals with JME should adopt lifestyle changes to maximize seizure control. This includes maintaining a regular eating and sleeping schedule, minimizing alcohol consumption, and maintaining a high percentage of medication compliance (Mantoan & Walker, 2011).

NURSING INTERVENTIONS, MANAGEMENT, AND IMPLICATIONS

There are several medication choices for the treatment of seizure disorders. Medication choice depends on seizure type, patient age, functional level, and comorbid conditions. Nursing intervention starts with the identification of the seizure. It is important to document how the patient looked at the start of the seizure, duration of the seizure, and duration until the child was back to baseline. Parental education is a crucial nursing function. There are several elements to seizure first aid and safety to be discussed with families. In addition to timing and noting the description of the event, parents should be instructed to lay the child down on a flat surface once the seizure starts. The child should be turned on his or her side to maintain a patent airway and prevent aspiration as the child may vomit during or immediately after the seizure. Keep the airway open and clear, and instruct the parents never to place anything, including their fingers, in the child's mouth. The child's glasses and nearby safety hazards should be removed. Safety issues for the child in the wheelchair are a bit different. These children are safer as they remain in the wheelchair. Make sure that the brakes of the wheelchair are engaged and that the seat belt is secured. Hold the wheelchair in place and upright while the child is seizing.

Nursing education of anticonvulsants includes more than discussing potential side effects. Compliance issues can be addressed by determining the route and frequency of medication administration that will work best for each patient. When checking anticonvulsant levels, instruct families to obtain levels first thing in the morning or late in the day as a trough level. A trough level may be more beneficial than obtaining a peak level. It is important for the nurse to know the reference range and parameters so that the lab value is interpreted correctly. A thorough medication history, including over-the-counter medications and herbal supplements, is done to determine any potential drug interactions.

Individuals with seizure disorders should be encouraged to take showers rather than baths, so the drain is always open, and standing water cannot accumulate. Nonskid strips on the tub or shower floor are often helpful in preventing falls, and bathroom doors should never be locked in the event an emergency occurs. Swimming needs to be supervised with an adult present who can remove the child from the water if a seizure occurs. Schools often require a seizure action plan for students with epilepsy. In addition to the student and parent's name, it should include several contact numbers for the family as well as for the treating provider. Medications, including routine and as needed (pro re nata [PRN]) rescue medications, as well as instruction for use are imperative. The plan needs to dictate when 911 is to be called as well as how to manage the child in the postictal period until able to return to the classroom.

The last restriction that should be discussed with the family is driving privileges. Each state has its protocol regarding getting and maintaining a license when there is a history of seizure disorders. The individual needs to demonstrate that he or she has been seizure free for at least 6 months. The individual needs to have a measurable blood level of his or her anticonvulsant(s). It is recommended that this level be checked randomly as a trough rather than at a scheduled or predetermined visit. The random check will give the provider a better sense of patient compliance rather than giving the patient the opportunity to take an oral load to catch up for missed doses. The state bureau of motor vehicle forms is completed every 6 to 12 months.

OUTCOMES

There are several medication choices for the treatment of seizure disorders. Medication choice depends on seizure type, patient age, functional level, and comorbid conditions. The outcome of medication treatment is to balance the therapeutic levels with toxic side effects. The patients' and families' quality of life will depend upon their perceived feeling of social difference and the cognitive, physical, and social development of the child.

Summary

Seizure disorders can affect individuals throughout their life spans, and the diagnosis can be challenging for both the patient and his or her family. It is imperative to provide support for the patient and all concerned. There are several community-based resources that can and should be made available to the family. The local Epilepsy Foundation (www.epilepsy.com) will provide additional educational materials as well as in-services for schools, day cares, and employers. The American Epilepsy Society (www.aesnet.org) can also provide helpful information. Prescription medication can be costly to families, and programs such as www.Rxassist.org should be discussed with the family. Finally, additional resources for insurance/coverage such as state health departments should be made available to families.

Fisher, R. S., Acevedo, C., Arzimanoglou, A., Bogacz, A., Cross, J. H., Elger, C. E., . . . Wiebe, S. (2014). ILAE official report: A practical clinical definition of epilepsy. *Epilepsia, 55*(4), 475–482. doi:10.1111/epi.12550

Kaddurah, A. (2017). Benign childhood epilepsy. In A. Kao (Ed.), *Medscape*. Retrieved from http://emedicine.medscape.com/article/1181649-overview#a1

Keddie, S., Angus-Leppan, H., Parker, T., Toescu, S., Nash, A., Adewunmi, O., & Liu, R. (2016). Discussing sudden unexpected death in epilepsy: Are we empowering our patients? A questionnaire survey. *Journal of the Royal Society of Medicine Open, 7*(9). doi:10.1177/2054270416654358

Mantoan, L., & Walker, M. (2011). Treatment options in juvenile myoclonic epilepsy. *Current Treatment Options in Neurology, 13*(4), 355–370. doi:10.1007/s11940-011-0131-z

Nickels, K. C., Wong-Kisiel, L. C., Moseley, B. D., & Wirrell, E. C. (2012). Temporal lobe epilepsy in children. *Epilepsy Research and Treatment, 2012*, 1–16. doi:10.1155/2012/849540

Park, J. T., Shahid, A. M., & Jammoul, A. (2015). Common pediatric epilepsy syndromes. *Pediatric Annals, 44*(2), e30–e35. doi:10.3928/00904481-20150203-09

Rossi, M. A. (2013). Juvenile myoclonic epilepsy: When will it end. *Epilepsy Currents, 13*(3), 148–149. doi:10.5698/1535-7511-13.3.148

Shinnar, R. C., & Shinnar, S. (n.d.). Febrile seizures. Retrieved from http://www.childneurologyfoundation.org/disorders/febrile-seizures

Tenney, J. R., & Glauser, T. A. (2013). The current state of absence epilepsy: Can we have your attention? *Epilepsy Currents, 13*(3), 135–140. doi:10.5698/1535-7511-13.3.135

Tomson, T., Surges, R., Delamont, R., Haywood, S., & Hesdorffer, D. C. (2016). Who to target in sudden unexpected death in epilepsy prevention and how? Risk factors, biomarkers, and intervention study designs. *Epilepsia, 57,* 4–16. doi:10.1111/epi.13234

Trinka, E., Cock, H., Hesdorffer, D., Rossetti, A. O., Scheffer, I. E., Shinnar, S., . . . Lowenstein, D. H. (2015). A definition and classification of status epilepticus—Report of the ILAE Task Force on Classification of Status Epilepticus. *Epilepsia, 56*(10), 1515–1523. doi:10.1111/epi.13121

Vrielynck, P. (2013). Current and emerging treatments for absence seizures in young patients. *Neuropsychiatric Disease and Treatment, 2013*(9), 963–975. doi:10.2147/NDT.S30991

■ SICKLE CELL DISEASE

Valerie Cachat

Overview

Sickle cell disease (SCD) is a group of chronic genetic disorders that affect an estimated 70,000 to 100,000 Americans (National Heart, Lung, and Blood Institute, 2014). SCD is characterized by an abnormal hemoglobin, called *hemoglobin S (HbS)* or *sickle hemoglobin*, in the red blood cells (RBCs). The most common form of SCD is homozygous (SS) allele. Other variants are the result of compound heterozygotes for HbS and other β-globin variants, including sickle cell (SC), Sβ+ thalassemia, and Sβ⁰ thalassemia. Patients with SCD are at high risk for acute and chronic complications that may result in disability or death.

Background

SCD is a group of inherited hemoglobinopathies associated with hemolytic anemia and vaso-occlusion complications. All forms of SCD are inherited in an autosomal recessive pattern. Normally, two β-globin chains combine with two α-globin chains to form the predominant normal Hb in adults (HBA). SCD involves a mutation in the β-globin genes. An amino acid substitution of valine from glutamic acid occurs (Piccone, 2011). In deoxygenated conditions, the polymerization of HbS results in the characteristic sickle shape of the red blood cells. These sickled cells are stiff and adhere to one another and the vasculature leading to occlusion of the microvasculature and cause decreased oxygen delivery to tissues. This impaired oxygen delivery affects multiple organ systems. Organ damage occurs because of the sickling of the RBCs and chronic hemolysis throughout the life span (Ware, 2010). Affected children in the United States now increasingly survive into adulthood because of increased knowledge and advances in disease therapy; however, the average life span remains 20 to 30 years less from those individuals without SCD (National Heart Lung and Blood Institute, n.d.). Although the life span has increased, SCD continues to cause significant morbidity and mortality. Acute complications such as sudden anemia, vaso-occlusive pain crisis (VOC), splenic sequestration, acute chest syndrome (ACS), and stroke occur. In addition, chronic hemolysis affects all organ systems and can lead to kidney, liver, and cardiac decompensation among other complications.

Clinical Aspects

SCD is now diagnosed based on newborn screen in the United States. Early diagnosis has led to a decrease in complications, in particular, the risk of sepsis. Patients with SCD have functional asplenia. Shortly after birth, they are diagnosed with SCD and antibiotic prophylaxis is started to decrease the risk of sepsis because of encapsulated organisms (*Streptococcus pneumoniae* in particular). Febrile illness in a patient with SCD is considered an emergency owing to the risk of bacterial sepsis. Fever may be the result of acute and sometimes life-threatening conditions such as ACS and osteomyelitis. Often, the cause of a fever is not clear. Patients with fever require evaluation including history and physical, complete blood count (CBC) with differential, reticulocyte count, blood culture, and urine culture when urinary tract infection is suspected. Patients presenting with respiratory symptoms or chest pain should have a chest radiograph done to rule out developing ACS. Prompt administration of empiric parenteral antibiotics with coverage for *S. pneumoniae* is necessary. Patients who appear ill should be hospitalized for observation and continued antibiotic administration, and intravenous fluids. Close attention should be paid to additional symptoms concerning the development of ACS including hypoxia, tachypnea, fever, increased work of breathing and osteomyelitis, including localized pain, fever, swelling, and erythema (Piccone, 2011).

ASSESSMENT

Pain is perhaps the hallmark of sickle cell disease, with both acute and chronic pain being a significant cause of morbidity. Occlusion of the microvasculature leads to poor perfusion causing hypoxia, ischemia, and ultimately, tissue damage (Ballas et al., 2012). Inflammation occurs as inflammatory mediators are released from damaged cells. In addition to the physical effects of dealing with pain, psychological well-being is often affected, particularly because of the unpredictable nature of the disease.

Some common triggers of VOC are illness, temperature changes, stress, dehydration, and high altitude. Often, there is no identifiable cause. One of the first presentations of pain in infants with SCD is called *dactylitis*, which is swelling of the hands and/or feet because of occlusion of the microvasculature. Pain can occur anywhere in the body and in more than one spot at a time. Although VOC is often the reason for pain, other differential diagnoses should be considered depending on the location of the pain. Most children are pain free between painful crises, but adolescents and adults may also suffer from ongoing chronic pain.

NURSING INTERVENTIONS, MANAGEMENT, AND IMPLICATIONS

Pain is best treated by a combination of nonsteroidal anti-inflammatory drugs (NSAIDs) and opiates. Patients should have a home-pain regimen established and attempt to manage pain at home with the use of NSAIDs, opiates if needed, and rest, hydration, and warmth. If they are unable to manage at home, they present to the hospital for further care including evaluation, administration of pain medications, hydration, and monitoring. Treatment with parenteral opioids can often lead to sedation, increasing the risk of developing ACS. A balance between adequate pain control and lack of sedation is needed. The nurse must closely monitor for oversedation when administering opiates for pain control. The nurse should also encourage ambulation, and bronchial hygiene should be used routinely to prevent atelectasis and decrease the risk of developing ACS (Ballas, Gupta, & Adams-Graves, 2012).

Patients with sickle cell disease live with chronic mild-to-moderate anemia. At times, they may present with severe anemia, which may be life threatening. Rapid hemolysis causes some episodes of anemia during a VOC. However, in children, the cause of severe anemia is often splenic sequestration or aplastic crisis.

Splenic sequestration is a serious and potentially life-threatening complication of SCD. Splenic sequestration is defined as a decrease in Hb with a rapidly enlarging spleen. Parents need to be educated during infancy on palpation of the spleen and symptoms of splenic sequestration to decrease morbidity and mortality (Piccone, 2011). Rapid enlargement of the spleen can lead to hypovolemic shock. Patients who present for anemia should be evaluated for splenic sequestration. A patient admitted with splenic sequestration should have frequent, regular assessment of the spleen size by palpation as well as laboratory monitoring of CBC. The nurse must remain vigilant to signs of worsening sequestration including tachycardia, pallor, hypotension, and altered mental status. Treatment may include fluid resuscitation and blood transfusion. Children with recurrent splenic sequestration may require chronic transfusions or splenectomy.

Aplastic crisis is another cause of acute anemia. This is usually caused by parvovirus B19 infection (also called *fifth disease*), a very common childhood illness. Patients with SCD are dependent on rapid replacement of red blood cells because of hemolysis. A virus such as a parvovirus B19, which causes reticulocytopenia, can lead to significant anemia in a patient with SCD. Patients present with pallor, headache, and fatigue and a marked decrease in their Hb with associated low reticulocyte count. Frequent laboratory assessment to evaluate for the return of reticulocytosis is necessary to determine the course of treatment. Patients may require red cell transfusion until bone marrow activity increases.

ACS is a potentially life-threatening complication of SCD. ACS is defined by respiratory symptoms (i.e., cough, chest pain), fever, and evidence of pulmonary infiltrate on chest radiography (Piccone, 2011). Patients admitted for pain management are at high risk of developing ACS because of decreased respiratory effort secondary to pain as well as sedation from parenteral opioids. Aggressive bronchial hygiene is needed for prevention of ACS. Treatment includes antibiotics, which would include the coverage of *S. pneumoniae* and atypical organisms. Patients with ACS require frequent and close monitoring of respiratory symptoms to identify when more aggressive treatment is required.

Stroke is a major complication of SCD, and approximately 11% of pediatric patients are at risk for this occurrence. The most common cause of pediatric stroke related to SCD is vaso-occlusive of the cerebral vasculature. Signs and symptoms may vary from very mild weakness to obvious hemiparesis, visual and speech disturbances, seizures, and altered mental status (Piccone, 2011). Patients presenting with symptoms of stroke require emergent evaluation. Treatment for patients with stroke is red blood cell transfusion to decrease the present HbS to less than 30%. Exchange transfusion is often used to avoid the risk of hyperviscosity that can lead to further cerebral injury.

Priapism, sometimes seen in patients with SCD, is defined as a sustained, painful penile erection. Priapism is caused by an obstruction of venous drainage from the penis. Prolonged priapism (greater than 3 hours) is considered an emergency requiring urological consultation. Treatment should include hydration and pain control, and medications such as α-agonists and β-agonists have been used, and prolonged episodes may require penile aspiration (Piccone, 2011).

Care for the child with sickle cell is ongoing. Children with SCD must stay up-to-date with childhood immunizations. Patients receive the 23-valent pneumococcal vaccine at age 2 years with a booster at age 5 years. They should also receive the flu shot annually. Penicillin prophylaxis is started shortly after birth and continued until the age of 5 years at a minimum. Daily folic acid supplementation of 1 mg/d is recommended to increase RBC production. Stroke screening begins at age 2 years with the use of transcranial Doppler ultrasonography (TCD). Those with abnormal velocities indicating risk for stroke will be initiated on a chronic transfusion protocol to decrease HbS and reduce the risk of stroke. Routine ophthalmologic exams should be done to evaluate for sickle retinopathy (National Heart, Lung, and Blood Institute, 2014).

OUTCOMES

Sickle cell disease affects every organ system. Owing to anemia and hemolysis, growth and puberty are often delayed. Avascular necrosis can occur, most often in the femoral and humeral head. Routine monitoring of kidney function, liver function, pulmonary function, and cardiac function are important. There are few treatments to decrease the severity of sickle cell disease. Hydroxyurea is a medication used to increase fetal Hb levels, therefore increasing oxygen-carrying capacity, decreasing sickled Hb levels, and reducing morbidity related to chronic hemolysis and hypoxia (Ware, 2010). Bone marrow transplant (BMT) is curative but has not become standard practice because of treatment-related complications and morbidities.

Summary

SCD has a variable presentation in pediatrics. Despite significant anemia, many patients are clinically well between acute complication episodes. Infection is the most common cause of mortality in the pediatric sickle cell population. Neonatal screening and early diagnosis, family education, and routine comprehensive care are necessary to reduce the morbidity and mortality associated with this chronic disease. Research is ongoing to identify ways to lessen the complications and cure this unpredictable disease.

Ballas, S. K., Gupta, K., & Adams-Graves, P. (2012). Sickle cell pain: A critical reappraisal. *Blood, 120,* 3647–3656. doi:10.1182/blood-2012-04-383430

National Heart, Lung, and Blood Institute. (2014). *Evidence-based management of sickle cell disease: Expert panel report, 2014.* Retrieved from https://www.nhlbi.nih .gov/health-pro/guidelines/sickle-cell-disease-guidelines

National Heart, Lung, and Blood Institute. (n.d.). What is sickle cell disease? Retrieved from https://www.nhlbi.nih.gov/health/health-topics/topics/sca

Piccone, C. M. (2011). Sickle cell disease. In T. A. Florin, S. Ludwig, P. Aronson, & H. Werner (Eds.), *Netter's pediatrics* (pp. 326–330). Philadelphia, PA: Elsevier.

Ware, R. E. (2010). How I use hydroxyurea to treat young patients with sickle cell anemia. *Blood, 115*(26), 5300–5311. doi:10.1182/blood-2009-04-146852

■ TRAUMATIC BRAIN INJURY

Elizabeth Wirth-Tomaszewski

Overview

Traumatic brain injury (TBI) is the leading cause of trauma-related death and disability worldwide, affecting both adult and pediatric populations significantly. The incidence in the United States is estimated at 1.36 million cases with 52,000 deaths, as well as 275,000 hospitalizations annually (Centers for Disease Control and Prevention, 2016). Worldwide, TBI remains the leading cause of morbidity and mortality in those aged younger than 45 years (Andersen, Gazmuri, Marin, Regueira, & Rovegno, 2015). TBI is a common and unfortunate cause of disability and death in infants and children. Unintentional causes of TBI include falls and motor vehicle accidents, while child abuse in infants and young children and assaults in adolescents are inflicted causes of TBI (Su, Raghupathi, & Huh, 2015). TBI encompasses a wide variety of conditions, ranging from mild to life threatening, and can best be described as an alteration in brain function and/or structure because of external forces such as blunt or penetrating trauma, or acceleration/deceleration forces (White & Venkatesh, 2016). Many types of TBI exist, such as concussions, hemorrhages, axonal injuries, and skull fractures to name a few. These injuries may further be designated as acute, subacute, chronic, or acute on chronic. TBIs also include primary and secondary injury classifications. Nursing implications include the assessment, identification of nursing problems, interventions, evaluation, and prevention of these injuries.

Background

TBI is defined as a pathological alteration in the function or structure of the brain by way of external forces. These forces can cause friction of the tissue, tearing of the vessels, or axonal injuries at the cellular level that cause impairment of function. Initial injuries are capable of causing secondary injuries, usually, because of cerebral edema, increased intracranial pressure (ICP), intracranial hypertension, oxidative stress, excitotoxicity, and seizures. Through assessment and intervention, the incidence of secondary brain injuries can be reduced (Andersen et al., 2015).

Prevalence of TBI varies by age. Children younger than 4 years of age, adolescents between 15 and 19 years of age, and adults older than 65 years are those most often diagnosed with TBI. Children younger than 14 years of age constitute approximately half of a million emergency department visits annually. Those older than 75 years are most likely to incur TBI-related hospitalization and death. TBI is a contributing factor to one third of all injury-related deaths in the United States. Mild TBIs constitute a majority of the reported injuries, with no available data on those who suffer mild TBIs and do not seek care. TBI is a costly public health issue, totaling approximately $60 billion per year when accounting for the direct and indirect costs (Centers for Disease Control and Prevention, 2016).

Mild TBIs, such as concussions, are most prominent at 80% of all TBIs. The leading cause of severe TBI is motor vehicle collisions, accounting for 30% to 50% of head injuries, with males aged 15 to 24 years being the most prominent demographic affected. Other risk factors include participation in contact sports, falls, advanced age (because of polypharmacy and sensory losses related to age), and failure to use safety devices, such as helmets, seat belts, and handrails (Garton & Lehmann, 2015). The structural pathology in TBI includes primary, secondary, Monro–Kellie Doctrine, and Cushing's triad phenomena.

Primary TBIs include skull fractures, hemorrhages, contusions, and diffuse axonal injury (DAI). Owing to extreme forces required, there exists high suspicion for concomitant cervical spine injury, and care should be taken to immobilize the spine. Skull fractures may require surgery to repair or may be medically managed by observation. Hemorrhages are treated differently, dependent on type and severity. Epidural hemorrhages are arterial, usually arising from a torn temporal artery and usually requiring surgical intervention. Subdural hemorrhages are venous in origin and may require evacuation if there is significant mass effect or deficits noted. Traumatic subarachnoid hemorrhages may require an external ventricular drain (EVD) to be placed to monitor bleeding and ICP monitoring. Contusions and DAI are medically monitored (Garton & Lehmann, 2015).

Secondary TBI includes cytotoxic and/or vasogenic cerebral edema, cellular ischemic injury, and loss of cerebral blood flow regulation, which occurs in response to the primary brain injury. Mechanisms include apoptosis, calcium-dependent cascades, and oxidative stress creating damage at the cellular level. Prevention of hypoperfusion of the brain and increased metabolic demands is key to limiting secondary brain injuries. (Andersen et al., 2015; Garton & Lehmann, 2015).

ICP is the result of three components within the skull: the brain tissue, cerebrospinal fluid, and blood. The brain can compensate for a small amount of tissue swelling, with a displacement of the cerebrospinal fluid (CSF) and blood. When the brain tissue becomes compressed related to its edema or mass effect from hematomas, blood supply is reduced leading to cerebral hypoperfusion and secondary brain injury. Untreated, this may lead to herniation through the foramen magnum (tonsillar herniation) or skull fractures (Garton & Lehmann, 2015).

The constellation of symptoms that accompanies herniation is known as Cushing's Triad. This includes bradycardia, hypertension, and respiratory irregularities. If the patient is intubated and on mechanical ventilation, many times the respiratory pattern goes unnoticed. The presence of Cushing's Triad is ominous and requires immediate attention by the neurosurgical provider. In severe cases of TBI with high ICPs and danger of herniation, decompressive craniectomy (removal of skull bone flap) may be required to allow expansion of the tissue to preserve life (Garton & Lehmann, 2015).

Clinical Aspects

ASSESSMENT

Obtaining an accurate history of the injury is important, as injury patterns may be identified. For instance, epidural hemorrhages are suspected when there is an initial loss of consciousness, a period of lucidity, and then the loss of consciousness once again. Amnesia, nausea, vomiting, headache, vertigo, nuchal rigidity, and vision disturbances are examples of significant findings in those with TBI (Garton & Lehmann, 2015).

Regarding physical assessment, frequent serial neurological examinations are key in those diagnosed with TBI. The consistency of those examinations among providers is extremely important and should be performed with both receiving and departing providers present to ensure continuity in method and examination findings. Components of the assessment should include airway patency, adequacy of breathing, blood pressure monitoring parameters, Glasgow Coma Scale scoring, protective reflexes (a cough, gag, corneal), pupillary size, equality and reaction, level of consciousness, as well as any focal deficits identified. Changes in examination should promptly be reported to the attending provider or neurosurgeon. Any impairment in airway patency (including loss of gag or cough reflex), ventilation, and/or depression in the level of consciousness with a Glasgow Coma score less than 8, requires emergency intervention for airway protection and mechanical ventilation (Garton & Lehmann, 2015).

Nursing problems associated with TBI include alteration in tissue perfusion, the potential for alteration in airway patency, the potential for seizures, the potential for infection (related to monitoring/drainage devices), malnutrition, alteration in skin integrity related to immobility, and alteration in mental status related to acute TBI.

NURSING INTERVENTIONS, MANAGEMENT, AND IMPLICATIONS

Nursing interventions for TBI center on supportive care, prevention of secondary brain injuries, and restoration of homeostasis. For those diagnosed with mild TBI, serial neurological examinations may be required for the first few days, with neurology follow-up. In moderate TBI, serial examinations and cardiovascular monitoring may be required for close observation. In severe TBI, serial examinations and cardiovascular monitoring are required, along with other possible modalities. Intracranial monitoring may be initiated by neurosurgery to facilitate monitoring of cerebral perfusion pressures (CPP) or EVD devices employed to monitor and treat elevated ICPs by way of removal of CSF through a conduit placed in the ventricle. EEG may be used if seizures are suspected. Nursing should institute seizure precautions, and neurology may order antiepileptic drugs on a prophylactic basis (Brain Trauma Foundation, 2016).

Maintenance of normal ventilation is essential in patients mechanically ventilated with severe TBI. Ventilation strategies are aimed at maintaining a normal level of carbon dioxide (CO_2; 35–45 mmHg). Lower CO_2 levels cause cerebral perfusion and ischemia, and higher CO_2 levels cause vasoconstriction and increased ICP.

Temperature-targeted therapy (therapeutic hypothermia) may be instituted to decrease metabolic demands and reduce cytotoxic events associated with cerebral edema. This type of therapy requires the critical care environment and is reserved for those with severe TBI. These patients are intubated, mechanically ventilated, and may require vasopressors to support a blood pressure sufficient enough to maintain cerebral perfusion (Andersen et al., 2015; Brain Trauma Foundation, 2016).

Cerebral edema may also be treated with hyperosmolar therapy in the form of mannitol or hypertonic saline. Both modalities employ osmolar pull to reduce edema in the brain by increasing the osmolality of the serum to pull fluid from this tissue. Mannitol has an additional diuretic component, which can ultimately affect blood pressure and reduce CPP. Hypertonic (3%) saline has been employed for the same osmotic effect, without diuretic properties (Brain Trauma Foundation, 2016).

Central diabetes insipidus is a condition related to antidiuretic hormone deficiency, characterized by large amounts of dilute urine output with low specific gravity, and high serum osmolality being noted. This condition leads to hypernatremia and is the body's attempt at hyperosmolar treatment. Desmopressin acetate may be required to control this phenomenon. (Fitzgerald, 2017).

OUTCOMES

Goals of therapy include stabilization of primary injury, minimization of secondary injury, and the return of homeostasis. Targets should include protecting airway patency and optimal ventilation, minimizing metabolic demands, providing nutrition support, and seizure precautions/prophylaxis. Measurable outcomes include maintaining a mean arterial pressure sufficient to provide cerebral perfusion pressure (CPP 60–70), measurable with monitoring devices such as intracranial bolts or EVDs. ICPs should ideally be maintained at 0 to 10 mmHg. Normoglycemia, fever prevention, and normocarbia are also measurable outcomes that benefit those diagnosed with TBI (Brain Trauma Foundation, 2016).

Prevention is the most valuable of all interventions. Nurses are at the forefront of public health and are in a position to provide the element of assessment and education to those identified at risk. Nurses should encourage the use of concussion guidelines in sports, promote the use of helmets and other safety devices, and assist in the provision of home safety, medication reconciliation, and sensory screening for elders.

Summary

TBI is a prevalent world health issue and carries a significant financial cost, as well as the morbidity and mortality associated with head injuries in many demographics. The long-term sequelae of TBI can last a lifetime, and prevention is key. The usage of safety devices and established guidelines in contact sports should be encouraged to all age groups.

TBI can be characterized as primary or secondary, by the acuity, and also by severity. Concussions, contusion, hemorrhages, and cellular injuries are some examples. Maintenance of cerebral perfusion and prevention of secondary injury is paramount in those with TBI. The goals of care are supportive and restorative, with guidelines in place by the Brain Trauma Foundation to guide providers in the care of these very complex patients. An ever-expanding wealth of knowledge is being gained in the area of TBI, and updates to these guidelines occur regularly.

Andersen, M., Gazmuri, J. T., Marin, A., Regueira, T., & Rovegno, M. (2015). Therapeutic hypothermia for acute brain injuries. *Scandinavian Journal of Trauma, Resuscitation, and Emergency Medicine, 23*, 42. doi:10.1186/s13049-015-0121-3

Brain Trauma Foundation. (2016). *Guidelines for management of traumatic brain injury* (4th ed.). Retrieved from https://braintrauma.org/uploads/03/12/Guidelines_for_Management_of_Severe_TBI_4th_Edition.pdf

Centers for Disease Control and Prevention. (2016). Get the stats on traumatic brain injury in the United States. Retrieved from https://www.cdc.gov/traumaticbrain injury/pdf/BlueBook_factsheet-a.pdf

Fitzgerald, P. A. (2017). Endocrine disorders. In M. A. Papadakis & S. J. McPhee (Eds.), *Current medical diagnosis and treatment* (56th ed., pp. 1113–1114). New York, NY: McGraw-Hill.

Garton, H., & Lehmann, E. (2015). Neurosurgery. In G. M. Doherty (Ed.), *Current diagnosis and treatment: Surgery* (14th ed., pp. 863–874). New York, NY: McGraw-Hill.

Su, F., Raghupathi, R., & Huh, J. (2015). Traumatic brain injury in children. In T. E. Corden (Ed.), *Medscape*. Retrieved from https://emedicine.medscape.com/article/909105-overview

White, H., & Venkatesh, B. (2016). Traumatic brain injury. In W. Kolka, M. Smith, & G. Citerio (Eds.), *Oxford textbook of neurocritical care* (pp. 210–224). Oxford, UK: Oxford University Press.

Neonatal Nursing

■ ABO INCOMPATIBILITY

Donna M. Schultz
Mary F. Terhaar

Overview

ABO incompatibility is the single, most common form of isoimmune hemolytic anemia in the Western world, occurring in 12% to 15% of all pregnancies (Roberts, 2008). The condition occurs when the maternal blood type differs from the fetal blood type. Most commonly, the condition arises in a blood type O mother who carries a blood type A or B fetus, although it can present in a blood type A or B mother who carries a fetus of a different blood type. In 3% to 4% of these pregnancies, maternal red blood cells (RBCs) cross the placenta and interact with fetal cells triggering complications, including anemia and hyperbilirubinemia (Basu, Kaur, & Kaur, 2011).

ABO incompatibility is one of the hemolytic anemias. Because of the antenatal administration of RhoGAM (anti-D gamma globulin), Rh isoimmunization decreases, leading to ABO incompatibility, one of the most common causes of hemolytic disease.

Background

Blood types are assigned to correspond to the surface antigen on the RBC. Type A blood carries A-antigens on the surface of the RBC along with anti-B antibodies. Type B blood carries B-antigens on the surface along with anti-A antibodies. Type AB blood carries both A- and B-antigens on the surface, but neither anti-A nor anti-B antibodies. Finally, type O blood carries neither A- nor B-antigens, but both anti-A and anti-B antibodies. Each blood type recognizes cells from the same type when they encounter corresponding antigens that match their own. Conversely, antibodies mobilize, clump, and hemolyze blood cells that carry antigens different from their own.

The reason why type O blood is the universal donor is that it carries no antigens to trigger hemolysis and rejection. The mother with type O blood has no antigens on the surface of her RBCs and so the fetus with a dissimilar blood type will not hemolyze maternal cells. However, her blood does carry anti-A and anti-B antibodies. When O negative cells of the mother cross into fetal circulation, the anti-A and anti-B antibodies they carry attack and hemolyze fetal cells, which lowers the RBC count and elevates the levels of waste products, including bilirubin. This is the mechanism by which ABO incompatibility leads to anemia and hyperbilirubinemia.

Clinical Aspects

ASSESSMENT

Actual, symptomatic hemolytic disease (HD) occurs in less than 1% of infants affected by ABO incompatibility. The primary symptom is hyperbilirubinemia and the presentation is generally mild, particularly if the Coombs direct antibody test (DAT) is negative.

Bilirubin causes jaundice, which is easily visible to the eye. However, visualization is an unreliable indicator of the severity of the disease or the risk. For this reason, routine screening is important, especially for infants with deeply pigmented skin (American Academy of Pediatrics Subcommittee on Hyperbilirubinemia, 2004).

Infants with ABO incompatibility should be closely monitored and their bilirubin levels plotted to determine their level of risk for hyperbilirubinemia. Diagnosis of ABO incompatibility can be quickly established shortly after birth. A blood type and DAT should be determined for all infants born to mothers with blood type O. Infants found to have a blood type of A or B, who also have a positive DAT, have a confirmed diagnosis of ABO incompatibility. However, a positive test does not indicate that severe hyperbilirubinemia will develop. It is important and necessary to evaluate the risk of HD. Serial bilirubin levels, a complete blood count (CBC), reticulocyte count, and a history of a sibling who was treated for significant hyperbilirubinemia are all predictors of HD (Bhat & Kumar, 2014).

Bilirubin levels for term newborns are typically drawn at the time of the metabolic screening and repeated at 8-hour intervals through discharge or initiation of phototherapy. However, with ABO incompatibility, hyperbilirubinemia is often seen within the first 24 hours of life. The bilirubin levels are plotted over hours of life and correlated with the risk of hyperbilirubinemia. The result is a four-zone risk stratification for newborns, where zone 1 is low risk, zone 2 is low-intermediate risk, zone 3 is high-intermediate risk, and zone 4 is high risk (Bhutani, Johnson, & Sivieri, 1999). Use of this nomogram is the best practice for monitoring newborns with hyperbilirubinemia (American Academy of Pediatrics Subcommittee on Hyperbilirubinemia, 2004).

Phototherapy is used for infants whose bilirubin levels rise to the moderate-to high-risk zone (Bhutani, Vilms, & Hamerman-Johnson, 2010). Bilirubin levels that are critical may require intravenous immunoglobulin (IVIG), or more rarely, an exchange transfusion (Smits-Wintjens et al., 2013).

Among newborns who receive phototherapy, roughly 50% will also have evidence of hemolysis on their complete blood count (CBC) analysis (Bhat & Kumar, 2012). Hemolytic anemia occurs when the infant's RBCs break down faster than normal in relation to the mother's antibodies. Maternal antibodies may remain in the infant for a few weeks after birth. As a result, the infant may require a blood transfusion.

NURSING INTERVENTIONS, MANAGEMENT, AND IMPLICATIONS

Nurses are integral to identifying and closely monitoring the risk factors for ABO incompatibility and hyperbilirubinemia. Mothers with blood type O need to be quickly identified so that their infants' blood can be typed and screened. The health care providers responsible for the infants' care need to be notified with the results of the lab work so that the infants can be closely monitored for hyperbilirubinemia and hemolysis (AAP Committee for Hyperbilirubinemia, 2004).

The infant with ABO incompatibility will benefit from breastfeeding early and at frequent intervals. For the infant whose mother who does not elect to breastfeed, small frequent feedings are beneficial. Both keep the infant well hydrated, which helps to clear the by-products of hemolysis and reduce the risk of kernicterus, which results from unmanaged hyperbilirubinemia.

Oral intake and urine output are monitored closely. The jaundiced infant may be fatigued, may have low muscle tone, and/or may have lethargy. All of these findings may contribute to difficulty with feeding and mild dehydration. Often, the baby may require intravenous (IV) fluid. The urine may be darker in color because the infant eliminates bilirubin in the urine as well as the stool.

Parents need to understand the importance of providing adequate fluid intake and recording urine and stool output. Because exclusively breastfed infants and those born before completing 38 weeks gestation face an increased risk of clinically significant hyperbilirubinemia, nurses need to teach families about the risks associated with hyperbilirubinemia. This understanding enables parents to advocate for their babies after they are discharged from the hospital (Centers for Disease Control and Prevention [CDC], n.d.).

Nurses must also be knowledgeable about the types of therapies used for the treatment of ABO incompatibility: phototherapy, IVIG administration, and exchange transfusion. Each treatment modality has risks associated with it and nurses must be aware of these risk factors so that symptoms can be identified early, if they occur.

OUTCOMES

Rarely does ABO incompatibility cause major sequelae in infants. Severe anemia, as a result of hemolysis, is known to occur. Kernicterus, as a result of extremely high bilirubin levels, is decreased with early and aggressive phototherapy.

Summary

Although ABO incompatibility is easily detected and primary treatment is close monitoring and phototherapy, it is important to ensure screening for HD. It is the most common type of isoimmune hemolytic anemia in the United States; can be diagnosed easily and early; and primary treatment, including adequate fluid intake and phototherapy, presents low risk and low cost. More severe forms of neonatal ABO incompatibility and hemolytic disease are rare, but easily detected and treated. Nursing plays an integral role in the identification of at-risk newborns. Guidelines should be in place so that nurses may track bilirubin levels against hours of life on the nomogram.

Best practices include development and adherence to evidence-based protocols for hyperbilirubinemia screening that include universal screening of all babies at 12 to 24 hours of life. Bilirubin levels (either transcutaneous or serum) should be plotted against hours of life on the nomogram to determine the risk (Cabra & Whitfield, 2005).

Nurses must also be aware of treatment modalities and their risk factors. In addition, nurses must prepare their families well by educating them on the risk factors of hyperbilirubinemia, treatment, and appropriate follow-up in the primary care setting until bilirubin levels start declining.

American Academy of Pediatrics Subcommittee on Hyperbilirubinemia. (2004). Management of hyperbilirubinemia in the newborn infant 35 or more weeks of gestation. *Pediatrics, 114*(1), 297–316. Retrieved from http://pediatrics.aappublications .org/content/114/1/297.long

Basu, S., Kaur, R., & Kaur, G. (2011). Hemolytic disease of the fetus and newborn: Current trends and perspectives. *Asian Journal of Transfusion Science, 5*(1), 3–7. doi:10.4103/0973-6247.75963

Bhat, R. Y., & Kumar, P. C. G. (2012). Morbidity of ABO haemolytic disease in the newborn. *Paediatrics and International Child Health, 32*(2), 93–96. doi:10.1179/20469 05512Y.0000000002

Bhat, R.Y., & Kumar, P. C. G. (2014). Sixth hour transcutaneous bilirubin predicting significant hyperbilirubinemia in ABO incompatible neonates. *World Journal of Pediatrics, 10*(2), 182–185. doi:10.1007/s12519-013-0421-5

Bhutani, V. K., Johnson, L., & Sivieri, E. M. (1999). Predictive ability of a predischarge hour-specific serum bilirubin for subsequent significant hyperbilirubinemia in healthy term and near-term newborns. *Pediatrics, 103*(1), 6–14. doi:10.1542/peds.103.1.6

Bhutani, V. K., Vilms, R. J., & Hamerman-Johnson, L. (2010). Universal bilirubin screening for severe neonatal hyperbilirubinemia. *Journal of Perinatology, 30*(Suppl.), S6–S15. doi:10.1038/jp.2010.98

Cabra, M. A., & Whitfield, J. M. (2005). The challenge of preventing neonatal bilirubin encephalopathy: A new nursing protocol in the well newborn nursery. *Baylor University Medical Center Proceedings, 18*(3), 217–219. doi:10.1080/08998280.20 05.11928070

Centers for Disease Control and Prevention. (n.d.). Jaundice & kernicterus: Guidelines and tools for health professionals. Retrieved from http://www.cdc.gov/ncbddd/ jaundice/hcp.html

Roberts, I. A. G. (2008). The changing face of haemolytic disease of the newborn. *Early Human Development, 84*(8), 515–523. doi:10.1016/j.earlhumdev.2008.06.005

Smits-Wintjens, V. E. H. J., Rath, M. E. A., van Zwet, E. W., Oepkes, D., Brand, A., Walther, F. J., & Lopriore, E. (2013). Neonatal morbidity after exchange transfusion for red cell alloimmune hemolytic disease. *Neonatology, 103*(2), 141–147. doi:10.1159/000343261

■ ACUTE RENAL FAILURE

Christine Horvat Davey

Overview

Acute renal failure (ARF), also known as *acute kidney injury*, is a reversible acute decline in renal function with rapid onset (Devarajan, 2017). ARF is marked by a decrease in the glomerular filtration rate, an inability of the kidneys to regulate fluid and electrolyte homeostasis as well as an increase in serum creatinine and blood urea nitrogen levels (Andreoli, 2009). The exact incidence of infant ARF is unknown. Nursing care for infants with ARF focuses on determination and treatment of the underlying cause with early medical management to decrease long-term sequelae.

Background

After birth, the kidneys undergo a maturation process and continue further to adapt, which is a vital element in the prevention and management of neonatal ARF (Nada, Bohachea, & Askenazi, 2017). The number of nephrons present at birth is attributed to the genetic and fetal environmental factors and range from 300,000 to 1.8 million per kidney (Nada et al., 2017). Premature infants with ARF can be at an increased risk of long-term kidney issues depending on the status of their nephrons (Nada et al., 2017). The incidence of ARF is rising in relation to the increased use of advanced medical technology for infants who are critically ill or experience chronic conditions (Devarajan, 2017).

ARF in infants is rarely caused by a primary renal issue, but rather by reversible prerenal failure owing to poor perfusion of kidneys, acute tubular necrosis, or cortical necrosis (Coulthard, 2016). Hypotension is the primary cause of poor perfusion and can be caused by cardiac failure, hypovolemia, vasodilation associated with sepsis, multiple organ failure, or a combination of these (Coulthard, 2016). There are several additional factors associated with an increased risk of the development of ARF in infants, including premature birth, birth weight, nephrotoxicity, genetics, hypoxia, ischemia, acute injury, or illness. Premature birth can lead to a low nephron count and incomplete nephrogenesis, contributing to an increased risk of the development of ARF. A low birth weight places infants at a higher risk of developing ARF (Arcinue, Kantak, & Elkhwad, 2015). Nephrotoxin-induced ARF is often related to hospitalization because hospitalization poses an increased risk of exposure to medications that are nephrotoxic (Sutherland et al., 2013). In addition to environmental factors, there may be genetic risk factors for ARF. Several candidate polymorphisms have shown an association with ARF (Andreoli, 2009).

The diagnosis of ARF is most often based on characteristic signs and symptoms: edema, decreased urine output, hematuria, and/or hypertension with abnormal laboratory results, especially abnormal serum creatinine levels.

A normal serum creatinine level for an infant is 0.2 to 0.4 mg/dL (18–35 μmol/L; Devarajan, 2017). However, the diagnostic use of serum creatinine levels can present issues. Following ARF, serum creatinine is an insensitive and delayed measure of decreased kidney function (Andreoli, 2009). Serum creatinine may not increase until a 50% or higher reduction in the glomerular filtration rate is present (Devarajan, 2017). In addition, if dialysis is initiated as a treatment, serum creatinine levels cannot be measured accurately. An abnormal urinalysis can also indicate ARF, though individuals with prerenal ARF may display a normal urinalysis. Urinalysis is most often utilized to determine the underlying cause of ARF. Regardless of the limitations posed by the serum creatinine levels in this diagnosis, it is presently the best laboratory test for the diagnosis of ARF in infants.

The ability to classify the causes of ARF can lead to early and targeted medical interventions. ARF in infants is often multifactorial. Causes of ARF can be prerenal, renal (intrinsic), and postrenal. Prerenal ARF signifies a functional alteration without actual kidney damage (Nada et al., 2017). This can present as a rise in the serum creatinine levels, nitrogen retention, and oliguria. Several factors can lead to prerenal ARF, including decreased renal perfusion, increased capillary permeability, decreased oncotic pressure, and medication exposure. Decreased renal perfusion can result from hypotension, decreased cardiac output, and decreased intravascular volume (Nada et al., 2017). Increased capillary permeability can be the result of sepsis. Exposure to certain medications prenatally or postnatally such as nonsteroidal anti-inflammatory drugs (NSAIDs) and angiotensin-converting enzyme (ACE) inhibitors can also contribute to prerenal ARF.

Renal ARF is characterized by persistent functional alterations that are not appropriately corrected and lead to kidney damage and acute tubular necrosis (Nada et al., 2017). Renal ARF can be caused by vascular compromise, renal artery thrombosis, renal infarction, or medications. Vascular compromise can be induced by bilateral renal vein thrombosis, which is often seen in umbilical artery catheter malposition (Nada et al., 2017). Medications known to induce renal ARF include antimicrobial medications such as aminoglycosides, gentamicin, acyclovir, intravenous immunoglobulin (IVIG), and radiocontrast agents.

Postrenal ARF is the least common form and is often caused by intrinsic obstructions, such as tumors, fungal balls, or may be congenital (Nada et al., 2017). Urethral strictures owing to traumatic bladder cauterization or malfunctioning indwelling urinary catheters can also cause postrenal ARF (Nada et al., 2017). Correction of the obstruction usually results in renal function improvement.

Clinical Aspects

ASSESSMENT

As soon as the diagnosis of known or suspected ARF is made, further assessment is dedicated to identifying the underlying cause. This evaluation includes an accurate record of an individual's physical assessment, medical history, and laboratory data. The physical assessment should focus on signs and symptoms related to alterations in renal function. These assessment findings include oliguria or anuria, edema, hematuria, and/or hypertension (Devarajan, 2017). Nursing responsibilities include accurate blood pressure measurement, assessment of edema or volume depletion (indicated by dry mucous membranes, decreased skin turgor, tachycardia, orthostatic falls in blood pressure, and decreased peripheral perfusion), recent weight gain, signs of system disease (rash or joint disease), enlarged palpable kidneys (may indicate renal vein thrombosis), and/or enlarged bladder (may indicate urethral obstruction; Devarajan, 2017).

An accurate history is essential because there is often a known etiologic factor that predisposes an infant to ARF. These factors include heart failure, shock, or a preceding streptococcal infection seen in patients with poststreptococcal glomerulonephritis (Devarajan, 2017). Laboratory data to monitor when there is a concern for alterations in renal function include elevation of serum creatinine and/or blood urea nitrogen levels, abnormal urinalysis, hyperkalemia, hyponatremia or less often hypernatremia, metabolic acidosis, hypocalcemia, and/or hyperphosphatemia. Renal imaging can also be performed or, on rare occasions, a kidney biopsy may be conducted to determine the underlying cause. Utilization of accurate physical assessment, medical history, and laboratory data can facilitate the initiation of proper and timely nursing care that can positively impact patient outcomes.

NURSING INTERVENTIONS, MANAGEMENT, AND IMPLICATIONS

Nursing care of infants with ARF should focus on the treatment of ARF and prevention of long-term sequelae. Nursing care includes monitoring of vital signs, including maintenance of proper blood pressure and daily weights; strict accurate measurement of intake and output; maintenance of proper electrolyte balance and nutrition; determination of underlying cause and correction of the cause; if necessary, initiation of treatment such as hemodialysis, peritoneal dialysis, or continuous renal reperfusion therapy (CRRT); monitoring of laboratory data; and psychological support for the family unit.

OUTCOMES

The anticipated outcomes of nursing evidence-based practice focus on the treatment of ARF and prevention of long-term sequelae. Early determination of ARF based on signs, symptoms, and laboratory data as well as prompt correction of the underlying cause facilitate positive outcomes. Urine output is a key indicator for the management of ARF in infants because of the fact that low urine volumes limit fluid administration and in turn restrict nutrition (Coulthard, 2016). A primary focus in reversing ARF is the correction of hypotension. Therefore, corrective measures include fluid resuscitation, cardiac inotropic support, correcting coagulopathies, and treating infections (Coulthard, 2016). It is vital to avoid fluid overload and inadequate nutrition. In addition to the correction of underlying causes of ARF and management of signs and symptoms, treatment options can include hemodialysis, peritoneal dialysis, and CRRT. Effective nursing care outcomes should result in the correction of ARF without long-term sequelae.

Summary

It is of utmost importance to recognize the early signs and symptoms of ARF as well as differentiating among prerenal, intrinsic, and postrenal failure. Morbidity and mortality are dependent on the etiology of the renal failure. Early recognition and medical management can facilitate positive outcomes and decrease incidence of long-term sequelae.

Andreoli, S. P. (2009). Acute kidney injury in children. *Pediatric Nephrology, 24*(2), 253–263. doi:10.1007/s00467-008-1074-9

Arcinue, R., Kantak, A., & Elkhwad, M. (2015). Acute kidney injury in ELBW infants (<750 grams) and its associated risk factors. *Journal of Neonatal–Perinatal Medicine, 8*(4), 349–357. doi:10.3233/NPM-15915022

Coulthard, M. G. (2016). The management of neonatal acute and chronic renal failure: A review. *Early Human Development, 102*, 25–29. doi:10.1016/j.earlhumdev.2016.09.004

Devarajan, P. (2017). Acute kidney injury: Still misunderstood and misdiagnosed. *Nature Reviews Nephrology, 13*(3), 137–138. doi:10.1038/nrneph.2017.9

Nada, A., Bonachea, E. M., & Askenazi, D. J. (2017). Acute kidney injury in the fetus and neonate. *Seminars in Fetal and Neonatal Medicine, 22*(2), 90–97. doi:10.1016/j.siny.2016.12.001

Sutherland, S. M., Ji, J., Sheikhi, F. H., Widen, E., Tian, L., Alexander, S. R., & Ling, X. B. (2013). AKI in hospitalized children: Epidemiology and clinical associations in a national cohort. *Clinical Journal of the American Society of Nephrology, 8*(10), 1661–1669. doi:10.2215/CJN.00270113

■ ANEMIA OF PREMATURITY

Barbara Greitzer Slone

Overview

Anemia of prematurity, anemia in preterm infants, or neonatal anemia is defined as a low hemoglobin or hematocrit concentration of more than two standard deviations below the mean for postnatal age. It is a major problem encountered in neonatal intensive care units (NICUs; Colombatti, Sainati, & Trevisanuto, 2016). Blood transfusions and administration of iron and erythropoiesis-stimulating agent are common nursing care measures in NICUs to address this clinical issue. There is also a role for the nurse in the promotion of delayed cord clamping for the prevention of anemia in this cohort of patients (Colombatti et al., 2016).

Background

Anemia of prematurity is an exaggerated drop in the hemoglobin (Hb)/hematocrit (Hct), more than that expected physiologically in these infants. Preterm infants are those at less than 37 weeks gestation (American Academy of Pediatrics and the American College of Obstetricians and Gynecologists, 2012). All infants experience a drop in their Hb/Hct levels after birth in the first few weeks of life. This is called *physiologic anemia of the newborn* and it may go unnoticed. In preterm infants, the anemia is more pronounced and the drop is faster, often presenting with symptoms, including pallor, tachypnea, poor feeding, poor growth, lethargy, and tachycardia, and frequently requiring treatment (Gardner, Carter, Hines, & Hernández, 2016). Anemia of prematurity is present in all preterm infants, but may not cause symptoms. Infants equal to or less than 32 weeks gestation often require blood transfusions; one citation estimates 80% of infants less than 32 weeks gestation require transfusion (Colombatti et al., 2016).

Anemia of prematurity presents with normocytic, normochromic, hyporegenerative anemia and this can be determined when evaluating the results of the complete blood count (CBC). The reticulocyte count is the index that reveals the bone marrow's response to anemia; a higher count would indicate that more new red blood cells are being manufactured.

Preterm infants, particularly those at 32 weeks and less, frequently require a myriad of medical interventions to assist them in breathing, digesting nutrients, and maintaining homeostasis. These medical interventions require frequent blood sampling to assess their adequacy. The preterm infant is ill equipped to respond to this demand for blood sampling. Preterm infants frequently are iron deficient, nutritionally deficient, and suffer from other chronic illnesses that contribute to their anemia.

Erythropoiesis or the making of new red blood cells in a newborn infant is a complex phenomenon and quite different from that of an adult. During human

gestation, blood formation occurs initially in the yolk sac; during the second trimester, this changes to the liver, spleen, and lymph nodes. Finally, in the last half
of gestation, the bone marrow takes over (Colombatti et al., 2016). Premature
infants are still in the process of switching over to erythropoiesis in the bone
marrow. Newborns are also born with a predominance of fetal hemoglobin,
which carries a higher affinity for oxygen and is necessary for intrauterine life.
The fetal hemoglobin has a shorter life span and in the first few weeks after birth
the newborn will switch over to adult hemoglobin, resulting in a more rapid
increase in the destruction of red blood cells. As the newborn transitions from
the hypoxic intrauterine environment to the oxygen-rich postnatal environment,
erythropoietin production is decreased, resulting in less production of red blood
cells. The preterm newborn in this physiologic milieu is predisposed to anemia.

Iron deficiency is an additional contributing factor to the severity of anemia
of prematurity. Iron stores at birth are largely obtained in the last trimester
of pregnancy. Children developing iron deficiency in the first year of life are
more at risk of developing neurocognitive sequelae, with poorer school performance and memory tasks (Kling & Coe, 2016). Factors that contribute to
decreased iron stores include prematurity; multiple gestation; male sex; small
size for gestational age; large size for gestational age; and maternal factors of
obesity, diabetes, placental dysfunction, stress, ethnicity, socioeconomic status,
and maternal iron-deficiency anemia (Kling & Coe, 2016).

Erythropoiesis-stimulating agents (erythropoietin), once widely used to aid
in the prevention of anemia of prematurity, have come into disfavor. There has
been an association between the use of these agents and cancers in adults (Hitti,
2007). In the newborn population, there is limited evidence for the efficacy of
this therapy and in a Cochrane review published in 2014, the authors concluded
that the administration of epoetin alfa did not significantly reduce or increase
any clinically important adverse outcomes (Ohlsson & Aher, 2014). These agents
are no longer being routinely used in most NICUs.

There is a growing body of evidence for delayed cord clamping in the delivery
room and its positive effect on decreasing the incidence and severity of anemia in
the preterm infant. This practice essentially provides the patient with additional
cells from the blood supply of the placenta (World Health Organiztion, 2013).
Here the nurse can educate the family and be supportive of his or her delivery
room colleagues.

Clinical Aspects

ASSESSMENT

The laboratory assessment of anemia of prematurity is largely done by obtaining a CBC of the infant. The evaluation of the hemoglobin and hematocrit (Hgb/
Hct) is dependent on the gestational age of the infant, chronological age of the
infant, and the need for oxygen therapy. The severity of the infant's illness also
needs to be considered. In general, the sicker the infant, the greater the need for
a higher Hgb/Hct.

NURSING INTERVENTIONS, MANAGEMENT, AND IMPLICATIONS

Nursing is integral to evaluate infants for anemia. On physical examination, pallor, increased work of breathing, substernal and intercostal retractions, tachycardia, or tachypnea can all be indicators of anemia. Anemia also frequently presents with apnea, bradycardia, desaturations, lethargy, poor feeding, or tachypnea after feeds, and poor growth.

An astute nurse can assess these symptoms and ensure that the patient is receiving appropriate treatment by describing the infant's vital signs, feeding tolerance, and changes in oxygen requirements to the care provider. In addition, the nurse should ensure that there is a regular, systematic surveillance of all the preterm infants to determine if intervention is required. Typically, in clinical practice, surveillance includes a CBC differential and a reticulocyte count.

Prevention of anemia is achieved by attentiveness to the necessity of all blood sampling for laboratory tests, careful attention to obtaining only the minimal amount of blood needed for each test, and vigilance during blood sampling to prevent extraneous loss. The mainstay of treatment is a blood transfusion. Packed red blood cells that are irradiated and leukocyte poor are used. They must be typed and cross-matched for each individual patient. Consent from the parent or guardian must be obtained. The usual dose is 15 mL/kg given over 3 hours intravenously. Exposure to multiple donors can be limited by the use of small aliquots of blood sourced from the same donor. In infants who are chronically ill with lung disease and who require ventilatory support, the transfusion can be followed by a dose of furosemide to minimize the effects of the additional fluid in the cardiovascular system of the patient. Transfusion-related gut injury concerns have led many practitioners to keep patients nil per os (NPO) for 3 hours before, during, and 3 hours posttransfusions. This requires that the nurse evaluate the blood sugar levels of the patient before, during, and after the infusion.

Iron supplementation is routinely given to infants who are able to tolerate full feeds. The iron may be in a liquid multivitamin form or may be given separately. The role of the nurse is to ensure that all infants are given iron supplementation in the nursery and provide parental education on the administration of the supplement and importance of continuing iron therapy at home.

OUTCOMES

Infants with anemia of prematurity may demonstrate apnea, poor growth patterns, and cardiovascular compromise if not treated. Anemia of prematurity is a transient, physiologic process that is exacerbated by multiple blood draws when the infant is ill and rapid growth during the recovery phase. Anemia of prematurity will resolve with good nutrition, careful monitoring of the hemoglobin and reticulocyte count, and iron supplementation.

Summary

Anemia of prematurity is a common problem in neonatal intensive care. Nurses can play a pivotal role in the prevention, recognition, and treatment of this problem. This can prevent both short-term and long-term consequences and neurodevelopmental sequelae in this patient population.

Buonocore, G. (2014). Erythropoietin use in the newborn. *Italian Journal of Pediatrics, 40*(Suppl. 2), A41. doi:10.1186/1824-7288-40-S2-A41

Colombatti, R., Sainati, L., & Trevisanuto, D. (2016). Anemia and transfusion in the neonate. *Seminars in Fetal and Neonatal Medicine, 21*(1), 2–9. doi:10.1016/j.siny.2015.12.001

Gardner, S. L., Carter, B. S., Hines, M. E., & Hernández, J. A. (Eds.). (2016). *Merenstein & Gardner's handbook of neonatal intensive care* (8th ed.). St. Louis, MO: Elsevier.

Hitti, M. (2007, November 8). Anemia drugs change black box warning. Retrieved from http://www.webmd.com/cancer/news/20071108/anemia-drugs-change-black -box-warning#1

Katheria, A. C., Truong, G., Cousins, L., Oshiro, B., & Finer, N. N. (2015). Umbilical cord milking versus delayed cord clamping in preterm infants. *Pediatrics, 136*(1), 61–69. doi:10.1542/peds.2015-0368

Kling, P. J., & Coe, C. L. (2016). Iron hemostatsis in pregnancy, the fetus, and the neo-nate. *NeoReviews, 17*(11), e657–e664. doi:10.1542/neo.17-11-e657

Ohlsson, A., & Aher, S. M. (2014). Early erythropoietin for preventing red blood cell transfusion in preterm and/or low birth weight infants. *Cochrane Database of Systematic Reviews, 2014*(4). doi:10.1002/14651858.CD004863.pub4

World Health Organization. (2013). *Delayed clamping of the umbilical cord to reduce infant anemia.* Geneva, Switzerland: Author. Retrieved from http://apps.who.int/iris/bitstream/10665/120074/1/WHO_RHR_14.19_eng.pdf

■ APNEA OF PREMATURITY

Amy Bieda

Overview

Apnea of prematurity (AOP) is a common clinical problem affecting premature infants and is related to developmental immaturity. By definition, it is the cessation of breathing for more than 15 to 20 seconds accompanied by bradycardia (heart rate less than 80 beats/min) and desaturations (SpO_2 less than 80%; Zhao, Gonzales, & Mu, 2011). AOP is inversely related to gestational age (Eichenwald & American Academy of Pediatrics Committee on Fetus and Newborn, 2016). The majority of infants with less than 1,000 g birth weight and less than 28 weeks gestational age at birth develop AOP (Morton & Smith, 2016). It is rarely experienced by infants born at greater than 37 weeks postmenstrual age (Fairchild et al., 2016). Neonatal intensive care unit (NICU) nurses are at the forefront of managing infants with AOP.

Background

Apnea is classified as central, obstructive, or mixed. Central apnea is the complete termination of respirations that occurs because of the immaturity of the brainstem and resultant poor control of the central respiratory drive. Obstructive apnea occurs when there is no airflow within the upper airway, particularly at the level of the pharynx, while the infant continues to have respiratory effort. Mixed apnea involves an event of central apnea that is directly followed by or preceded by an obstructive apnea event. The majority of premature infants experience mixed apnea, which occurs as an episode of apnea and bradycardia with desaturation. AOP needs to be distinguished from periodic breathing in which pauses in respiration last for as long as 20 seconds and alternate with breathing. Newborns of all gestational ages have periodic breathing that is a normal variant of respiration in the neonate. However, if the respiratory pause lasts more than 20 seconds, it is considered apnea and requires ongoing observation and may require treatment.

Due to the immaturity of the respiratory system, premature infants have an altered response to hypoxia and hypercapnia. In response to hypoxia, infants experience ventilatory depression that is a transient increase in respiratory rate followed by a decrease in spontaneous respirations below the infant's baseline respiratory rate. This pattern may recur over several weeks. Various neurotransmitters are involved in hypoxic ventilatory depression. In response to hypercapnia, premature infants have a decreased respiratory rate and prolonged exhalation unlike adults, who increase their respiratory rate when hypercapnic (Darnall, 2010). Hypercapnic ventilatory response is mediated primarily by central chemoreceptors.

The laryngeal chemoreflex is involved in the control of breathing. This reflex protects the lungs from aspiration. However, in the premature infant, an exaggerated response to stimulation of the laryngeal mucosa can lead to apnea, bradycardia, and hypotension. The passage of a feeding tube or vigorous suctioning of an infant are examples of stimulation that can trigger a bradycardic episode, followed by apnea. As infants mature, the laryngeal chemoreflex matures to respond more often by coughing and less often by apnea and swallowing (Thach, 2007). This laryngeal chemoreflex is mediated through superior laryngeal nerve afferents.

Although AOP is primarily attributed to physiologic immaturity, other factors may contribute. Functional residual capacity (the air left in the lung after an exhalation) is decreased because of pulmonary immaturity and increased chest wall compliance. This results in increased work of breathing for the infant, the development of diaphragmatic fatigue, and apnea. Apnea occurs more often during rapid eye movement (REM) sleep when infants have more paradoxical breathing than during quiet sleep. The mechanism of sucking, swallowing, breathing, and esophageal function is complex and requires physiologic maturity lacking in premature infants (Lau, 2015). Premature infants have difficulty coordinating this process with resultant apneic episodes during feeds.

Infants are traditionally obligate nose breathers. Irritation of the mucus membranes from a nasogastric tube and frequent suctioning of the nares contributes to swelling of the mucus membranes of the nasal passages with resultant obstruction of the nares. This, in turn, may cause apnea.

Clinical Aspects

ASSESSMENT

AOP may be idiopathic. However, it is also a symptom of multiple pathologic conditions in the infant, including infection, intraventricular hemorrhage, seizures, electrolyte imbalance, inborn errors of metabolism, congestive heart failure, patent ductus arteriosus, anemia, necrotizing enterocolitis, and temperature instability. The association between gastroesophageal reflux (GER) and AOP is controversial. Although there is a temporal relationship, cause and effect has not been established.

In premature infants, pathologic conditions may present concurrent with apnea, cyanosis or pallor, and hypotonia and this is called *secondary apnea*. It is critical that the evaluation of an infant occurs in a timely manner, whether an infant develops apnea or has increased apneic events.

In addition to the physical evaluation, it is important to read both the mother's and the infant's birth history to determine if there are any factors that predispose to apnea. A complete blood count (CBC) and C-reactive protein (CRP) assess for infection and anemia. A lumbar puncture may be necessary if the infant's history and current condition clinically indicate it. Electrolytes should be evaluated to assess for possible metabolic causes. A head ultrasound (HUS) may be needed to rule out intraventricular hemorrhage (IVH). A chest x-ray is done to assess respiratory and cardiac status.

NURSING INTERVENTIONS, MANAGEMENT, AND IMPLICATIONS

The nurse at the bedside is instrumental in the care of the infants with AOP. Cardiorespiratory and pulse oximetry monitors assist the nurse in monitoring apneic events. Documentation of apnea, bradycardia, and desaturation episodes is paramount. The nurse needs to document any event that occurs before the apnea; the length of the apnea; if the apnea is associated with bradycardia, including how low the heart rate falls; if a desaturation occurred, how low the desaturation fell, as well as how long the desaturation lasted; any change in color; what intervention the nurse performed; and the infant's response to that intervention. Infants usually respond to gentle stimulation if they become apneic. In the event that the infant does not respond to the stimulation, the nurse needs to initiate bag-and-mask ventilation.

Positioning of the infant is extremely important. The nurse must assess the infant's alignment and keep the head at midline without extension or flexion of the neck. Term and healthy preterm infants should be placed supine, but it is not known if preterm infants may benefit from prone or side-lying positions to help decreased apneic events (Bredemeyer & Foster, 2012).

Keeping premature infants in a neutral thermal environment is a basic tenet of neonatal nursing. Rapid changes in temperature have resulted in apneic events in infants (Gardner, Carter, Enzman Hines, & Hernández, 2016). Keeping an infant in the lower end of the neutral thermal environment, rather than the upper end, may help decrease the number of apneic events.

Respiratory support is commonly required. A number of noninvasive support measures, including high-flow nasal cannula, synchronized nasal intermittent positive-pressure ventilation (SNIPPV), nasal bi-level positive airway pressure (N-BiPAP), nasal continuous positive airway pressure (CPAP), and bubble CPAP may be required for an infant who does not respond to gentle stimulation or bag-and-mask ventilation. Sicker infants may require mechanical ventilation.

Medications are commonly used. Methylxanthines, such as caffeine citrate, aminophylline, and theophylline are pharmacologic treatment modalities for AOP. Caffeine citrate is preferred because it requires only daily dosing, has a longer half-life, and a wider therapeutic index. Nurses should give caffeine in the morning to prevent disruption of sleep–wake patterns. Nurses need to be cognizant of the side effects of caffeine citrate therapy, such as jitteriness, tachycardia, and feeding intolerance. Doxapram is another medication that has been used for the treatment of AOP for over four decades in Europe, but is not used in the premature infant population in the United States because it contains benzyl alcohol.

Anemia may play a role in AOP. Increase in apneic events may occur at the time the premature infant's hemoglobin has fallen to its physiologic nadir. Treatment for AOP with packed red blood cell transfusions is controversial. Blood transfusions are usually reserved for infants with severe anemia who are having multiple apneic events daily.

OUTCOMES

Nurses play a critical role in the prevention and treatment of AOP. The sophisticated monitoring equipment available today alerts nurses when an infant's status is changing, but medical device alarm safety is a major patient safety issue. The majority of the equipment used in the hospital has some type of alarm system. Because of the number of false alarms triggered, nurses, as well as all members of the health care team, have become sensory overloaded and desensitized. This is known as *alarm fatigue* (Sendelbach & Funk, 2013). As a result, health care team members may ignore, override, or turn off alarms (Tanner, 2013). Alarm fatigue has resulted in avoidable deaths. Most NICUs have set parameters for cardiorespiratory and pulse oximetry monitors. However, education needs to be ongoing to ensure safe patient care.

Summary

AOP is a common clinical problem and reflects physiologic immaturity. Current treatment modalities include xanthine therapy and noninvasive ventilator support. As infants mature, the number of apneic events and the interval between apneic events should be decreased in order to discharge the infant home safely. Parents need extensive education, including infant CPR. Close, accurate monitoring and documentation of all apneic events are an important component of infant care and the ultimate responsibility of the bedside nurse.

Bredemeyer, S., & Foster, J. (2012). Body positioning for spontaneously breathing preterm infants with apnoea. *Cochrane Database of Systematic Reviews, 2012*(6), Art. No.: CD004951. doi:10.1002/14651858.CD004951.pub2

Darnall, R. A. (2010). The role of CO_2 and central chemoreception in the control of breathing in the fetus and the neonate. *Respiratory Physiology and Neurobiology, 173*(3), 201–212. doi:10.1016/j.resp.2010.04.009

Eichenwald, E. C., & American Academy of Pediatrics Committee on Fetus and Newborn. (2016). Apnea of prematurity. *Pediatrics, 137*(1), e20153757. doi:10.1542/peds.2015-3757

Fairchild, K., Mohr, M., Paget-Brown, A., Tabacaru, C., Lake, D., Delos, J., ... Kattwinkel, J. (2016). Clinical associations of immature breathing in preterm infants: Part 1—Central apnea. *Pediatric Research, 80*(1), 21–27. doi:10.1038/pr.2016.43

Gardner, S., Carter, B., Enzman Hines, M., & Hernández, J. (2016). *Merenstein & Gardner's handbook of neonatal intensive care* (8th ed., pp. 647–673). St. Louis, MO: Elsevier.

Lau, C. (2015). Development of suck and swallow mechanisms in infants. *Annals of Nutrition and Metabolism, 66*(5), 7–14. doi:10.1159/000381361

Sendelbach, S., & Funk, M. (2013). Alarm fatigue: A patient safety concern. *AACN Advanced Critical Care, 24*(4), 378–386. doi:10.1097/NCI.0b013e3182a903f9

Tanner, T. (2013). The problem of alarm fatigue. *Nursing for Women's Health*, 17(2), 153–157. doi:10.1111/1751-486X.12043

Thach, B. (2007). Maturation of cough and other reflexes that protect the fetal and neonatal airway. *Pulmonary Pharmacology and Therapeutics*, 20(4), 365–370. doi:10.1016/j.pupt.2006.11.011

Zhao, J., Gonzalez, F., & Mu, D. (2011). Apnea of prematurity: From cause to treatment. *European Journal of Pediatrics*, 170(9), 1097–1105. doi:10.1007/s00431-011-1409-6

■ BRONCHOPULMONARY DYSPLASIA

Amy Bieda

Overview

Bronchopulmonary dysplasia (BPD) is a multifactorial disorder that evolves in infants born prematurely. These infants require some degree of mechanical ventilation and have an oxygen requirement because of respiratory distress (Davidson & Berkelhamer, 2017). Extremely premature infants are at the highest risk of developing BPD because it usually occurs at a pivotal stage of lung development. With the advent of postnatal corticosteroids, surfactant therapy, and improved ventilator management, the survival rate has increased, resulting in infants with this long-term morbidity. Infants with BPD may have prolonged hospitalizations and multiple hospital readmissions, especially during the first year of life. Approximately 10,000 to 15,000 infants are diagnosed yearly in the United States with a prevalence of males over females (Jensen & Schmidt, 2014).

Background

Northway, Rosan, and Porter (1967) first described BPD in a group of moderate to late premature infants who developed pulmonary changes on chest radiograph with respiratory failure related to long-term mechanical ventilation and prolonged exposure to high levels of oxygen. These changes included areas of atelectasis and marked scarring with hyperinflation, pulmonary fibrosis, and smooth muscle hypertrophy in the pulmonary vasculature. This description is referred to as "classic" BPD.

The introduction of surfactant therapy in the early 1990s, increased use of antenatal steroids, and improvements in ventilator technology changed the clinical presentation of BPD (Jensen & Schmidt, 2014) and a new pathophysiology emerged. In this group of infants, alveoli formation may stop or there may be a decrease in alveolar growth. Lung changes include less pulmonary fibrosis, inflammation, and smooth muscle hypertrophy with an increase in lung fluid and damage to vascular development. These changes are derived from an interruption in lung development rather than barotrauma and volutrauma from mechanical ventilation and was labeled the "new" BPD.

In 2001, the National Institute of Child Health and Human Development (NICHD) proposed a change in the definition of BPD in infants less than 32 weeks gestational age. This definition was based on the severity of lung disease and the need for supplemental oxygen at 28 days of life and/or method of ventilatory support at 36 weeks postmenstrual age. However, because of the wide practice variations in neonatal intensive care units (NICUs) and the spectrum of the severity of this disease, the new definition has limitation (Davidson & Berkelhamer, 2017).

Antenatal risk factors, such as chorioramnionitis, lack of antenatal steroids, and fetal growth restriction have been implicated as prenatal risks for the development of BPD. The risk factor of chorioramnionitis is controversial because of its complex nature. Empirical research suggests that inflammation increases surfactant production and promotes lung maturation (Davidson & Berkelhamer, 2017), whereas animal models suggest lung injury. There are multiple confounders making it difficult to determine a causal relationship.

Antenatal steroids are a primary prophylactic treatment of women who are in preterm labor (American College of Obstetricians and Gynecologists, 2011) and their use has contributed to decreased respiratory distress syndrome (RDS) and morbidities common in premature infants. Although antenatal steroids stimulate lung maturation in the fetus, they have not decreased the rate of BPD.

Low birth weight is a robust predictor of BPD especially in infants less than 28 weeks gestational age. Increased rates of BPD and aberrant pulmonary outcomes have also been demonstrated in preterm infants who are small for gestation age (SGA) or have intrauterine growth restriction (IUGR) at delivery (Poindexter & Martin, 2015).

Clinical Aspects

ASSESSMENT

Infants born extremely premature are in the canalicular stage of lung growth and mechanical ventilation interferes with normal lung development. Mechanical ventilation can contribute to volutrauma (increased lung volume or lung stretching) and barotrauma (excessive ventilator pressures) resulting in lung overdistention. As a result, there is a cycle of continuous injury to the lung with healing and rehealing (Gardner, Hines, & Nyp, 2016).

In addition, very sick infants may be exposed to high levels of supplemental oxygen therapy for prolonged periods of time. Hyperoxia causes acute pulmonary injury to the developing lung resulting in inflammation, pulmonary edema, and thickening of the alveolar membrane. In addition to hyperoxia, preterm infants lack antioxidant mediators contributing to cytotoxic oxygen free radical production resulting in oxidative stress and further lung injury (Glen & Kinsella, 2011).

Infants with a patent ductus arteriosis (PDA) and persistent left to right (systemic to pulmonary) shunting of blood may have increased pulmonary circulation resulting in increased interstitial fluid. Increased interstitial fluid results in impaired pulmonary function and prolongs the need for mechanical ventilation as well as increases the need for supplemental oxygen, which contribute to the pathology of BPD (Glen & Kinsella, 2011). Infants with severe BPD may also develop pulmonary hypertension and cor pulmonale (right-sided heart failure).

An increased incidence of BPD has also been associated in infants with RDS who receive large volumes of fluid in the first few days of life. In a Cochrane review (Bell & Acarregui, 2014), careful regulation of fluid intake in premature infants may reduce the risk of BPD.

BPD in premature infants has been associated with postnatal nosocomial infection. Gram positive and gram negative bacteria, cytomegalovirus (CMV), and adenovirus have been shown to increase the systemic inflammatory response in the lungs resulting in the production and release of proinflammatory cytokines. Prolonged antibiotic use especially during the first week of life has also been implicated (Novitsky et al., 2015).

NURSING INTERVENTIONS, MANAGEMENT, AND IMPLICATIONS

In addition to surfactant therapy, which decreases the duration of mechanical ventilation and reduces the incidence of BPD, multiple modes of noninvasive respiratory modalities that do not require intubation/mechanical ventilation are available. Often infants are given surfactant via the endotracheal tube and then extubated to continuous positive airway pressure (CPAP), high-flow nasal cannula (HFNC), bi-level positive airway pressure (BiPAP), or nasal intermittent positive pressure ventilation (NIPPV). Permissive hypercapnia is a strategy that may reduce the risk of lung injury by accepting higher values of $PaCO_2$ while using lower tidal volumes and inspiratory pressures. This is to evade pulmonary overdistention.

Corticosteroids such as dexamethasone, which reduce lung inflammation and improve gas exchange, may judiciously be used in the treatment of infants. Corticosteroids facilitate weaning and extubation from mechanical ventilation but the medication has side effects, including hyperglycemia, hypertension, infection, and gastrointestinal bleeding especially if given in the immediate postnatal period. Longitudinal studies have established that corticosteroids contribute to smaller head growth and abnormal neurological outcomes including cerebral palsy (CP; Khetan, Hurley, Spencer, & Bhatt, 2016). The type of corticosteroid, dose, and timing of initiation of therapy have not been determined (Onland, De Jaegere, Offringa, & van Kaam, 2017).

Other pharmacologic agents can be used in the treatment of BPD. Intravenous (IV) caffeine, if started in the first 3 days of life, helps in decreasing the incidence of BPD. Diuretics, such as furosemide (IV and oral), are loop diuretics used to treat the interstitial alveolar edema that is commonly seen. Thiazides, such as chlorothiazide and spironolactone, are also used. There is less electrolyte imbalance with the use of thiazides, which may decrease the need for furosemide.

Bronchodilators, such as albuterol and ipratropium bromide, can also be used to reduce reactive airway disease and help increase lung compliance. Premature infants at birth have low body stores of vitamin A, an antioxidant that is important in surfactant synthesis and the repair of lung epithelial cells. The administration of vitamin A starting after delivery may be useful in reducing oxygen use at 36 weeks postmenstrual age.

A PDA is usually treated either by surgical ligation, coil occlusion performed in a cardiac catheterization laboratory, or medically with either IV indomethacin or IV ibuprofen. All treatment modalities have associated risks. Current controversy exists whether to treat a PDA as the majority of them close spontaneously.

Many centers are using a more cautious approach that includes clinical assessment of the infant, fluid restriction, and diuretic therapy.

Nutrition is an integral component in the management of premature infants. Postnatal growth is slower in infants with BPD and many have failure to thrive. These infants have high energy expenditure coupled with poor caloric intake, feeding difficulties (including oral aversion), and complications of respiratory disease, and may be fluid restricted on diuretic therapy resulting in poor linear growth and inadequate weight gain. Early enteral nutrition and increased protein in calorie dense formula or fortified maternal breast milk are of prime importance in improving lung growth, lung repair, decreasing the risk and severity of BPD, and improving neurologic outcomes (Poindexter & Martin, 2015).

Caring for the infant with BPD requires a strong interdisciplinary team of neonatologists, pulmonologists, nurses, nutritionists, physical therapists, occupational therapists, social workers, and child life specialists. Nurses must have in-depth knowledge of the pathophysiology of BPD, arterial and capillary blood gases, medications, oxygen therapy, ventilator management, nutrition, and growth and development.

This group of infants can be challenging to care for and should have a dedicated core of nurses who understand not only the infants' physiologic status and recognition of any changes from baseline, but must also understand the infants' nuances in behavior and responses to treatment.

Parental education is an ongoing process because these infants can be in the hospital for an extended period of time. Nurses must not only promote parent–infant bonding, but also help parents engage in socialization, language development, and emotional support of their infants.

Summary

BPD is a chronic condition that affects primarily premature infants. Current treatment modalities, such as noninvasive respiratory support, gentle ventilation, pharmacologic agents, and optimal nutrition are imperative. However, the prevention of BPD is challenging and at the core of this is preventing premature birth.

American College of Obstetricians and Gynecologists Committee on Obstetric Practice. (2011). Opinion No. 475: Antenatal corticosteroid therapy for fetal maturation. *Obstetrics and Gynecology, 117*(2, Pt. 1), 422–424. doi:10.1097/AOG.0b013e31820eee00

Bell, E., & Acarregui, M. (2014). Restricted versus liberal water intake for preventing morbidity and mortality in preterm infants. *Cochrane Database of Systematic Reviews, 2014,* 1–26. doi:10.1002/14651858.CD000503.pub3

Davidson, L., & Berkelhamer, S. (2017). Bronchopulmonary dysplasia: Chronic lung disease of infancy and long-term pulmonary outcomes. *Journal of Clinical Medicine, 6*(1), 4. doi:10.3390/jcm6010004

Gardner, S., Hines, M., & Nyp, M. (2016). Respiratory diseases. In S. Gardner, B. Carter, M. Hines, & J. Hernández (Eds.), *Merenstein and Gardner's handbook of neonatal intensive care* (8th ed., pp. 565–643). St. Louis, MO: Elsevier.

Gien, J., & Kinsella, J. P. (2011). Pathogenesis and treatment of bronchopulmonary dysplasia. *Current Opinion in Pediatrics, 23*(3), 305–313. doi:10.1097/MOP.0b013e328346577f

Jensen, E. A., & Schmidt, B. (2014). Epidemiology of bronchopulmonary dysplasia. *Birth Defects Research. Part A, Clinical and Molecular Teratology, 100*(3), 145–157. doi:10.1002/bdra.23235

Khetan, R., Hurley, M., Spencer, S., & Bhatt, J. M. (2016). Bronchopulmonary dysplasia within and beyond the neonatal unit. *Advances in Neonatal Care, 16*(1), 17–25; quiz E1. doi:10.1097/ANC.0000000000000251

Northway, W. H., Rosan, R. C., & Porter, D. Y. (1967). Pulmonary disease following respirator therapy of hyaline-membrane disease—Bronchopulmonary dysplasia. *The New England Journal of Medicine, 276*(7), 357–368. doi:10.1056/NEJM196702162760701

Novitsky, A., Tuttle, D., Locke, R. G., Saiman, L., Mackley, A., & Paul, D. A. (2015). Prolonged early antibiotic use and bronchopulmonary dysplasia in very low birth weight infants. *American Journal of Perinatology, 32*(1), 43–48. doi:10.1055/s-0034-1373844

Onland, W., De Jaegere, A. P. M. C., Offringa, M., & van Kaam, A. (2017). Systemic corticosteroid regimens for prevention of bronchopulmonary dysplasia in preterm infants. *The Cochrane Database of Systematic Reviews, 2017*(1), CD010941. doi:10.1002/14651858.CD010941.pub2

Poindexter, B. B., & Martin, C. R. (2015). Impact of nutrition on bronchopulmonary dysplasia. *Clinics in Perinatology, 42*(4), 797–806. doi:10.1016/j.clp.2015.08.007

■ DECREASED PULMONARY BLOOD FLOW

Jennifer Johntony
Jodi Zalewski

Overview

Decreased pulmonary blood flow results from the shunting of deoxygenated blood from the right side of the heart to the oxygenated left side of the heart (Nelson, Hirsch-Romano, Ohye, & Bove, 2015). Infants born with heart defects that cause a decrease in pulmonary blood flow present with cyanosis and hypoxemia because of a lack of blood flow to the lungs. The systolic and diastolic pressures on the right side of the heart exceed those on the left because of some form of obstruction to pulmonary blood flow, leading to this right-to-left shunting. Congenital heart defects (CHDs) that result in decreased pulmonary blood include tetralogy of Fallot (TOF), pulmonary atresia, tricuspid atresia, and pulmonary stenosis.

Background

TOF accounts for approximately 4% of CHDs (Nelson et al., 2015). The classic description of TOF includes (a) the presence of a ventricular septal defect (VSD), (b) some form of right ventricular outflow track obstruction, (c) overriding of the aorta, and (d) right ventricular hypertrophy (Hockenberry & Wilson, 2015). The degree of cyanosis is often determined by the severity of the right ventricular outflow tract obstruction. The obstruction to the right ventricular outflow tract in TOF patients can start below the pulmonary valve and extend all the way out to the branches of the pulmonary arteries. If the obstruction is severe and degree of cyanosis is significant in the neonatal period, a palliative or temporizing procedure is often performed to increase oxygen saturation and therefore increase pulmonary blood flow (Hockenberry & Wilson, 2015). Complete repairs are generally performed in the first year of life. The operative mortality for total correction of TOF is less than 3% (Hockenberry & Wilson, 2015).

Pulmonary atresia is a relatively rare defect and accounts for approximately 1% of all congenital heart lesions (Park, 2016). In this disorder, the pulmonary valve is absent or atretic and the intraventricular septum can be either intact, or accompanied by a VSD. This particular anatomy, where the intraventricular septum is intact, leads to an absence of blood exiting the right ventricle into the main pulmonary artery (Nelson et al., 2015). Patients born with this disorder must have an interatrial communication (either atrial septal defect or patent foramen ovale) or the presence of a patent ductus arteriosus (PDA) to allow for adequate pulmonary blood flow and cardiac output after birth. To maintain patency of the ductus arteriosus, intravenous prostaglandin E1 (PGE1) is administered (Park, 2016). The size of the right ventricle and pulmonary arteries determines the type and success of surgical repair. If the size of the right ventricle and pulmonary arteries is adequate, a two-ventricular repair can be performed. If the size or function of the right ventricle is inadequate, a single ventricle palliative approach may be necessary (Nelson et al., 2015). The survival rate of pulmonary atresia varies and is determined by a biventricular repair, single ventricle palliation, or cardiac transplantation.

Tricuspid atresia accounts for 1% to 3% of all CHDs (Park, 2016). Tricuspid atresia, a complete lack of a tricuspid valve, results in the absence of direct communication between the right atrium and right ventricle (Nelson et al., 2015). Pulmonary blood flow is achieved when deoxygenated blood flows or shunts across an atrial septal defect from the right atrium to the left atrium, then to the left ventricle, through a VSD and out to the lungs (Hockenberry & Wilson, 2015). The complete mixing of oxygenated and unoxygenated blood in the left atrium results in systemic desaturations and hypoxemia (Hockenberry & Wilson, 2015). This particular lesion is treated in three stages. The first-stage palliation for the majority of patients occurs in the newborn period and is the placement of a systemic to pulmonary artery shunt (modified Blalock–Taussig shunt) to maintain adequate pulmonary blood flow. The second procedure, referred to as the *Glenn procedure*, connects the superior vena cava directly to the pulmonary artery. In the third procedure, the Fontan, a direct connection between the inferior vena cava and pulmonary artery is created, thus completing the full separation of oxygenated and deoxygenated blood. All blood flow to the lungs is now passive and the single ventricle is solely responsible for pumping oxygenated blood to the body. The overall survival for tricuspid atresia is approximately 83% at 1 year, 70% at 10 years, and 60% at 20 years (Nelson et al., 2015).

Isolated pulmonary stenosis accounts for 10% of all CHDs and is defined as a thickening of the pulmonary valve at the entrance of the main pulmonary artery (Jone, Darst, Collins, & Miyamoto, 2016). This thickened pulmonary valve leads to variable levels of obstruction to pulmonary blood flow resulting in an increase in the right ventricular pressure that can be potentially life threatening (Jone et al., 2016). Neonates with severe pulmonary valve obstruction and minimal pulmonary blood flow present with cyanosis at birth (Jone et al., 2016). To minimize the patient's degree of cyanosis, the patency of the ductus arteriosus must be established with prostaglandins. Then the decision to treat the patient with either a balloon angioplasty of the pulmonary valve or surgical treatment with the placement of a modified Blalock–Taussig shunt is made. Long-term outcomes after balloon valvuloplasty are favorable; however, restenosis or valve incompetence may occur later in life (Hockenberry & Wilson, 2015).

Clinical Aspects

ASSESSMENT

Patients born with TOF can either present with cyanosis at birth, or develop it over time as the subvalvular obstruction increases (Jone et al., 2016). The patient's physical examination is positive for a grade II to IV/VI systolic ejection murmur that is heard best at the left sternal border in the third intercostal space and radiates to the lungs. Extreme cyanosis or hypoxic episodes occur causing severe "blue spells" or "tet spells." Hypercyanotic spells are defined as a sudden onset of cyanosis or deepening of cyanosis. Infants have dyspnea, alterations in consciousness, from irritability to syncope with a decrease or disappearance of the systolic murmur (Jone et al., 2016).

Infants with pulmonary atresia present with cyanosis at birth and as the ductus arteriosus closes, they will become more cyanotic (Jone et al., 2016). These patients have a continuous murmur because of the PDA (Park, 2016). To maintain pulmonary blood flow, patency of the ductus must be achieved with infusion of prostaglandins until surgery can be performed (Jone et al., 2016).

Infants with tricuspid atresia usually present with cyanosis at birth as well as tachycardia, tachypnea, and increased work of breathing (Hockenberry & Wilson, 2015). If there is a significant increase in pulmonary blood flow, they may develop symptoms of congestive heart failure, such as sweating, tachypnea, poor oral intake and increased time to orally feed, resulting in poor weight gain (Jone et al., 2016). A grade III/VI systolic murmur from the VSD is often heard at the lower left sternal border (Park, 2016).

Patients with pulmonary stenosis have variable presentations. Those with mild pulmonary stenosis are usually asymptomatic. Infants with severe pulmonary stenosis present often with hypoxic spells, failure to thrive, and right-heart failure (Nelson et al., 2015). The murmur of valvular pulmonary stenosis is an ejection click heard best at the upper left sternal border. A low-pitched murmur indicates less severe pulmonary stenosis (Park, 2016). Those patients may be followed symptomatically with mild to moderate pulmonary stenosis. Catheter-based intervention or surgical intervention should be considered for a gradient higher than 50 mmHg, progressive ventricular hypertrophy, or new tricuspid regurgitation.

NURSING INTERVENTIONS, MANAGEMENT, AND IMPLICATIONS

Nursing-related issues for infants with decreased pulmonary blood flow can vary depending on the lesion. These infants can experience cyanosis, dyspnea, tachycardia, irritability, and feeding difficulties.

It is important to become informed about the infant's cardiac anatomy and baseline clinical presentation in order to intervene when changes occur. The nurse should assess and record heart rate, respiratory rate, breath sounds, blood pressure, and pulse oximetry readings. Oxygen administration and nasopharyngeal suctioning may be required to maintain appropriate pulse oximetry and reduce respiratory distress. Any prescribed cardiac medications need to be given at the scheduled time and monitored for any side effects or signs and symptoms of toxicity, which should be reported and documented (Hockenberry & Wilson, 2016).

The nurse can decrease cardiac demands by minimizing unnecessary stress and stimulation. Nursing interventions must focus on providing maximum rest and comfort care such as offering nonnutritive sucking and swaddling. In order to promote energy conservation, nursing must organize activities that allow for uninterrupted sleep (Hockenberry & Wilson, 2016). In order to provide adequate nutrition, infants should be fed in a semi-upright position and be offered small, frequent feedings.

Cyanotic infants must be well hydrated in order to maintain good cardiac output and to minimize their risk for cerebral vascular accidents because of polycythemia (Hockenberry & Wilson, 2016). Infants with decreased pulmonary blood flow are at risk for hypercyanotic spells, which occur suddenly and are typically observed in the setting of extreme agitation or painful stimulation. The interventions to reverse hypercyanotic spells center around promoting an increase in pulmonary blood flow and include the following: place infant in a knee–chest position, calm the infant with comfort measures, administer 100% oxygen, give intravenous morphine, begin fluid replacement and volume expansion (Hockenberry & Wilson, 2016).

In any patient born with a cardiac defect, alteration in parenting related to the perception of the infant as vulnerable may be present. These families experience periods of shock, followed by tremendous anxiety and oftentimes fear that their child may die (Hockenberry & Wilson, 2016). Nurses are instrumental in dealing with parental stress; providing support and education; and participating as an interdisciplinary team member in order to care for both the infants and their families.

OUTCOMES

Patients with congenital heart disease have outcomes specific to evidence-based nursing practice that focus on assisting the patient to demonstrate an improvement in cardiac function, a decrease in cardiac demands, and optimal blood flow to the lungs (Hockenberry & Wilson, 2016). Improvement in cardiac function occurs when there is a decrease in the afterload of the heart, thereby increasing the overall cardiac output.

Summary

Infants born with TOF, pulmonary atresia, tricuspid atresia, and pulmonary stenosis are at increased risk for decreased pulmonary blood flow because of an interruption of blood flow leaving the right side of the heart and entering the lungs. They may experience cyanosis, feeding issues, and inadequate weight gain. Many of these infants undergo palliative or corrective surgery within the first few weeks of life. Understanding each specific patient's cardiac anatomy is imperative to caring for the infant effectively. Providing efficient and holistic nursing care to hospitalized infants with congenital heart disease results in increased survival and quality of life in this vulnerable patient population.

Hockenberry, M., & Wilson, D. (2015). *Wong's nursing care of infants and children* (10th ed.). St. Louis, MO: Elsevier Mosby.

Jone, P.-N., Darst, J. R., Collins, K. K., & Miyamoto, S. D. (2016). Cardiovascular diseases. In W. W. Hay Jr., M. J. Levin, R. R. Deterding, & M. J. Abzug (Eds.), *Current diagnosis & treatment pediatrics* (23rd ed., pp. 550–610). New York, NY: McGraw-Hill. Retrieved from http://accessmedicine.mhmedical.com/content.aspx?bookid=1795&Sectionid=125741666

Nelson, J. S., Hirsch-Romano, J. C., Ohye, R. G., & Bove, E. L. (2015). Congenital heart disease. In G. M. Doherty (Ed.), *Current diagnosis & treatment: Surgery* (14th ed., pp. 423–454). New York, NY: McGraw-Hill.

Park, M. (2016). *The pediatric cardiology handbook* (5th ed.). Philadelphia, PA: Elsevier Saunders.

■ EXTREMELY LOW-BIRTH-WEIGHT INFANT

Jenelle M. Zambrano

Overview

Extremely low-birth-weight (ELBW) infants are defined as infants weighing less than 1,000 g at birth (Mandy, 2016; Sherman, 2014). In 2013, 8% of the approximate 550,000 preterm infants born in the United States were low-birth-weight infants (Mandy, 2016). Less than 1% of the low-birth-weight infant population consists of ELBW infants (Mandy, 2016; Morris, 2015). Although ELBW infants account for a small percentage of overall births, they are generally the most critically ill and at the highest risk for death and disability (Glass et al., 2015; Sherman, 2014). Care of the ELBW infant is complex and requires understanding the ELBW subgroups and the pathophysiologic processes associated with each subgroup (Papageorgiou & Pelausa, 2014). Care for these infants requires expert management beginning in the delivery room and continuing in the neonatal intensive care unit (NICU). Careful consideration is necessary when providing respiratory, thermoregulatory, and nutritional support, and neuroprotective care (Morris, 2015; Sherman, 2014).

Background

Prematurity, defined as birth before 37 weeks of gestation, is a significant contributor to infant and child morbidity and mortality and is associated with one third of all infant deaths in the United States (Glass et al., 2015). The rate of premature births in the United States had been on a steady rise during the 1990s and early 2000s, but had begun to decrease annually in the early 2010s. However, in 2015, the U.S. premature birth rate increased for the first time in 8 years from 9.57% to 9.63% (March of Dimes, 2016). Major risk factors for preterm births include multiple births (e.g., twins or triplets), history of preterm delivery, stress, infection, smoking and/or illicit drug use, and extremes in maternal age (e.g., mothers younger than 16 years old, mothers older than 35 years old; Mandy, 2016; Morris, 2015).

Of the 450,000 to 500,000 preterm births in the United States each year, fewer than 1% of these infants are ELBW (Mandy, 2016; Morris, 2015). ELBW infants can be classified into two subgroups: The first ELBW group consists of extremely premature infants who are appropriate for gestational age, and the second ELWB group consists of intrauterine growth–restricted infants who are small for gestational age, but not necessarily very premature (i.e., less than 27 weeks gestational age; Papageorgiou & Pelausa, 2014). Understanding the differences between these two subgroups is essential as the different pathophysiologic processes associated with each group may yield different responses and outcomes to the care provided.

Although perinatal care, technology, and understanding of the pathophysiology and needs of the ELBW infant have improved, ELBW infants remain at high risk for death with 30% to 50% mortality and high risk for severe impairment with 20% to 50% long-term morbidity in survivors (Glass, 2015; Papageorgiou & Pelausa, 2014; Sherman, 2014). The risk of death increases with decreasing birth weight and gestational age, and both are associated with increasing immaturity. The infant mortality rates per 1,000 live births in the United States in 2013 were 124.6 for infants weighing 750 to 999 g, 394.3 for those weighing 500 to 749 g, and 853 for those weighing less than 500 g (Mandy, 2016). Risk factors for death and severe neurodevelopmental impairment in ELBW infants are bronchopulmonary dysplasia (BPD), brain injury, severe retinopathy of prematurity (ROP), infection, and cardiopulmonary resuscitation (CPR) in the delivery room. ELBW infants who received CPR in the delivery room were more critical with higher pneumothorax, grade III and IV intraventricular hemorrhage (IVH), and BPD rates compared to those who did not receive CPR (Mandy, 2016). Therefore, successful management of the ELBW infant must begin in the delivery room.

Clinical Aspects

ASSESSMENT

A standardized, team approach, ideally consisting of an experienced neonatologist, nursing, respiratory, and social worker in a level III facility, is essential for the proper management and care of the ELBW infant (Morris, 2015; Papageorgiou & Pelausa, 2014). This team approach should begin from the prenatal consultation and continue in the delivery room management of the ELBW infant and care in the NICU. Prenatal consultation should involve similar information, incorporating both national and hospital outcomes, open and honesty dialogue, and understanding of family expectations in order to be supportive of the family's decisions, regardless of the members who constitute the team conducting the consultation (Morris, 2015; Sherman, 2014).

NURSING INTERVENTIONS, MANAGEMENT, AND IMPLICATIONS

In the management of the ELBW infant in the delivery room and in the NICU, it is important to be aware of the in utero environment from which the infant came and would have stayed in had the infant not been born prematurely. The infant's environment changes from a warm, fluid-filled, quiet, dark environment where movements are slow and supported to one that is bright, loud, invasive, exposed, and full of stimulation where the infant's movement is no longer supported (Morris, 2015). The initial stages of care during the first few hours after birth determine the outcome of the ELBW infant. Umbilical cord clamping should be delayed 30 to 60 seconds after birth with the infant at a level below the placenta. Delayed cord clamping has been shown to improve transitional circulation, establish better red blood cell volume, reducing the need for blood transfusion as well as potentially reducing the risk of an IVH by 50% (Sherman, 2014).

A majority of ELBW infants require resuscitation. The goal of delivery resuscitation is to efficiently deliver the least amount of intervention needed to support normal gas exchange and decrease the potential for lung injury. Current practice recommendations for administering supplemental oxygen to the ELBW infant include basing administration on objective preductal oxygen saturation monitoring, using blended oxygen, and administering positive pressure for persistent cyanosis (Sherman, 2014). If positive pressure ventilation is necessary, low inspiratory pressure should be provided to avoid overinflation of the lungs and potential lung injury. Debate over the administration of surfactant in the first few minutes of an ELBW infant's life is still ongoing. In the NICU, most ELBW infants require respiratory assistance, ranging from nasal continuous positive airway pressure (CPAP) to intubation, to survive. Progressive weaning protocols that provide respiratory assistance on low peak inspiratory pressures and rates are thought to be more efficacious and help with nutrition advancement.

Thermoregulation is another important aspect in ELBW infant care. Owing to their structurally and functionally immature skin and large body surface area, these infants lose heat quickly and are prone to cold stress, which can affect glucose, oxygenation, and acid–base balance. Neonatal Resuscitation Program recommendations include increasing delivery room temperature to 77°F to 80°F, preheating the radiant warmer, using a polyethylene bag without first drying the skin, and using a portable warming mattress (Morris, 2015). In the NICU, ambient humidity of 70% or higher for ELBW infants is recommended to decrease transepidermal water loss and heat loss. The fragility of the skin places the ELBW infants at risk for experiencing skin shearing and denuding and increases their risk of infection. Therefore, skin integrity preservation must be incorporated into their daily care and must include frequent skin condition assessments and repositioning of the infants a minimum of every 4 hours.

Nutritionally, ELBW infants have limited reserves, immature nutrient absorption and metabolic pathways, and have higher nutrient needs, which can cause them to rapidly enter into a catabolic state (Papageorgiou & Pelausa, 2014; Sherman, 2014). Introducing parenteral nutrition early as soon as these infants are stabilized prevents them from experiencing metabolic shock. In addition, early trophic feeds using colostrum, then breast milk, or donor milk and standardized feeding guidelines are recommended to improve feeding tolerance, stimulate gut motility and maturity, shorten the time to full feeds, and decrease length of stay (Morris, 2015).

OUTCOMES

Because ELBW infants are at increased risk for developing severe cognitive and motor impairments, modifications to the NICU environment are necessary to limit exposure to negative stimuli. Strategies to promote a neuroprotective environment include decreasing ambient light and noise, clustering care and minimal handling to allow for periods of uninterrupted sleep, and using positioning aids for containment (Sherman, 2014). These considerations, along with the respiratory, thermoregulatory, and nutritional considerations constitute the care necessary to successfully manage the ELBW infant.

Summary

ELBW infants are generally the sickest infants with the highest rates of mortality and morbidity than other infants. Care of the ELBW infant is complex and requires an expert team approach from the beginning at delivery. The goal of resuscitation is to efficiently deliver the least amount of intervention needed to support normal gas exchange and reduce the potential for lung injury. Strategies to promote respiratory, thermoregulatory, nutritional, and neuroprotective support must be consistently practiced to ensure comprehensive care of the ELBW infant and to improve his or her chances of survival.

Glass, H. C., Costarino, A. T., Stayer, S. A., Brett, C. M., Cladis, F., & Davis, P. J. (2015). Outcomes for extremely premature infants. *Anesthesia and Analgesia, 120*(6), 1337–1351. doi:10.1213/ANE.0000000000000705

Mandy, G. T. (2016). Incidence and mortality of the preterm infant. In M. S. Kim (Ed.), *UpToDate*. Retrieved from https://www.uptodate.com/contents/incidence-and-mortality-of-the-preterm-infant

March of Dimes. (2016). Preterm birth increases in the U.S. for the first time in eight years: 2016 March of Dimes premature birth report card reveals underlying geographic, racial/ethnic disparities. Retrieved from http://www.marchofdimes.org/news/preterm-birth-increases-in-the-us-for-the-first-time-in-eight-years.aspx

Morris, M. (2015). Care of the extremely low birth weight infant [PowerPoint slides]. Retrieved from https://www.anymeeting.com/WebConference/RecordingDefault.aspx?c_psrid=E950DF86884E31https://www.anymeeting.com/WebConference/RecordingDefault.aspx?c_psrid=E950DF86884E31

Papageorgiou, A., & Pelausa, E. (2014). Management and outcome of extremely low birth weight infants. *Journal of Pediatric and Neonatal Individualized Medicine, 3*(2), 1–6. doi:10.7363/030209

Sherman, J. (2014). Care of the extremely low birth weight (ELBW) infant. In M. T. Verklan & M. Walden (Eds.), *Core curriculum for neonatal intensive care nursing* (5th ed., pp. 427–438). St. Louis, MO: Elsevier Saunders.

■ GASTROESOPHAGEAL REFLUX

Suzanne Rubin

Overview

Gastroesophageal reflux (GER) refers to uncomplicated, recurrent spitting and vomiting in healthy infants that resolves without intervention. It is considered physiologic and usually resolves before 12 months of life. GER occurs commonly in healthy infants and is a frequent area of discussion with pediatricians, especially during the first several months of life. Symptoms include frequent non-bilious "spit up" after feedings that does not seem to cause problems. Weight gain, attainment of developmental milestones, and general contentment are noted. Clinical interventions for parents at this stage involve education and reassurance that resolution is likely by 12 months of life. Gastroesophageal reflux disease (GERD) is a more complicated, pathological form of reflux that causes alarming symptoms or leads to medical complications and may occur at any age. The esophageal manifestations of GERD can include heartburn, frequent regurgitation, and mucosal injury of the esophagus.

Background

Historical literature search shows a relative lack of reference to this disease process before the mid-19th century. Most likely this represents a lack of anatomical understanding of the disease process and identification. How and where the reflux condition initiated was not well understood before the invention of the rigid endoscopy and the first barium upper gastrointestinal radiologic studies in the 1960s (Modlin, Kidd, & Lye, 2003). At this time, major access to the esophageal lumen was developed and the understanding of anatomy and physiology began. Following use of this procedure, the development of pressure manometers and pH probes helped to document the relationship of acid secretion as well as esophageal–gastric structure, physiology, and pathology. Understanding normal maturational changes in the infants' stomach and esophagus contributed to a better understanding of these processes. The association of infants with colic, feeding disorders, and regurgitation followed. Increasing awareness has permitted the development of additional diagnostic studies and treatment. GER is common in infants and usually is not pathological (Martin & Hibbs, 2016).

Clinical Aspects

GER is common in infants with regurgitation present in 50% to 70% of all infants, peaking at age 4 to 6 months, and typically resolving by 1 year. A small minority of infants with GER develop other symptoms suggestive of GERD, including irritability, feeding refusal, hematemesis, anemia, respiratory symptoms, and failure to thrive (Martin & Hibbs, 2016).

ASSESSMENT

Premature infants are at increased risk when compared to full-term infants for GER because of immaturity of feeding skills as well as immature or impaired anatomic and physiologic factors that limit reflux (e.g., transient relaxation of the lower esophageal sphincter). GER is more common in healthy preterm infants where gastric fluids reflux into the esophagus as often as 30 or more times daily (Martin & Hibbs, 2016). Nursing assessment includes close monitoring of growth parameters, feeding and vomiting history, history of irritability, and other findings that may be related to pathologic reflux.

Older children may also experience GER, with symptoms described similar to adults. They may complain of heartburn, swallowing difficulty, or regurgitation into the oral cavity. Some syndromes have increased incidence of the disease because of anatomical differences, such as asthma, cystic fibrosis, hiatal hernia, developmental delays, or prior chest surgery. Weakened chest muscles or increased frequency of coughing can increase intraabdominal pressure in the stomach, causing movement of stomach acids to the esophagus.

NURSING INTERVENTIONS, MANAGEMENT, AND IMPLICATIONS

Pediatric GER clinical guidelines for management of pediatric GER in clinical practice were published by the North American Society for Pediatric Gastroenterology, Hepatology, and Nutrition (NASPGHAN) and the European Society for Pediatric Gastroenterology, Hepatology, and Nutrition (ESPGHAN). These guidelines were adopted in 2009 by the American Academy of Pediatrics (AAP). Evidence-based progressive interventions start with a complete history and physical by the infant or child's primary pediatrician. If clinical findings include persistent vomiting/regurgitation and poor weight gain, further investigation may include calorie and diet counseling. When GER is accompanied by increasing symptoms, the consideration of thickened formula, allergen elimination diet (including mothers who breastfeed for most common offenders such as milk and eggs) may be an effective strategy to address GER in many patients. In particular, the AAP adopted guidelines emphasizing that milk protein allergy can cause a clinical presentation that mimics GERD in infants. Therefore, a 2- to 4-week trial of a maternal exclusion diet that restricts at least milk and egg is recommended in breastfeeding infants with GERD symptoms, whereas an extensively hydrolyzed protein or amino acid–based formula may be appropriate in formula-fed infants (Neu, Corwin, Lareau, & Marcheggiani-Howard, 2012).

Teaching families about the resolution of uncomplicated disease, possible etiology, and home interventions for GER can enhance adherence to recommended infant care. Because parents note different signs associated with reflux (fussiness, irritability, spitting up, arching of back), it may be difficult to know whether symptoms are caused by reflux or another discomfort such as gas or pain. Although many published reviews are available, there is lack of agreement in the scientific community as to the best intervention for infants. Symptoms most frequently monitored include irritability and spitting up of feeds.

Specific interventions may vary from infant to infant. Combination interventions may be nonpharmacologic or pharmacologic. Activities aimed at soothing the infants include patting, touching, holding, massaging, or placing them in an infant swing. Feeding modifications such as thickened formulas, hydrolyzed formulas, elimination diet in breastfeeding mothers, upright positioning after feeding, or small frequent feedings may be initiated. Tobacco-smoke elimination from home may be helpful. At this time, meta-analysis of all interventions does not show an advantage in one single intervention. It appears that the passage of time was the only consistent factor reducing irritability and spitting up, usually after 6 months of life (Neu et al., 2012). More research is needed in addition to anticipatory guidance for families of infants with GER and GERD.

When dietary management does not improve symptoms, consultation with a pediatric gastroenterologist may be required. Failure of caloric management should initiate complete blood count, urinalysis, and celiac disease screening (if infant older than 6 months). If any diagnostic findings are positive, management of these disease states is recommended.

Pharmacologic support, including buffering agents, oral acid suppression therapy, or prokinetics can be trialed for effectiveness. Increasing severity may result in hospitalization for intensive feeding therapy or nasogastric (NG)/nasojejunal (NJ) feedings.

Pharmacological therapy involves two major classes of pharmacologic agents. These include acid suppressants and prokinetic agents. Acid suppressants include antacids, histamine-2 receptor antagonists (H2-blockers), and proton pump inhibitors (PPIs). The goal is to increase the pH of stomach secretions and reduce chemical trauma to esophageal mucosa. Prokinetic agents strengthen the lower esophageal sphincter and aid in the stomach content emptying faster. These agents seems to be effective for longer episodes of reflux.

Antacids do not have a strong record of efficacy of relieving symptoms of GERD among infants and they may promote adverse events such as aluminum toxicity. Histamine-2 receptor antagonists can be effective against GERD, but decreasing response can develop within 6 weeks of initiation of treatment. These medications appear less effective than PPIs.

OUTCOMES

An alternative treatment for severe GERD may be surgical intervention. The indications for surgical treatment are controversial. Generally, if all prior dietary and pharmacological treatments have been unsuccessful and chronic airway distress is persisting, a procedure called a *fundoplication* may benefit some infants. The most commonly performed procedure is the Nissen fundoplication in which the fundus of the stomach is wrapped around the lower esophagus. This procedure may be done laparoscopically. Infants with severe reflux may be the most vulnerable population with GERD, because of the risk of aspiration and subsequent poor airway protection (Wakeman, Wilson, & Warner, 2016). Although the outcome of a successful fundoplication may diminish future reflux episodes and aspiration, this population is generally more vulnerable as a surgical candidate and risk–benefit ratio should be calculated.

Summary

The establishment of standardized guidelines adopted by the AAP has emphasized evaluation and treatment using best practices for use by general pediatricians and pediatric subspecialists. The infant with uncomplicated recurrent regurgitation may be physiologic and require only conservative management. Parental education and anticipatory guidance may be all that is required. Weight gain and progression of developmental attainment of milestones is reassuring. Infants with recurrent regurgitation and symptoms, such as weight loss or apparent pain, may benefit from individual comfort or dietary interventions. When comfort or dietary adjustments are inadequate, there may be some efficacy in the use of pharmacological agents. Consultation with pediatric gastrointestinal specialty may be required, where additional diagnostic evaluation and pharmaceutical or surgical options may be further pursued. Current research is inconclusive as to a single most effective treatment.

Lightdale, J., Gremse, D., & Section on Gastroenterology, Hepatology and Nutrition. (2013). Gastroesophageal reflux: Management guidance for the pediatrician. *Pediatrics, 131*(5), e1684–e1695. doi:10.1542/peds.2013-0421

Martin, R., & Hibbs, A. M. (2016). Gastroesophageal reflux in premature infants. In A. G. Hoppin (Ed.), *UpToDate*. Retrieved from https://www.upto date.com/contents/gastroesophageal-reflux-in-premature-infants

Modlin, I. M., Kidd, M., & Lye, K. D. (2003). Historical perspectives on the treatment of gastroesophageal reflux disease. *Gastrointestinal Endoscopy Clinics of North America, 13*, 19–55. doi:10.1016/S1052-5157(02)00104-6

Neu, M., Corwin, E., Lareau, S. C., & Marcheggiani-Howard, C. (2012). A review of nonsurgical treatment for the symptom of irritability in infants with GERD. *Journal for Specialists in Pediatric Nursing, 17*, 177–192. doi:10.1111/j.1744-6155.2011.00310.x

Wakeman, D. S., Wilson, N. A., & Warner, B. W. (2016). Current status of surgical management of gastroesophageal reflux in children. *Current Opinion in Pediatrics, 28*(3), 356–362. doi:10.1097/MOP.0000000000000341

■ GASTROSCHISIS AND OMPHALOCELE

Beverly Capper

Overview

Defects in the abdominal wall occur during the early stages of fetal development. Interruption in the normal development of the abdomen between 6 and 10 weeks of gestation prevents normal closure of the abdomen and allows the abdominal organs to float freely in amniotic fluid (Lepigeon, Van Miegham, Maurer, Giannoni, & Baud, 2014). Abdominal wall defects increase neonatal mortality and morbidity, as well as the risk of preterm delivery, neonatal surgery, infection, digestive issues, and prolonged hospitalization. Gastroschisis and omphalocele are the two most common types of congenital abdominal wall defects in newborns (Corey et al., 2014). Gastroschisis occurs once in every 12,000 live births, and omphalocele occurs once in every 4,000 live births (Corey et al., 2014). The increase in incidence of gastroschisis over the past 10 years is concerning and unexplained (Bergholz, Boettcher, Reinshagen, & Wenke, 2014). Currently there is no fetal intervention for gastroschisis or omphalocele and a large number of these pregnancies result in preterm birth (Lepigeon et al., 2014). Surgical correction of gastroschisis and omphalocele is imminent after birth and best managed with a team of specialists (Insigna et al., 2014). Delivery ideally occurs in a center equipped to perform surgery and care for the newborn in a neonatal intensive care unit.

Background

The formation of the abdomen occurs during weeks 6 to 10 of fetal development. During this time, the abdomen lacks sufficient room to accommodate the growth of organs so the intestines naturally protrude into the umbilical cord and then at week 11 recede back into the abdomen (Rubarth & Van Woudenberg, 2016). Failure of the organs to recede prevents closure and allows organs to form outside the abdomen. Gastroschisis and omphalocele are both characterized by herniation of abdominal organs that may include the intestines, spleen, liver, or other organs (Corey et al., 2014). The presence of gastroschisis or omphalocele is generally detected prenatally on a routine ultrasound and an elevated maternal serum alpha fetoprotein (AFP; Lepigeon et al., 2014). Once a defect is identified, repeated ultrasounds are recommended throughout the remainder of the pregnancy to monitor the growth and well-being of the fetus (Lepigeon et al., 2014).

Although the etiology is unknown, there is evidence linking environmental factors and maternal smoking and alcohol ingestion, genitourinary infection during the first trimester, use of selective serotonin-reuptake inhibitors (SSRIs), and poor prenatal care (Insigna et al., 2014). The risk of gastroschisis is highest among women younger than 20 years of age, whereas the risk for omphalocele is noted in advanced maternal age.

A gastroschisis is herniation typically located to the right of the umbilicus and lacks a membrane or sac to cover the exposed organs. The defect is not associated with chromosomal defects and classified as simple or complex. Simple gastroschisis has intestines or other organs outside the abdomen, whereas complex gastroschisis has additional pathologies of intestinal atresia, perforation, necrotic segments, or volvulus (Bergholz et al., 2014). Complex gastroschisis requires a longer hospitalization and is associated with more feeding complications.

The omphalocele is a midline abdominal wall defect located near the base of the umbilical cord with a thin membrane or sac covering the exposed organs. Omphalocele is frequently associated with trisomy 13, 18, and 21 chromosomal defect, Beckwith–Wiedeman syndrome, and other congenital anomalies (Corey et al., 2014). Although the prevalence of omphalocele is lower than gastroschisis, it carries a higher mortality rate thought to be related to the associated congenital anomalies.

Perinatal treatment strategies for the timing and mode of the delivery remain controversial, but Lepigeon et al. (2014) reported evidence from a study that showed a decreased risk of sepsis and organ damage with induction of labor at 37 weeks. There is little evidence demonstrating a benefit of cesarean section over vaginal delivery. Surgical correction is needed shortly after birth to restore the integrity of the abdominal wall and prevent damage to exposed organs (Insigna et al., 2014). Three surgical approaches described by Wu, Lee, and DeUgarte (2016) include a nonoperative strategy, primary closure, and a staged repair using a silo that contains eviscerated intestines. The nonoperative procedure is a newer strategy, and is performed at the bedside by placing an umbilical flap to cover the opening in the abdomen. Primary closure is the preferred procedure and places the intestines and other organs back in the abdomen in one surgery. Staged repair may be necessary if swelling and inflammation of the intestines prevent a primary closure. The intestines remaining outside the abdomen are covered with a mesh silo and suspended over the abdomen. The intestines recede by gravity, and the silo is tightened daily to gently push the intestines into the abdomen.

Clinical Aspects

ASSESSMENT

Essential components for nursing care for the newborn include obtaining a thorough maternal history that includes the pregnancy and mode of delivery, as well as physical assessment of the newborn, laboratory data, and echocardiogram. These assessments help to properly identify risk factors and medications that may have had adverse effects on the newborn. The physical assessment of the newborn is focused on respiratory function and alterations that result from preterm delivery, low birth weight, and intrauterine growth retardation (IUGR). Of particular concern is the respiratory compromise attributable to increased intraabdominal pressure, cold stress from heat loss through exposed organs, and changes in heart rate because of extreme fluid loss. The initial assessment confirms the differential diagnosis between gastroschisis and omphalocele based on the presence or absence of a sac surrounding the exposed organs. Caution is needed to protect the integrity of the organs themselves with both defects and specifically the sac in presence of an omphalocele. Laboratory data are monitored to evaluate electrolytes for the effectiveness of fluid resuscitation. After initial stabilization, physical assessment findings are evaluated for additional congenital anomalies and heart function is evaluated with a fetal echocardiogram.

NURSING INTERVENTIONS, MANAGEMENT, AND IMPLICATIONS

Nursing care of the newborn with gastroschisis or omphalocele is focused on prevention of complications during the immediate stabilization and throughout the neonatal recovery period. Nursing problems include maintaining thermoregulation, fluid resuscitation to maintain vascular perfusion and adequate ventilation, protection of herniated abdominal organs to maintain sac integrity and prevent organ damage, administration of broad spectrum antibiotics, decreased cardiac output from increased abdominal pressure following primary closure, optimization of gastric function to prevent ileus and long-term feeding problems, and provision of support for parents and family during a prolonged hospitalization.

Immediately after birth the exposed organs are covered with a nonadherent dressing and clear plastic bag to prevent heat and fluid loss, drying of organs, and to promote visualization. Use of a radiant warmer or the warm humidified environment of an isolette assists with thermoregulation. Fluid replacement may require volumes at twice the normal maintenance amounts and placement of an oral or nasogastric tube is needed for decompression and also to decrease the risk of aspiration. Enteral feedings may be delayed for several weeks requiring the insertion of a peripherally inserted central catheter (PICC) or central venous line to infuse total parental nutrition. Maternal or donor breast milk is the preferred nutrition and tolerance of human milk may help gain faster attainment of full enteral feeds. Postoperative care includes pain management, infection prevention, and feeding. Discharge preparation begins early, engaging the parent(s) in caring for their newborn and teaching normal newborn care and care specific to the comorbidities or congenital anomalies.

OUTCOMES

Prognosis is determined by the severity of the defect. Newborns with gastroschisis have an excellent recovery and the majority have no long-term health problems. Complex gastroschisis has greater feeding difficulties, and 4% to 10% of infants experience bowel obstruction requiring additional surgery and possibly resulting in short gut (Lepigeon et al., 2014). Omphalocele has a higher morbidity and mortality rate reflective of associated congenital anomalies. Parents may need counseling for future pregnancies and support for future hospitalizations.

Summary

Early prenatal diagnosis and delivery at a tertiary care center optimizes the stabilization and surgery for the newborn diagnosed with gastroschisis or omphalocele. Treatment is prolonged for complex gastroschisis and omphalocele averaging more than 1 month with costs exceeding $100,000 (Wu et al., 2016). Further research is needed to determine the etiology of gastroschisis and omphalocele.

Bergholz, R., Boettcher, M., Reinshagen, K., & Wenke, K. (2014). Complex gastroschisis is a different entity to simple gastroschisis affecting morbidity and mortality—A systematic review and meta-analysis. *Journal of Pediatric Surgery, 49,* 1527–1532. doi:10.1016/j.jpedsurg.2014.08.001

Corey, K. M., Hornik, C. P., Laughon, M. M., McHutchinson, K., Clark, R. H., & Smith, P. B. (2014). Frequency of anomalies and hospital outcomes in infants with gastroschisis and omphalocele. *Early Human Development, 90,* 421–424.

Insigna, V., Lo Verso, C., Antona, V., Cimador, M., Ortolano, R., Carta, M., . . . Corsello, G. (2014). Perinatal management of gastroschisis. *Journal of Pediatric Neonatal Individual Medicine, 3*(1), e030113. Retrieved from http://www.jpnim.com/index.php/jpnim/article/view/129

Lepigeon, K., Van Mieghem, T., Maurer, S. V., Giannoni, E., & Baud, D. (2014). Gastroschisis—What should be told to parents. *Prenatal Diagnosis, 34,* 316–326. doi:10.1002/pd.4305

Rubarth, L. B., & Van Woudenberg, C. D. (2016). Development of the gastrointestinal system: An embryonic and fetal review. *Neonatal Network, 35*(3), 156–158. doi:10.1891/0730-0832.35.3.156

Wu, X. J., Lee, S. L., & DeUgarte, D. A. (2016). Cost modeling for management strategies of uncomplicated gastroschisis. *Journal of Surgical Research, 205,* 136–141. doi:10.1016/j.jss.2016.06.039

■ HIRSCHSPRUNG'S DISEASE

Anne M. Modic

Overview

Hirschsprung's disease (HD) is also referred to as *congenital aganglionic megacolon* or *meconium plug syndrome*. Meconium plug syndrome is a broader diagnosis that correlates with a 13% incidence of Hirschsprung's (Keckler et al., 2008). HD is most often found in the sigmoid colon of the large intestine preventing normal contraction of the affected area and subsequently normal expulsion of stool.

Background

HD is a congenital disease in which ganglion nerve cells in the myenteric and submucosal plexi responsible for peristalsis and smooth muscle movement of the gut are absent from the intestine. This results from failure of the ganglion cells to migrate in a craniocaudal direction during the fifth through the 12th week of gestation (Keckler et al., 2008). As a result, there is a continual state of contraction of the aganglionic segment of bowel and the internal anal sphincter preventing normal expulsion of stool.

Short-segment HD is defined by the absence of nerve cells in the sigmoid colon (Keckler et al., 2008). In long-segment disease, there is an absence of nerve cells throughout most or all of the large intestines, occasionally part of the small intestine, and rarely the entire intestinal tract. The proximal bowel subsequently becomes dilated because of normal function in an effort to pass stool. The incidence is approximately one in 5,000 live births. Occurrence of this disease is a 4:1 male to female ratio (Moore, 2016). HD accounts for 20% to 25% of intestinal obstruction in the neonatal period.

Historically, this was a fatal disease. In 1886, Hirschsprung, a Danish pediatrician, presented two cases of infants at the Berlin Conference of German Society Pediatrics (Sergi, 2015). The infants' similar symptoms included absence of spontaneous bowel movements, abdominal distention, and episodes of diarrhea. Treatment consisted of laxatives and daily enemas. Both children died. The autopsies showed rectal narrowing, dilated loops of bowel as well as some ulceration of the mucosa associated with thickening of the bowel wall (Sergi, 2015).

Significant HD research looking at the enteric nervous system (ENS) has been the focus of developmental neurobiologists and geneticists (Heanue & Pachnis, 2007; Moore, 2016). The ENS is the part of the parasympathetic nervous system that regulates smooth muscle movements and peristalsis of the gut. Developmental neurobiologists have been uncovering the molecular process of the migration, proliferation, and differentiation of neural crest cells responsible for the creation of the normal ENS. Geneticists have found a number of genetic expressions related to the development of HD. Biologic and genetic advances in HD have brought the focus to exploration for ENS stem cells.

Clinical Aspects

Clinical presentation of HD may occur from early in the neonatal period to 2 or 3 years of life and beyond. Older children often present with chronic constipation or enterocolitis. However, in 80% to 90% of cases, symptoms occur in the neonatal period (Barksdale, Chwals, Magnuson, & Parry, 2011).

ASSESSMENT

The neonate fails to pass meconium in the first 24 to 48 hours of life with varying symptoms of abdominal distention, poor feeding, vomiting, and occasionally enterocolitis. The physical examination varies from an abdomen that is soft and nondistended to tense with significant abdominal distention. A rectal examination may produce notable gas and explosive stool. Abdominal radiographs with contrast show dilated loops of bowel with lack of air in the rectum. A full thickness or suction rectal biopsy is performed for histology to determine the presence or absence of ganglion cells. Bowel decompression is done followed by surgical intervention. The level of surgical repair is determined by ascending serial biopsies and frozen section biopsy to ascertain presence of ganglion cells.

The aganglionic portion of the bowel is resected; the normal bowel is attached to the anus in a primary pull-through procedure known as a "single-stage pull-through" (SSPT). The Swenson, Soave, and Duhamel are the most common techniques used. Each of these procedures differs in how the connection between bowel and rectum is created. When there is long segment, higher level disease, enterocolitis or other bowel damage such as perforation, the aganglionic bowel is removed and an ostomy is created at the level of normal bowel in a multistage-pull-through (MSPT). An ostomy takedown is done after the bowel is sufficiently healed and the healthy bowel is connected to the rectum. In general, SSPT is associated with improved outcomes (Sulkowski et al., 2014).

NURSING INTERVENTIONS, MANAGEMENT, AND IMPLICATIONS

Nurses are instrumental both in the diagnosis and care of infants with HD. Nurses must pay close attention to gastrointestinal (GI) status, including feeding tolerance and stooling patterns, particularly in the first 48 hours of life. Close monitoring by nurses is important because of the concern for perforation with intestinal distention proximal to the aganglionic area. Abdominal decompression with a nasogastric tube is critical. The inability of the neonate to orally feed and possible subsequent vomiting require clinicians to follow electrolytes, hydration status, and nutritional needs closely. Total parenteral nutrition is standard nutritional support. Neonates should be closely monitored for sepsis or enterocolitis. Symptoms include temperature instability, abdominal distention, vomiting, explosive diarrhea that may be foul smelling or bloody, and, in advanced cases, septic shock. Treatment includes antibiotics, observation for signs of septic shock, nothing by mouth, and intravenous fluid support. Rectal saline washout is required before surgery when enterocolitis is present (Bucher, Pacetti, Lovvorn, & Carter, 2016).

In addition to normal postoperative care, the nurse must be diligent in monitoring electrolytes, maintaining hydration and nutrition, monitoring the abdominal status and/or ostomy site, and preventing infection. Nurses are at the forefront of pain control for these infants. Opioids are generally used for immediate postop pain control with transition to acetaminophen. Parental nutrition and abdominal decompression are provided until GI function has been reestablished. Feeds can then be slowly initiated with close monitoring of feeding tolerance. At times, tolerance of elemental formula is better than standard formula. However, breast milk and breastfeeding are strongly recommended. Stooling patterns should be observed for normalcy. Significant constipation or diarrhea around areas of constipation may be indicative of strictures.

The presence of strictures requires rectal dilation. Hegar dilators are used with the size of the dilator increased over time. Symptoms include constipation or diarrhea around areas of significant constipation. Postoperative antibiotics are prescribed prophylactically for enterocolitis. Establishment and tolerance of enteral feeds as well as family education are necessary prerequisites before safe discharge. Family education for rectal dilation, symptoms of enterocolitis, and, if needed, ostomy care should be provided (Malcolm, 2015).

OUTCOMES

Persistent constipation can occur with unresected areas of aganglionosis that may require further surgical intervention to remove the abnormal segment of bowel. HD patients generally are followed for at least 1 year postop. Ongoing issues require long-term follow-up and intervention. This may include enterocolitis and/or chronic bowel dysfunction. Enterocolitis can occur at any time. Treatment includes antibiotics and rectal washout. In severe cases, an ostomy may be needed. In a review of patients with HD reported by Moore (2016), 68% of HD patients had normal bowel function after postoperative repair, 10.3% had soiling, and 21.7% needed laxatives or enemas for chronic, significant constipation. Possible causes may be sphincter achalasia, ENS dysganglionosis, or other areas of aganglionosis. Some patients experience enuresis, incontinence, or dysuria and may require bowel management programs. The focus of follow-up care includes stool softeners, laxatives, and enemas in addition to diet, exercise, and bowel training.

Summary

HD was historically a terminal disease for infants and children. Great progress has been made in the identification and treatment of HD. Neurobiology and genetic research is ongoing with a number of genetic expressions related to development of HD identified. Stem cell therapy is at the forefront of current research and brings hope of treatment without the need for surgical intervention.

Awareness of symptoms in the early neonatal period is crucial in identifying HD and nurses play an important role in the identification, care, and family education of these infants. Close follow-up of bowel function, growth, nutrition, and early identification of enterocolitis maximizes the potential for best long-term outcomes.

Barksdale, E. M., Jr., Chwals, W. J., Magnuson, D. K., & Parry, R. L. (2011). The gastrointestinal tract. Part 3: Selected gastrointestinal anomalies. In R. J. Martin, A. A. Fanaroff, & M. C. Walsh (Eds.) *Fanaroff and Martin's neonatal-perinatal medicine: Diseases of the fetus and newborn* (9th ed., pp. 1400–1430). St. Louis, MO: Elsevier.

Bucher, B., Pacetti, A., Lovvorn, H., III, & Carter, B. (2016). Neonatal surgery. In S. Gardner, B. Carter, M. Hines, & J. Hernández (Eds.), *Merenstein & Gardner's handbook of neonatal intensive care* (8th ed., pp. 786–819). St. Louis, MO: Elsevier.

Heanue, T. A., & Pachnis, V. (2007). Enteric nervous system development and Hirschsprung's disease: Advances in genetic and stem cell studies. *Nature Reviews. Neuroscience, 8*(6), 466–479. doi:10.1038/nrn2137

Keckler, S. J., St. Peter, S. D., Spilde, T. L., Tsao, K., Ostlie, D. J., Holcomb, G. W., III, & Snyder, C. L. (2008). Current significance of meconium plug syndrome. *Journal of Pediatric Surgery, 43*(5), 896–898. doi:10.1016/j.jpedsurg.2007.12.035

Malcolm, W. (2015). *Beyond the NICU: Comprehensive care of the high-risk infant* (pp. 492–494, 735). New York, NY: McGraw-Hill.

Moore, S. (2016). Hirschsprung disease: Current perspectives. *Open Access Surgery, 9,* 39–50. doi:10.2147/OAS.S81552

Sergi, C. (2015). Hirschsprung's disease: Historical notes and pathological diagnosis on the occasion of the 100th anniversary of Dr. Harald Hirschsprung's death. *World Journal of Clinical Pediatrics, 4*(4), 120–125. doi:10.5409/wjcp.v4.i4.120

Sulkowski, J. P., Cooper, J. N., Congeni, A., Pearson, E. G., Nwomeh, B. C., Doolin, E. J., . . . Deans, K. J. (2014). Single-stage versus multi-stage pull-through for Hirschsprung's disease: Practice trends and outcomes in infants. *Journal of Pediatric Surgery, 49*(11), 1619–1625. doi:10.1016/j.jpedsurg.2014.06.002

■ HYDRONEPHROSIS

Charlene M. Deuber

Overview

Hydronephrosis is one of the most common fetal anomalies, detected in 1% of pregnancies. A sign rather than a diagnosis, hydronephrosis references significant dilation of the upper urinary tract. Common causes of hydronephrosis include physiologic hydronephrosis, ureteropelvic or ureterovesical junction (UVJ) obstruction, posterior urethral valves (PUVs), Eagle–Barrett (prune belly) syndrome, and vesicoureteral reflux (VUR; Martin, Fanaroff, & Walsh, 2011).

Prenatal diagnosis is highly correlated with postnatal findings (Policiano et al., 2015). The goal of prenatal ultrasound is reduction in the incidence of postnatal urinary tract infection (UTI) and prevention of acquired renal damage in asymptomatic patients. Early identification of the finding affords the opportunity for prenatal consultation with nephrology or urology specialists, facilitating postnatal care coordination. Prenatal interventions are limited in efficacy and associated with increased risk of preterm labor and chorioramnionitis. Expectant prenatal management prevails, with fetal surgical intervention rarely indicated (Liu, Armstrong, & Maizels, 2014).

Background

Occurring unilaterally or bilaterally, hydronephrosis is characterized by enlargement of the renal collecting system, including renal calyces and pelvis. The etiology is varied although it may be obstructive in origin. Prenatal hydronephrosis may be transient or secondary to clinically significant abnormalities of the kidney and urinary tract. As much as 15% of prenatally detected hydronephrosis occurs because of delayed fetal ureter maturation independently of anatomic abnormalities of the upper urinary tract (physiologic hydronephrosis) and typically resolve spontaneously before birth or by 2 years of age. The incidence of significant urinary tract disease in identified cases of hydronephrosis has been estimated at 0.2% to 0.4% (Aslan, 2005).

Ultrasound-guided prenatal grading of unilateral or bilateral hydronephrosis informs prenatal and postnatal management. The grading system of the Society of Fetal Urology (grades I–V) describes the degree of calyceal dilatation and renal parenchymal thickness.

Grading may be used as a guideline to describe the degree of hydronephrosis. Measuring the greatest dimension of the renal pelvis has also gained favor for defining hydronephrosis. An unfavorable outcome, including need for postnatal surgery, has been associated with a renal anteriorposterior (AP) diameter of 7 mm or more in the third trimester and the presence of urinary tract anomalies (Plevani et al., 2014).

Prenatal ultrasonography findings, including increased renal echogenicity, bilateral disease, and oligohydramnios may be associated with long-term renal dysfunction and deserve additional prenatal consultation with nephrology or urology specialists (Vogt & Dell, 2011). Despite improvements in technique, prenatal imaging may not detect all defects of the urinary tract.

Clinical Aspects

The majority of cases of hydronephrosis are unilateral and mild, necessitating postnatal follow-up with serial ultrasonography beginning at 7 to 10 days of age to resolution (or progression) of findings. Newborns with a normal ultrasound in the first week of life should undergo a repeated study at 4 to 6 weeks of age to eliminate an initial false-negative study owing to relative dehydration or low glomerular filtration rate (GFR). Two normal postnatal ultrasound examinations exclude the presence of significant renal disease.

Sencan et al. (2014) describe a low incidence of UTI and VUR in children with mild antenatal hydronephrosis (ANH) at 2 weeks through 3 months of age, suggesting that routine voiding cystourethrogram (VCUG) and long-term antibiotic prophylaxis should be initiated only in symptomatic children presenting with UTI. Moderate to severe unilateral hydronephrosis prompts postnatal study, including ultrasonography followed by a VCUG and a functional renal scan (diuretic renography) to identify etiology precisely.

Mild isolated bilateral hydronephrosis should similarly be followed with sequential ultrasound examination. Causes of bilateral hydronephrosis include UVJ obstruction, referring to a blockage in the region of the UVJ where the ureter meets the bladder. The obstruction impedes flow of urine down to the bladder, causing the urine to back up into and dilate the ureters and kidney, appreciated on ultrasound as megaureter (dilated ureter) and hydronephrosis. Moderate to severe bilateral hydronephrosis may indicate potential obstructive uropathy and requires prompt, detailed evaluation postnatally, particularly in male infants who have an increased risk of PUVs.

In cases of severe bilateral hydronephrosis (greater than 15-mm AP diameter in third trimester), postnatal ultrasonography should be completed in the first 48 hours of life and prophylactic antibiotic therapy initiated. A VCUG follows with the continuation of antibiotic therapy or additional renal scans to complete diagnostic evaluation and determine presence and location of obstruction.

ASSESSMENT

Trending the blood pressure is important to monitor for hypertension as well as temperature to monitor for sepsis. Strict intake and output (I&O) is crucial and need to be calculated every 4 hours. Infants may need intravenous (IV) fluids to maintain hydration and IV antibiotics to prevent infection in the bladder or kidneys. If the hydronephrosis is severe, the infant may need a Foley catheter to keep the kidneys drained. Proper nutrition for growth and development is important and mothers should be encouraged to provide breast milk although there is a special commercial formula available.

NURSING INTERVENTIONS, MANAGEMENT, AND IMPLICATIONS

Treatment of all infants with hydronephrosis has the same goal, which is to preserve renal function. Nurses must be able to assess infant renal function and inform the other members of the health care team of any acute or subtle changes they observe in the infant.

In addition, nurses must understand normal and abnormal laboratory values. Serial renal function panels are performed to determine kidney function. Waste products, urea/blood urea nitrogen (BUN), and creatinine (Cr) can accumulate in the blood causing serious damage to the kidneys.

Parent education is of primary importance even if the parents are aware of the diagnosis prenatally. The different tests their infant may undergo must be reinforced to them at a level they can understand. No matter what degree of hydronephrosis, it remains a frightening experience and parents need support. An important aspect is the need for follow-up with a pediatric nephrologist and continuation of antibiotics if required.

OUTCOMES

Spontaneous resolution of mild hydronephrosis is greater than moderate or severe hydronephrosis. Infants with moderate/severe hydronephrosis are at greater risk for a UTI (Conkar, Memmedov, & Mir, 2016), but still may be treated conservatively.

Summary

Neonatal hydronephrosis is often self-limiting, but may signal obstructive pathology of the lower or upper urinary tract. Prenatal diagnosis is important in guiding postnatal follow-up and management, with the goal of amelioration of acquired renal damage. Nursing care focuses on identification of prenatal diagnosis and implementation of postnatal follow-up. Preparation for procedures necessitates parental education and support.

Aslan, A. (2005). *Neonatal hydronephrosiss (UPJ obstruction) and multicystic dysplastic kidneys*. In L. S. Baskin (Ed.), *Handbook of pediatric urology* (pp. 123–130). Philadelphia, PA: Lippincott Williams & Wilkins.

Conkar, S., Memmedov, V., & Mir, S. (2016). Outcomes of antenatal hydronephrosis. *Annals of Clinical and Laboratory Research,* 4(1), 1–5. Retrieved from http://www.aclr.com.es/clinical-research/outcome-of-antenatal-hydronephrosis.pdf

Liu, D. B., Armstrong, W. R., & Maizels, M. (2014). Hydronephrosis: Prenatal and postnatal evaluation and management. *Clinics in Perinatology,* 41(3), 661–678. doi:10.1016/j.clp.2014.05.013

Martin, R., Fanaroff, A., & Walsh, M. (2011). *Fanaroff and Martin's neonatal-perinatal medicine* (9th ed.). St. Louis, MO: Elsevier Mosby.

Plevani, C., Locatelli, A., Paterlini, G., Ghidini, A., Tagliabue, P., Pezzullo, J. C., & Vergani, P. (2014). Fetal hydronephrosis: Natural history and risk factors for postnatal surgery. *Journal of Perinatal Medicine, 42*(3), 385–391. doi:10.1515/jpm-2013-0146

Policiano, C., Djokovic, D., Carvalho, R., Monteiro, C., Melo, M. A., & Graça, L. M. (2015). Ultrasound antenatal detection of urinary tract anomalies in the last decade: Outcome and prognosis. *The Journal of Maternal-Fetal & Neonatal Medicine, 28*(8), 959–963. doi:10.3109/14767058.2014.939065

Sencan, A., Carvas, F., Hekimoglu, I. C., Caf, N., Sencan, A., Chow, J., & Nguyen, H. T. (2014). Urinary tract infection and vesicoureteral reflux in children with mild antenatal hydronephrosis. *Journal of Pediatric Urology, 10*(6), 1008–1013. doi:10.1016/j.jpurol.2014.04.001

■ HYPERBILIRUBINEMIA

Donna M. Schultz
Mary F. Terhaar

Overview

Destruction of old red blood cells (RBCs) is a normal and adaptive process in newborns as it is across the life span. When RBCs die, they are lysed and bilirubin is released as a by-product. Under certain conditions, the rate of RBC destruction exceeds the body's ability to eliminate bilirubin, which results in excess levels of the waste product circulating in the bloodstream. This condition is called hyperbilirubinemia, or jaundice. Jaundice is the yellow coloration of skin and sclera that results when excessive bilirubin levels accumulate in skin and mucous membranes.

During pregnancy, the placenta, attached to the fetus, removes bilirubin along with other waste from the fetal bloodstream. Once delivery is complete and the umbilical cord is cut, the newborn must activate his or her own hepatic pathways to conjugate and eliminate bilirubin along with other wastes through the gastrointestinal system (Cohen, Wong, & Stevenson, 2010). It is the imbalance of RBC destruction and hepatic function that produces hyperbilirubinemia.

Background

Hyperbilirubinemia has two distinct presentations, physiologic and pathologic, which are distinguished by the timing, etiology, and severity of the jaundice. Approximately 60% to 85% of all term newborns will develop clinical signs of hyperbilirubinemia (Azzuqa & Watchko, 2015).

Physiologic jaundice in the newborn is a normal, adaptive process; commonly it is self-correcting, time-limited, and lacking in clinical significance. The condition results during normal transition to extrauterine life when the newborn breaks down fetal RBCs even as the kidneys, liver, and gastrointestinal system are assuming responsibility for elimination of waste. This increase in waste product generation precedes functional capacity for elimination. Bilirubin levels usually peak between 3 and 5 days of life and start to decrease by the end of the first week. This is the presentation of physiologic jaundice.

Pathologic jaundice occurs in a relatively small group of newborns. The jaundice presents before 24 hours of life, with total bilirubin levels rising to exceed 5 mg/dL, or greater than the 95th percentile on the Bhutani nomogram (Bhutani, Vilms, & Hamerman-Johnson, 2010). Multiple factors increase the risk for pathologic jaundice, including prematurity, polycythemia, hemolytic disease, genetic abnormalities such as G6PD or Gilbert's disease, sepsis, blood cell irregularities, extensive bruising, abnormal pooling of blood as seen in cephalohematoma, family history of jaundice, inefficient feeding, and dehydration. Newborns of Asian, Arabic, or Mediterranean ethnicity face greater risk as well.

A thorough medical history from the mother is important so that health care providers can identify risk factors and monitor the baby for pathologic jaundice (Cohen et al., 2010).

The first cases of jaundice, *icterus neonatorum*, were described in the late 19th century as a benign and self-limiting yellowing of the skin and the sclera that generally disappeared by the end of the baby's stay in the hospital (which was 10–14 days in the late 19th century; Cashore, 2010). A second, more severe form of jaundice *icterus gravis* was associated with significant anemia, neurologic abnormalities, and increased mortality (Cashore, 2010). The acute phase of this condition is named bilirubin-induced encephalopathy (BIND) and the resultant long-term sequelae are identified as kernicterus. Bilirubin is a neurotoxin in large doses. Both BIND and kernicterus result when bilirubin levels become too high, allowing the toxin to cross the blood–brain barrier and deposit in the basal ganglia producing serious neurologic damage (American Academy of Pediatrics [AAP] Subcommittee on Hyperbilirubinemia, 2004). Kernicterus has not been reported in infants with peak TSB levels less than 20 mg/dL (Bhutani et al., 2004). However, it has not been determined at what level kernicterus can occur.

Because length of hospital stay for the mother–baby dyad has radically decreased, careful monitoring for hyperbilirubinemia is key to newborn well-being. In the case of spontaneous vaginal delivery, mother and newborn are commonly discharged to home by 48 hours after the birth. In the case of birth by cesarian section, mother and newborn are commonly discharged to home at approximately 72 hours. In both cases, discharge takes place before bilirubin levels can be expected to peak. This discrepancy motivated The Joint Commission to issue a sentinel event detailing the rise in BIND and kernicterus. In response, the AAP revised guidelines for the management of hyperbilirubinemia and rates began to decline (2004). As a result, The Joint Commission retired their sentinel alert. Best practice now calls for all newborns to be screened for hyperbilirubinemia before discharge to home.

Clinical Aspects

ASSESSMENT

Early assessment of risk for hyperbilirubinemia is essential. Family history, maternal history, and progression of the pregnancy and labor are all relevant to risk assessment. It is important to make note of any discrepancy between maternal, paternal, and newborn blood and Rh type; use of antibiotics or oxytocin during pregnancy or labor; prolonged second stage of labor; use of mechanical assistance with delivery (vacuum or forceps); any trauma or bruising to the fetus or newborn; as well as presence of cephalohematoma. Each of these findings is associated with increased risk.

A transcutaneous bilirubin (TcB) level is routinely obtained within the first 12 to 24 hours of life. TcB measurements are a noninvasive way to obtain a cutaneous bilirubin level and to determine if a serum bilirubin level needs to be drawn (Maisel, Coffey, & Kring, 2015). Abnormal values are brought to the attention of the responsible health care provider.

Use of the Bhutani nomogram for infants 35 or more weeks gestational age, with the four risk-zone stratification, is best practice for monitoring newborns with hyperbilirubinemia (AAP Committee on Hyperbilirubinemia, 2004). Infants whose total bilirubin levels are plotted in the high-risk zone should receive phototherapy. The number of banks of lights is determined by the bilirubin level. An infant's discharge should be delayed until a pattern of declining bilirubin levels is documented (Bhutani et al., 2010).

Infants whose bilirubin levels rise to the high–intermediate risk zone should be sent home only if feeding, voiding, and stooling appropriately. A bilirubin level at discharge must be documented. A follow-up appointment should be scheduled for the following day after discharge with the family's primary care provider (PCP) to monitor the bilirubin level.

Phototherapy promotes conjugation of bilirubin, which allows it to be eliminated in urine and stool. Aside from hydration and monitoring, phototherapy is the most commonly used intervention for the jaundiced newborn (American Academy of Pediatrics, 2004). Blue to green light (wavelengths 460–490 nm) most effectively facilitates conjugation of bilirubin and is used in treatment of the newborn (Muchowski, 2014). Fluorescent or halogen lights and light emitting diodes (LED) are commonly used (Muchowski, 2014). Exposure to these lights with as much skin exposed as possible for as much time as possible maximizes effect. Eye shields are used to protect the infant and need to be placed carefully to prevent them from becoming loose, leaving the eyes unprotected. Phototherapy can lead to burns, retinal damage, temperature instability, dehydration, rashes, and loose stools.

NURSING INTERVENTIONS, MANAGEMENT, AND IMPLICATIONS

Frequent breastfeeding (or bottle feeding if the parents choose) is key. A delay in breast milk production can lead to mild dehydration in the infant. Skin-to-skin contact between mother and newborn is begun in the delivery room or birthing suite and continued unless the newborn or maternal conditions prohibit the practice. Monitoring of urine and stool output helps to determine sufficiency of intake.

Care pathways and electronic health record (EHR) documentation systems, which incorporate checklists, help assure proper identification of all risk factors and support provision of individualized care. These approaches have been established as effective means to reduce errors of omission and promote early identification of newborns who require vigilant monitoring and careful discharge planning. Care pathways and the EHR should capture and report the initial transcutaneous bilirubin (TcB) level within the first 12 to 24 hours of life. Abnormal values documented over time, measured in hours of life, should be brought to the attention of the responsible health care provider.

Educating families about hyperbilirubinemia by nursing is key. Families need to understand the need for phototherapy and to be supported as they experience separation from the infant during treatment (Muchowski, 2014). Parents should understand the importance of close primary care follow-up, because often the infant should be discharged before normal bilirubin peak levels. Families must require understanding about the effects of hyperbilirubinemia such as sleepiness, decreased wet diapers, stooling, and feeding as well as when to call their PCP.

OUTCOMES

Parents should be given a copy of the infant's discharge summary and the bilirubin nomogram so the PCP has accurate information to transition the baby into the primary care setting and develop an appropriate plan of care. Parents should be provided with education and resources to consult after discharge to home. Many health care systems provide home health team visits and lactation support.

Early identification of risk, early detection of rising bilirubin levels, and early treatment are key to, and timely resolution of, the problem. These same elements of care are key to avoiding readmissions.

Summary

Hyperbilirubinemia is one of the most common complications seen in newborn infants. Hydration, monitoring, and phototherapy are usual practices. Nonetheless, the evidence to support phototherapy is based largely on consensus and expert opinion. Limited strong evidence is available to support the current practice. Research is needed to support meaningful risk assessment and to evaluate treatment options. More important, little evidence is available to predict risk for severe hyperbilirubinemia, kernicterus, or readmission.

American Academy of Pediatrics Subcommittee on Hyperbilirubinemia. (2004). Clinical practice guideline: Management of hyperbilirubinemia in the newborn infant 35 or more weeks of gestation. *Pediatrics, 114*(1), 297–316. doi:10.1542/peds.114.1.297

Azzuqa, A., & Watchko, J. F. (2015). Bilirubin concentrations in jaundiced neonates with conjunctival icterus. *The Journal of Pediatrics, 167*(4), 840–844. doi:10.1016/j.jpeds.2015.06.065

Bhutani, V. K., Vilms, R. J., & Hamerman-Johnson, L. (2010). Universal bilirubin screening for severe neonatal hyperbilirubinemia. *Journal of Perinatology, 30*(Suppl.), S6–S15. doi:10.1038/jp.2010.98

Cashore, W. (2010). A brief history of neonatal jaundice. *Medicine and Health, Rhode Island, 93*(5), 154–155. Retrieved from http://www.rimed.org/medhealthri/2010-05/2010-05-154.pdf

Cohen, R. S., Wong, R. J., & Stevenson, D. K. (2010). Understanding neonatal jaundice: A perspective on causation. *Pediatrics and Neonatology, 51*(3), 143–148. doi:10.1016/S1875-9572(10)60027-7

Maisels, M. J., Coffey, M. P., & Kring, E. (2015). Transcutaneous bilirubin levels in newborns <35 weeks' gestation. *Journal of Perinatology, 35*(9), 739–744. doi:10.1038/jp.2015.34

Muchowski, K. E. (2014). Evaluation and treatment of neonatal hyperbilirubinemia. *American Family Physician, 89*(11), 873–878. Retrieved from https://www.aafp.org/afp/2014/0601/p873.html

■ HYPERTENSION

Mary F. Terhaar

Overview

Hypertension in neonates may present insidiously as feeding difficulty, irritability, tachypnea, apnea, or lethargy; may be identified on routine screening; or may present more acutely as congestive heart failure or cardiogenic shock (Flynn, 2000). In infants, as in adults, hypertension is dangerous, particularly when undetected or undermanaged. Preventing organ damage, maintaining healthy function of organ systems, and promoting healthy development depend on early detection and careful management (Kaelber et al., 2016).

Background

Blood pressure (BP) in neonates increases with gestational age, neonatal age, birthweight, and time. Evidence-based BP charts that describe ranges of pressure over time have made it possible to standardize expectations for BP values and help clinicians identify hypertension more consistently and with greater confidence (Flynn, 2000; Flynn & Rosenkrantz, 2016).

Normotension in the neonate is defined as a BP within the 95th percentile on those charts. Conversely, hypertension in the neonate is defined as elevation in systolic BP (on three separate occasions) above the 95th percentile for age, weight, and gender (Watkinson, 2002). By definition then, 5% of all neonates are hypertensive, although in practice, the incidence is closer to 0.2% to 3.0% (Dionne, Abibtol, & Flynn, 2012).

Neonatal hypertension may result from several different causes. It can develop as a result of congenital conditions, including aortic coarctation or structural defects of the renal system; as a consequence of renal disease, including parenchymal or vascular disease; as sequelae to bronchopulmonary dysplasia; as an unintended outcome of medical care, following administration of certain medications, accompanying endocrine disorders such as congenital adrenal hyperplasia and hyperthyroidism; or develop from thromboembolism following umbilical catheterization (Flynn, 2000; Flynn & Rosenkrantz, 2016). Hypertension can progress to cardiovascular disease, kidney disease, and stroke in the adult without proper diagnosis and management (Nickavar & Assadi, 2014).

Among 398,079 children receiving well child care between the ages of 3 and 18 years, 3.3% met diagnostic criteria and were identified as hypertensive and another 10.1% were prehypertensive. These findings agree with prevalence projections described earlier. Regardless, American Academy of Pediatrics recommended treatment was not initiated for the 2,813 infants diagnosed as hypertensive (Kaelber et al., 2016).

A careful history, including both the pregnancy and the neonatal period, is key to evaluating risk, detecting disease, effectively managing the condition, and preventing complications. Family history of renal disease or hypertension, in utero exposure to cocaine or other street drugs, and clinical history of broncho-pulmonary dysplasia are highly correlated with development of hypertension in the newborn (Flynn & Rosenkrantz, 2016).

Clinical Aspects

ASSESSMENT

Head-to-toe assessment establishes findings to confirm or rule out hypertension. Organ systems impacted by sustained elevated BP are particularly relevant for assessment because microvascular changes in these organs lead to symptoms throughout the body (Nickavar & Assadi, 2014). Important findings include bluish or pale coloration to the skin and rapid respirations, which indicate poor perfusion and oxygenation.

In the primary care setting, weight gain that does not correspond to post-natal age and failure to meet developmental milestones indicate compromised perfusion and oxygenation to vital organs and systems over an extended period. Frequent urinary tract infections point to structural or vascular abnormalities associated with hypertension. Symptoms of pronounced or advanced disease include irritability, seizures, difficulty in breathing, feeding intolerance, and vomiting (Kaelber et al., 2016).

In the neonatal intensive care unit (NICU), routine assessment of respiratory rate and function, heart rate, perfusion, liver function, and oxygenation, as well as systolic, diastolic, and pulse pressures provide useful information to complement BP readings. Observation of the wave formation from arterial lines, urine output, and perfusion to lower extremities provides a picture of vascular conditions. Umbilical arterial lines that are commonly used in the NICU must be discontinued at any sign of complications, including presence of blood in the urine, change in location of the catheter tip on radiography, or compromised perfusion.

Because hypertension in the neonate is defined by three discrete BP measurements that fall above the 95th percentile on standard BP charts, repeated measurement of BP, respiratory rate, heart rate, and pulse oximetry inform the diagnosis (Flynn, 2000; Flynn & Rosenkrantz, 2016). In practice, hypertension is most commonly diagnosed and treated when the BP persistently exceeds the 99th percentile. These data, in combination with the aforementioned clinical findings, indicate need for and effectiveness of the treatment regimen, which is adjusted to the severity and responsiveness of the clinical presentation.

NURSING PROBLEMS, INTERVENTIONS, AND MANAGEMENT

Care for the hypertensive infant in the NICU focuses on promoting comfort, managing medications, monitoring fluid status and renal function, and parent education. Comfort is promoted through careful positioning, providing opportunities for nonnutritive sucking, clustering care to allow time for rest, administration of analgesics as indicated, providing skin-to-skin experiences with parents, and maintaining a restive environment. Medications are administered as prescribed. Fluid status is assessed by checking for edema in the extremities and face, strict monitoring of intake and output, testing specific gravity, and monitoring blood urea nitrogen (BUN), creatinine levels, and hematocrit.

In the NICU, pain, agitation, renal output, underlying conditions, interventions such as ventilators and phlebotomy, and medications can influence BP. Pain can complicate assessment and exaggerate the presentation of hypertension. Meticulous pain management is an essential component of treatment especially when hypertension is a consequence of prematurity, which requires a stay in critical care or in the case of congenital anomalies that require surgical intervention.

BP measurements are essential for management of hypertension in the NICU and primary care. Readings can be influenced by many factors, including behavioral state, pain, hunger, and agitation. In order for data to be meaningful, it is useful to measure the BP with the infant in a quiescent state and to note any condition that may have altered the reading at any given time. Proper fit of the cuff to the size of the infant is essential (Nickavar & Assadi, 2014).

In the primary care setting, a variety of medications are prescribed to manage neonatal hypertension, which commonly resolves in the short term in the instance where it presents as a complication of acute illness or medical management. In a meta-analysis of clinical trials conducted on hypertensive infants, angiotensin-converting enzyme inhibitors and angiotensin receptor blockers were most commonly prescribed (35%) followed by diuretics in 22% of the children, calcium channel blockers in 17%, and beta-blockers in another 10% (Kaelber et al., 2016). Infant weight, heart rate, respirations, and BP complete the assessment here as well. Insufficient weight gain may indicate failure to thrive as a result of hypertension and excessive weight gain that presents with edema can also indicate poor BP control.

In cases where hypertension results from renal vascular or parenchymal disease, medications should focus on those disease processes. Management of hypertension that results from kidney disease commonly requires more prolonged treatment under the supervision of a renal specialist.

Lifestyle changes, including diet and exercise, which are among the most effective approaches for adults with hypertension, are ill suited for infants. Evidence supports pharmacologic interventions as most effective for this age group (Chaturvedi, Lipszyk, Licht, Craig, & Parekh, 2014). However, until recently few clinical trials have provided robust data to describe efficacy and long-term outcomes and guide management. This is the reason careful monitoring of BP and other clinical data are very important.

Medications are frequently used to manage hypertension. In a study of more than 2,000 hypertensive children and infants, angiotensin-converting enzyme inhibitors and angiotensin receptor blockers were most commonly prescribed (35%); 22% received diuretics; 17% received calcium channel blockers; and another 10% received beta-blockers (Kaelber et al., 2016).

Parents of infants with hypertension require support and education. Parents must have a clear understanding of the medications they administer, the side effects each may cause, and potential interactions between medications and foods. Parents need to understand the importance of follow-up visits, target respiratory rate, goals for growth and development, as well as the symptoms that indicate that the medications and plan of care are effective or failing. Parents must understand the nature of the disease and long-term consequences for their infants. Just as hypertension in adults is a silent disease, so too the negative consequences of hypertension in the infant may be advanced before signs and symptoms are recognizable. For this reason, screening and management are key.

OUTCOMES

Management of hypertension is the priority in avoiding long-term complications, which result from end organ and vascular damage. Such complications include left ventricular hypertrophy, encephalopathy, and retinopathy (Nickavar & Assadi, 2014). Failure to gain weight and failure to thrive can also result when hypertension is not recognized or managed.

Summary

Effective treatment of hypertension in the NICU and in the primary care setting depends on careful assessment, early diagnosis, understanding of the disease, and a familiarity with the evidence. In the case when hypertension results from hospitalization in the NICU and associated conditions, parents need education and support to manage. The same is true when hypertension extends beyond the NICU stay. In both cases, the goal is to prevent end organ damage that can have life-long negative impact. Just as hypertension is a silent disease in adults, so it is for infants. In both situations, vigilance as well as compliance with medication regimens and lifestyle modifications are associated with best outcomes.

Chaturvedi, S., Lipszyc, D. H., Licht, C., Craig, J. C., & Parekh, R. S. (2014). Cochrane in context: Pharmacological interventions for hypertension in children. *Evidence-Based Child Health: A Cochrane Review Journal, 9*(3), 581–583. doi:10.1002/ebch.1975

Dionne, J. M., Abitbol, C. L., & Flynn, J. T. (2012). Hypertension in infancy: Diagnosis, management and outcome. *Pediatric Nephrology, 27*(1), 17–32. doi:10.1007/s00467-010-1755-z

Flynn, J. T. (2000). Neonatal hypertension: Diagnosis and management. *Pediatric Nephrology, 14*(4), 332–341. Retrieved from http://med.stanford.edu/content/dam/sm/pednephrology/documents/secure/5neonatalhypertension.pdf

Flynn, J. T., & Rosenkrantz, T. (2016). Neonatal hypertension. *Theheart.org Medscape.* Retrieved from https://emedicine.medscape.com/article/979588-overview

Kaelber, D. C., Liu, W., Ross, M. Localio, A. R., Leon, J. B., Pace, W. D., . . . Fiks, A. G. (2016). Diagnosis and medication treatment of pediatric hypertension: A retrospective cohort study. *Pediatrics*, e20162195. doi:10.1542/peds.2016-2195

Nickavar, A., & Assadi, F. (2014). Managing hypertension in the newborn infants. *International Journal of Preventive Medicine, 5*(Suppl. 1), S39–S43. Retrieved from https://www.ncbi.nlm.nih.gov/pmc/articles/PMC3990926

Watkinson, M. (2002). Hypertension in the newborn baby. *Archives of Disease in Childhood—Fetal and Neonatal Edition, 86*(2), F78–F81.

■ HYPOGLYCEMIA

Tina Di Fiore

Overview

Hypoglycemia is the most common metabolic problem seen in newborn infants. The overall incidence of neonatal hypoglycemia varies from 1.3 to 3 per 1,000 live births (Adamkin & American Academy of Pediatrics, 2011). This variability is seen due in part to the controversial definition of neonatal hypoglycemia in addition to the different populations, different method and timing of feeding, and different types of glucose testing. For example, serum glucose levels are higher than whole blood values. The controversial definition is reinforced by the American Academy of Pediatrics statement, which notes that "there has been no substantial evidence-based progress in defining what constitutes clinically important neonatal hypoglycemia particularly regarding how it relates to brain injury, and that monitoring for, preventing, and treating neonatal hypoglycemia remain largely empirical." In other words, the level or duration of hypoglycemia that is harmful to an infant's developing brain is not known.

Background

The laboratory value used to define neonatal hypoglycemia varies in part because of the normal physiologic changes a newborn experiences as he or she transitions to extrauterine life. The healthy neonate demonstrates a drop in the blood glucose concentrations to approximately 30 mg/dL within 1 to 2 hours after birth, and typically returns to more than 45 mg/dL with normal feeding within 12 hours (Cornblath et al., 2000).

Neonatal hypoglycemia is a result of an imbalance between glucose supply and the metabolic needs of the neonate, which may be because of inadequate glycogen stores, inappropriate changes in insulin secretion, inadequate muscle stores as a source of amino acids for gluconeogenesis, or inadequate lipid stores for the release of fatty acids, or increased glucose utilization from sepsis or other illnesses (Deshpande & Ward Platt, 2005). Excluding infants who are receiving insulin therapy, almost all hypoglycemia in the neonate occurs during fasting. Postprandial hypoglycemia is rare in neonates but may be seen with hyperinsulinism, or persistent hyperinsulinemic hypoglycemia of infancy (PHHI). PPHI is the most common cause of hypoglycemia in the first 3 months of life. It is well recognized in infants of mothers with diabetes. The etiology for hyperinsulinism is the fetal response to elevated maternal glucose by producing elevated levels of insulin. Following birth, the insulin concentrations are inappropriately elevated and lead to neonatal hypoglycemia. Most cases of hyperinsulinism are transient; however, prolonged neonatal hyperinsulinism, also known as "congenital hyperinsulinism," is most commonly associated with an abnormality of beta-cell regulation throughout the pancreas. In rare cases, surgical treatment is necessary for the neonate who is unresponsive to conventional therapy. Surgical treatment involves resection of 80% to 90% of the pancreas (Garg & Devaskar, 2006).

Clinical Aspects

ASSESSMENT

The clinical presentation of neonatal hypoglycemia is nonspecific and can vary from infant to infant. In addition, infants in the first or second day of life may be asymptomatic or may have life-threatening central nervous system (CNS) or cardiopulmonary disturbances. The most common clinical manifestations include lethargy, hypotonia, poor feeding, weak or high pitched cry, tachypnea or respiratory distress, and hypothermia or temperature instability. Other symptoms may also be seen, including tremors, jitteriness, cyanosis, apnea, irritability, and exaggerated Moro reflex or seizures, a serious sign that usually occurs late in severe neonatal hypoglycemia (Jain, 2008).

To assist with the identification of the high-risk infant, a review of the maternal history should be obtained on all infants. The history review should focus on identifying at-risk infants. Assessment with frequent and vigilant monitoring of infants with known risk factors remains key in the diagnosis, management, and treatment of neonatal hypoglycemia. High-risk groups who need screening for hypoglycemia in the first hour of life include newborns who weigh more than 4 kg or less than 2 kg and large for gestational age (LGA) infants who are above the 90th percentile in weight for their gestational age. Small for gestational age (SGA) infants below the 10th percentile for their gestational age, infants with intrauterine growth restriction (IUGR), and infants less than 37 weeks gestation are at a higher risk of hypoglycemia because of decreased glycogen stores and larger brain size.

Infants at high risk for hypoglycemia include newborns suspected of having sepsis or born to a mother suspected of having chorioramnionitis; newborns with symptoms suggestive of hypoglycemia, including jitteriness, tachypnea, hypotonia, poor feeding, apnea, temperature instability, seizures, and lethargy; infants with respiratory distress because of their increased glucose utilization; discordant twins with weight differences greater than 20%; infants with perinatal stress, significant hypoxia, asphyxia, hypoxic–ischemic encephalopathy; infants with hypothermia (cold stress); infants with hyperviscosity syndrome/polycythemia (central hematocrit greater than 70%); mothers who have received terbutaline or infants born to mothers with type 1, type 2, or gestational diabetes (Straussman & Levitsky, 2010)

NURSING INTERVENTIONS, MANAGEMENT, AND IMPLICATIONS

If neonatal hypoglycemia is suspected, the plasma or blood glucose level should be determined by laboratory method. However, a long delay in processing the specimen can result in a falsely low concentration as erythrocytes in the sample metabolize the glucose in the plasma. This problem can be avoided by transporting the blood in tubes that contain a glycolytic inhibitor such as fluoride. If recurrent hypoglycemia occurs, then further laboratory testing needs to be done, including obtaining serum insulin levels, evaluating for urine ketones, analyzing the urine for organic acids abnormalities, and screening for metabolic errors.

Management efforts are directed toward the immediate normalization of glucose levels and the identification and treatment of the various causes. It is important to note that feeding infants early decreases the incidence of hypoglycemia. Therefore, the nurse should identify the at-risk neonate and focus on early feeding in the newborn. Infants at high risk for hypoglycemia should be treated as soon as possible to prevent long-term complications. In the breastfed infant, early feeding may be problematic because of decreased breast milk supply and difficulty with breastfeeding initiation. Supplementation with infant formula or oral glucose gel may be used.

If the mother wishes to exclusively breastfeed, glucose gel has been demonstrated to safely treat hypoglycemia while decreasing the separation of the mother and infant. Using a dose of 0.2 g of glucose per kilogram administered orally, using the commercially available 40% oral glucose gel given into the buccal mucosa in combination with feedings, has been demonstrated as another treatment for neonatal hypoglycemia (Harris, Weston, Signal, Chase, & Harding, 2013). In the newborn with respiratory distress or other suspected illness, treatment should focus on the use of intravenous (IV) glucose administration. IV fluids should be started with a solution containing 10% dextrose and administered at a rate of 60 to 80 mL/kg/d. Frequent monitoring of blood glucoses with adjustment in the IV rate or an increase in dextrose concentration should occur if needed.

OUTCOMES

Sustained or repetitive hypoglycemia in infants has a major impact on normal brain development and function. Evidence suggests that hypoxemia and ischemia potentiate hypoglycemia cause brain damage that may permanently impair neurologic development. Therefore, neonates who have comorbidities should be monitored closely for hypoglycemia even when they are out of the immediate newborn period (Deshpande & Platt, 2005).

It is nursing's responsibility to be vigilant in monitoring infants with hypoglycemia. Most newborn nurseries and neonatal intensive care units have specific hypoglycemia protocols to follow. Encourage mothers to breastfeed frequently (every 1–2 hours). Education of parents is extremely important especially if the infant is being monitored in the NICU, which increases parental stress and anxiety.

Summary

Neonatal hypoglycemia can lead to major long-term sequelae, including neurologic injury resulting in mental retardation, recurrent seizure activity, developmental delay, and possibly impaired cardiovascular function. It is imperative for nurses to monitor infants closely and to be able to recognize and promptly treat hypoglycemia.

Adamkin, D. H., & American Academy of Pediatrics Committee on Fetus and Newborn. (2011). Postnatal glucose homeostasis in late-preterm and term infants. *Pediatrics, 127, 575–579.* doi:10.1542/peds.2010-3851

Cornblath, M., Hawdon, J. M., Williams, A. F., Aynsley-Green, A., Ward-Platt, M. P., Schwartz, R., & Kalhan, S. C. (2000). Controversies regarding definition of neonatal hypoglycemia: Suggested operational thresholds. *Pediatrics, 105*(5), 1141–1145. doi:10.1542/peds.105.5.1141

Deshpande, S., & Platt, M. (2005). The investigation and management of neonatal hypoglycemia. *Seminars in Fetal and Neonatal Medicine, 10,* 351–361. doi:10.1016/j.clp.2006.10.00

Garg, M., & Devaskar, S. (2006). Glucose metabolism in the late preterm infant. *Clinics in Perinatology, 33*(4), 853–870. doi:10.1016/j.clp.2006.10.001

Harris, D. L., Weston, P. J., Signal, M., Chase, J. G., & Harding, J. E. (2013). Dextrose gel for neonatal hypoglycemia (the Sugar Babies Study): A randomised, double-blind, placebo-controlled trial. *Lancet, 382*(9910), 2077–2083. doi:10.1016/S0140-6736(13)61645-1

Jain, A. (2008). Hypoglycemia in the newborn. *Indian Journal of Pediatrics, 75*(1), 63–66. doi:10.1007/s12098-008-0009-6

Straussman, S., & Levitsky, L. (2010). Neonatal hypoglycemia. *Current Opinion in Endocrinology, Diabetes & Obesity, 17,* 20–24. doi:10.1097/MED.0b013e328334f061

■ HYPOXIC ISCHEMIC ENCEPHALOPATHY

Ke-Ni Niko Tien

Overview

Hypoxic ischemic encephalopathy (HIE) is impaired gas exchange caused by a decrease in cerebral blood flow that results in hypoxemia (low blood oxygen levels), hypercarbia (elevated CO_2 levels), and severe consequence of global cerebral ischemia (Karlsen, 2013; Zanelli, Kaufman, & Stanley, 2016). HIE can also lead to neurologic injuries, seizures, and death. Intrauterine asphyxia, such as clotting of placental arteries, placental abruption, inflammatory process or perinatal infarction are the most common mechanism of hypoxic injury in term infants (Fatemi, Wilson, & Johnston, 2009). Evidence has shown that providing advanced quality care may reduce the incidence and severity of outcome of neonatal encephalopathy by half (Graham, Ruis, Hartman, Northington, & Fox, 2008).

Currently, the most promising therapy is neuroprotective/therapeutic hypothermia as indicated by intentional head or body cooling (Karlsen, 2013; Price-Douglas & Fernandes, 2015). However, cooling is primarily limited to levels III and IV neonatal intensive care units (NICUs), because of complex care issues that the infant may have. The infant may need to be transported to a tertiary care center (Barks, 2008; Price-Douglas & Fernandes, 2015). It is critical for health care providers at delivery to recognize newborns with HIE who may be candidates for cooling.

Background

The incidence of HIE is one in four cases per 1,000 live births in the United States (Wayock et al., 2014; Zanelli et al., 2016). Worldwide, there are approximately 840,000 neonatal deaths as a result of perinatal asphyxia (Zanelli et al., 2016). Severe hypoxemia may lead to the production of lactic acid during anaerobic glycolysis that results in metabolic acidosis (a low pH and an elevated base deficit), which is the most objective assessment of perinatal HIE (Graham et al., 2008; Karlsen, 2013). In addition, studies have shown an increase in seizures if the umbilical arterial pH is less than 7.0, as well as a significant increase in neurologic morbidities (Fatemi et al., 2009; Graham et al., 2008).

The criteria identified in determining intrapartum asphyxia in an infant are late decelerations on fetal monitoring or meconium/meconium-stained fluid at delivery; delayed respiratory effort after birth; arterial cord blood pH less than 7.1; Apgar score less than 7 at 5 minutes of age and multiorgan injury (Graham et al., 2008). However, studies have shown that numerous factors can contribute to low Apgar scores, such as intrapartum maternal sedation or anesthesia, congenital malformation, the appearance of infection, and the effectiveness of resuscitation. Therefore, the Apgar score alone is not the most reliable predictor for perinatal hypoxemia (Graham et al., 2008).

Severe HIE can lead to clinical seizures, epileptic activity seen on electroencephalogram (EEG), hypotonia, lack of gag reflex, poor feeding, and a prolonged depressed consciousness status. Infants who survive a birth asphyxia insult may develop neurologic sequelae such as cerebral palsy, mental retardation, learning difficulties, cognitive and motor deficits, as well as other disabilities (Karlsen, 2013; Zanelli et al., 2016).

Several clinical trials have shown the promising results of intentional hypothermia therapy (Fatemi et al., 2009). Clinical investigations have demonstrated an overall reduction in mortality and disability for infants who received hypothermia therapy (cooling) within the first 24 hours of life. Hypothermia therapy reduces cerebral metabolism and the inflammation process triggered by ischemic events (Fatemi et al., 2009). Currently, hypothermia therapy has become a standard of care in moderate to severe HIE treatment.

Accurately predicting the prognosis and severity of long-term complications of HIE is difficult. The lack of spontaneous respiratory effort for 20 to 30 minutes after birth; presence of frequent and uncontrollable seizure activity; prolonged abnormal clinical neurologic findings, including abnormal muscle tone and posture; abnormal background activity on EEG; persistent feeding difficulties because of abnormal sucking and swallowing and poor head growth are the most helpful indicators in determining possible long-term outcomes of HIE (Zanelli et al., 2016).

Clinical Aspects

ASSESSMENT

There are three levels of HIE: mild, moderately severe, and severe (Zanelli et al., 2016). Mild hypertonia, poor feeding, and irritability present during the first few days of life is categorized as mild HIE. Hypotonia, diminished grasp and gag, Moro reflex and suck, seizure activity, and apneic episodes may be seen when HIE is moderately severe. These symptoms may resolve within 1 to 2 weeks and lead to a better long-term outcome. In infants with severe HIE, seizures can be delayed, severe, and show resistance to conventional anticonvulsant therapy. Other symptoms of severe HIE may also include stupor or coma, respiratory failure requiring mechanical ventilation, generalized hypotonia and depressed reflexes, abnormal ocular motion such as nystagmus, dilated or fixed pupils, and arrhythmia as well as hypotension. These symptoms may worsen during the rewarming period and even cause death.

Therapeutic hypothermia/cooling therapy is the most promising treatment for HIE. The gold standard is to initiate cooling within 6 hours of birth to maximize an optimal outcome (Karlsen, 2013). Once cooling therapy is determined, passive (turning off the radiant warmer) or active cooling (placing an infant on a cooling blanket or head cooling) should be implemented.

All neonates who qualify for cooling therapy are cooled to a rectal temperature of 33.5°C or 92.3°F for 72 hours (Burton et al., 2015; Wayock et al., 2014; Zanelli et al., 2016). The criteria to determine whether or not to initiate cooling are a gestational age greater than or equal to 36 weeks and a birth weight greater than or equal to 1,800 g; umbilical cord blood gas or arterial blood gas obtained in the first hour of life with a pH less than or equal to 7.0; or base deficit greater than 16 mmol/L. Cooling also requires a neurologic examination denoting seizures, level of consciousness, spontaneous activity when awake or aroused, posture, tone, primitive reflexes, heart rate, respiratory rate, and reaction of pupils to light.

Seventy-two hours after being placed on a cooling blanket or cooling hat, a slow and controlled rewarming process should be cautiously performed and monitored. At present, there is limited evidence to indicate the safest way and speed to rewarm severely hypothermic infants. Based on the recommendation, rewarming speed should not exceed 0.5°C per hour to prevent sudden vasodilation, hypotension, and other clinical deterioration (Holton, 2014; Karlsen, 2013). During the rewarming period, vital signs, level of consciousness, neurologic examination, and blood gases should be closely monitored.

NURSING INTERVENTIONS, MANAGEMENT, AND IMPLICATIONS

It is critical for the nurse to closely monitor heart rate and rhythm, blood pressure, pulses, perfusion, respiratory rate and effort, oxygen saturation, acid–base status, and blood glucoses during both cooling and rewarming phases. Monitoring the rectal temperature is helpful, because the skin temperature of the infant is higher than the rectal temperature during the rewarming period. If an infant deteriorates rapidly during either the cooling or rewarming period, the nurse must be prepared to perform a full cardiopulmonary resuscitation.

It is important to monitor closely for any seizure activity. Continuous EEG monitoring is normally placed during the duration of cooling. A full montage EEG and an MRI should be obtained after an infant is rewarmed and stable.

It is essential to perform a complete neurologic examination with hands-on care, including pupils, level of consciousness, and any signs or symptoms of increased intracranial pressure. It is important to ensure appropriate sedation during cooling therapy to optimize comfort and efficacy of the cooling. Inadequate sedation increases metabolic rate and decreases the effectiveness of cooling.

It is critical to monitor intake and output closely as fluid is normally restricted to avoid fluid overload and cerebral edema. Infants who undergo cooling therapy are at risk for renal impairment and electrolyte imbalance, which requires frequent monitoring and correction of any imbalance.

Infants who receive cooling often are treated with antibiotics for possible infection. It is vital to monitor any signs and symptoms of infection. It is also important to monitor for any signs of coagulopathy such as petechiae. Infants may require transfusions because of coagulopathy induced by hypothermia and decreased platelet function.

It is critical to frequently assess the skin for possible subcutaneous fat necrosis. Erythematous nodules and plaques over boney areas such as the back, arms, buttocks, and thighs are the characteristic areas of subcutaneous fat necrosis that may worsen during cooling and can be very painful.

Families are an integral part of care for an infant admitted to the NICU. Continuous updates and support are essential to families while their babies undergo cooling therapy. It is important to encourage bonding by allowing parents to touch their baby and help with care.

OUTCOMES

Perinatal HIE is a major health issue globally. It can lead to neurologic deficits, neurodevelopmental disabilities, long-term functional impairments, and significant learning difficulties later on in a child's life. Although there are no effective pharmacologic therapies to treat HIE currently, intentional cooling therapy has been the most promising and has become the standard of care for moderate to severe HIE. All cooling criteria and a sound neurologic examination need to be carefully reviewed to determine if the infant is a candidate for this therapy.

Close monitoring of an infant, including thorough frequent assessments, is critical during the cooling and rewarming phase. It is important to understand and recognize any potential side effects. It is also vital to include parents and family in nursing care. Families must understand the reasons behind cooling therapy, the expected length of treatment, and the potential for long-term morbidities.

Summary

Current research supports the efficacy of intentional cooling treatment for infants who are more than or equal to 36 weeks gestation and more than or equal to 1,800 g. However, there has been significant research in HIE for multimodal therapeutic approaches, and many clinical trials are in the process to prove that cooling used on infants who are younger than 36 weeks is applicable and effective as well.

Barks, J. (2008). Technical aspects of starting a neonatal cooling program. *Clinics in Perinatology, 35*(4), 765–775. doi:10.1016/j.clp.2008.07.009

Fatemi, A., Wilson, M. A., & Johnston, M. V. (2009). Hypoxic-ischemic encephalopathy in the term infant. *Clinics in Perinatology, 36*(4), 835–858. doi:10.1016/j.clp.2009.07.011

Graham, E. M., Ruis, K. A., Hartman, A. L., Northington, F. J., & Fox, H. E. (2008). A systematic review of the role of intrapartum hypoxia-ischemia in the causation of neonatal encephalopathy. *American Journal of Obstetrics & Gynecology, 199*(6), 587–595. doi:10.1016/j.ajog.2008.06.094

Holton, T. (2014). Clinical guidelines (nursing): Therapeutic hypothermia in the neonate. *The Royal Children's Hospital Melbourne*. Retrieved from http://www.rch.org.au/rchcpg/hospital_clinical_guideline_index/Therapeutic_hypothermia_in_the_neonate

Karlsen, K. A. (2013). *The S.T.A.B.L.E. program: Pre-transport/post-resuscitation stabilization care of sick infants guidelines for neonatal healthcare providers* (6th ed.). Salt Lake City: UT: The S.T.A.B.L.E. Program.

Price-Douglas, W., & Fernandes, C. J. (2015). Infants with hypoxic-ischemic encephalopathy may need to be transported for therapeutic cooling. *AAP News, 36*(10). doi:10.1542/aapnews.20153610-15

Wayock, C. P., Meserole, R. L., Saria, S., Jennings, J. M., Huisman, T. A. G. M., Northington, F. J., & Graham, E. M. (2014). Perinatal risk factors for severe injury in neonates treated with whole-body hypothermia for encephalopathy. *American Journal of Obstetrics & Gynecology, 211*(1), 41.e1–41.e8. doi:10.1016/j.ajog.2014.03.033

Zanelli, S. A., Kaufman, D. A., & Stanley, D. (2016). Hypoxic-ischemic encephalopathy. In T. Rosenkrantz (Ed.), *Medscape*. Retrieved from http://emedicine.medscape.com/article/973501-overview

■ INCREASED PULMONARY BLOOD FLOW

Jennifer Johntony
Jodi Zalewski

Overview

Increased pulmonary blood flow may result in leakage of fluids into the interstitial space with subsequent pulmonary edema because of increased pulmonary pressures and congestion (Capozzi & Santoro, 2011). In patients with acyanotic congenital heart disease, this increase in pulmonary blood flow occurs in heart defects with left to right shunts. Cardiac shunting occurs when there is a diversion of normal blood flow. The type and location of the shunt, as well as the pathophysiology of the defect, determine the risk of potential complications from increased pulmonary blood blow. These complications include pulmonary bleeding, pulmonary hypertension, and eventually irreversible parenchymal lung disease. The most common congenital cardiac lesions related to increased pulmonary blood flow are patent ductus arteriosus (PDA), atrial septal defect (ASD), ventricular septal defect (VSD), and atrioventricular canal (AVC) defect also known as *endocardial cushion defect*.

Background

The PDA accounts for approximately 10% of newborns with cardiac defects, and is a normal part of fetal circulation (Park, 2016). In utero, oxygenated blood from the placental circulation bypasses the nonaerated fetal lungs and is delivered directly to the fetus's lower body organs (Capozzi & Santoro, 2011). The PDA is a vascular communication between the main pulmonary artery and the descending aorta. The degree of left to right shunting is determined by the size of the PDA, which includes measurement of the diameter, length, and level of pulmonary vascular resistance (Park, 2016). The PDA functionally closes within 48 hours after birth and by 2 weeks of age closes anatomically (Delaney, Baker, Bastardi, & O'Brien, 2015).

Isolated ASD accounts for 5% to 10% of all congenital heart defects and is most common in females (Park, 2016). ASDs are openings in the atrial septum that allow blood flow to shunt from the left side of the heart to the right side, leading to right atrial dilatation, right ventricular volume overload, and increased pulmonary blood flow (Jone, Darst, Collins, & Miyamoto, 2016).

There are four types of ASDs that can be distinguished by their location within the atrial septum: ostium secundum, sinus venosus, ostium primum, and coronary sinus. The type and location of the defect and/or enlargement of the right heart chambers determine what intervention is needed.

VSDs are the most common forms of congenital heart disease, accounting for 15% to 20% of all pediatric heart surgeries (Park, 2016). VSDs are openings in the ventricular septum that allow for blood flow to shunt from the left side of the heart to the right side, leading to left atrial dilation, left ventricular volume over-load, and increased pulmonary blood flow. If left to right shunting is significant at the ventricular level, there will be excessive pulmonary blood flow leading to pulmonary edema and tachypnea (Nelson et al., 2015). The effects of increased pulmonary blood flow depend on the size and number of defects and resistance to flow through the lungs.

There are three types of VSDs that can be distinguished by their location within the ventricular septum: perimembraneous, infundibular, and muscular defects. Infants with small VSDs usually do not require surgery. Infants with a large VSD are usually repaired by 1 year of age.

AVC defects account for 2% of all congenital heart diseases and 30% of these defects occur in children with Trisomy 21 (Park, 2016). AVC defects consist of three components: ostium primum ASD, an inlet VSD, and clefts in the mitral valve leaflet and the septal leaflet of the tricuspid valve (Park, 2016). AVC defects can be delineated into two categories: complete or partial. A complete AVC consists of an ASD, large VSD, and single atrioventricular valve; infants may have ventricular asymmetry which is categorized as an unbalanced AVC (Nelson et al., 2015). A partial AVC consists of an ASD with a cleft in the anterior leaflet of the left atrioventricular valve, no VSD, and two atrioventricular valves present (Nelson et al., 2015). The level of left to right shunting depends on several factors: the shunt can be interatrial and/or interventricular; if there is atrioventricular (AV) valve regurgitation present; or if there is a LV-RA shunt. The increase in left to right shunting increases atrial and ventricular volume overload with resultant increased pulmonary blood flow leading to congestive heart failure (CHF; Park, 2016).

Clinical Aspects

ASSESSMENT

The size and degree of shunting of the PDA determine symptoms (Delaney et.al, 2015). Patients with a small ductus usually are asymptomatic. However, if the defect is large with significant left to right shunting, infants can show signs of CHF (Park, 2016). Typical symptoms are tachypnea, tachycardia, and poor feeding. A widened pulse pressure and bounding pulses are also present owing to extra blood flow from the aorta to the pulmonary arteries (Delaney et al., 2015). The classic murmur of a PDA is a continuous "machinery" murmur heard best along the left upper sternal border (Nelson et al., 2015). Indications for surgical closure of a PDA are hemodynamic instability. PDAs can be closed by surgical repair or transcatheter closure in the cardiac catheterization laboratory (Park, 2016).

Patients with ASDs are usually asymptomatic but can develop signs of heart failure later in life if the ASD is undiagnosed (Delaney et al., 2015). The majority of ASDs can close spontaneously, but, if left untreated, infants are at risk for atrial dysrhythmias, pulmonary vascular obstructive disease, and emboli formation owing to increased pulmonary blood flow (Delaney et al., 2015). The classic physical findings in infants with ASDs include widely split and fixed S2 and a grade 2–3/6 systolic ejection murmur heard best at the left upper sternal border. This occurs because of increased flow across a normal pulmonary valve (Park, 2016). The three main interventions of choice are no therapy, if the right side of the heart is not enlarged; surgical closure; or transcatheter device closure; which has become the treatment of choice.

Patients with small VSDs are asymptomatic and the defect usually closes within the first 2 years of life. A VSD typically has a grade 2–5/6 holosystolic murmur that is best heard at the left lower sternal border. Small VSDs have louder murmurs because of restrictive blood flow (Park, 2016). Larger VSDs can cause symptoms of CHF, which include tachypnea, hepatomegaly, poor feeding, and failure to thrive (Nelson et al., 2015). If the infant has significant heart failure, diuretics as well as digoxin and beta-blockers may be initiated until surgical closure of the VSD can be performed.

Patients with AVC present early in infancy with signs and symptoms of CHF when there is both atrial-level and ventricular-level shunting (Nelson et al., 2015). Infants, on physical examination, have a hyperactive precordium with a prominent thrill. A grade III to IV/VI holosystolic murmur can be heard best at the left sternal border (Park, 2016). Infants can be optimized on heart failure medications until they are ready for surgical repair (Nelson et al., 2015).

NURSING INTERVENTIONS, MANAGEMENT, AND IMPLICATIONS

Nursing-related problems specific to infants with increased pulmonary blood flow focus on the management of pulmonary overcirculation and CHF. Infants with increased pulmonary blood flow can experience impaired myocardial function, pulmonary congestion, and systemic venous congestion (Delaney et al., 2015).

Due diligence by nursing with respect to the infant's cardiac anatomy and baseline clinical presentation is vital in order to intervene when changes occur. The nurse must assess and record heart rate, respiratory rate, breath sounds, blood pressure, and pulse oximetry readings. Infants with myocardial dysfunction present with tachycardia, diaphoresis, and irritability. Improvement in cardiac function includes the administration of digitalis glycosides (digoxin) and angiotensin-converting enzyme (ACE) inhibitors (Delaney et al., 2015). Prescribed cardiac medications need to be given at the scheduled time and any side effects or signs and symptoms of toxicity should be reported and documented (Delaney et al., 2015). Nurses must assess and document signs of pulmonary overcirculation such as tachypnea, retractions, nasal flaring, grunting, and wheezing because of decreased lung compliance. Administration of oxygen may assist in improving gas exchange. Increased blood flow to the heart and lungs may result in orthopnea, which can be alleviated by placing the infant in the recumbent position. Increased pressure and pooling of blood in the venous circulation are caused by systemic venous congestion because of right-sided heart failure and may result in hepatomegaly, edema, and fluid retention (Delaney et al., 2015). The nurse must monitor laboratory results, document frequent intake and output measurements, and assess for clinical signs of fluid overload, including periorbital and peripheral edema, and increased work of breathing. The administration of diuretics is the standard treatment to eliminate excess water and salt from the body. The most commonly used diuretic for treatment of right-sided heart failure in infants is furosemide.

In any infant born with a cardiac defect, alteration in parenting related to the perception of the infant as vulnerable may be present. Clear communication between all members of the health care team and the family is paramount. In addition, it is the nurses' responsibility to provide knowledge and skills to these families. This includes newborn care and adequate nutrition; safe administration of medications; learning signs of heart failure, possible complications, and when to call their primary care provider.

OUTCOMES

Infants with congenital heart disease that result in an increase in pulmonary blood flow have outcomes specific to evidence-based nursing practice that focuses on assisting the infant in having improvement in cardiac function, reduction in accumulated fluid and sodium, a decrease in cardiac demands, improvement in tissue oxygenation, and a decrease in oxygen consumption (Delaney et al., 2015).

Improvement in cardiac function occurs when there is a decrease in the afterload of the heart, thereby increasing the overall cardiac output. ACE inhibitors reduce afterload on the heart, allowing for it to pump more easily and its ability to contract is improved with the administration of digoxin. In infants with increased pulmonary blood flow and right-sided heart failure, management of fluid and sodium retention consists of diuretic therapy. The overall goal for infants with pulmonary overcirculation is to decrease cardiac demands. The nurse can facilitate this by performing interventions that decrease the work load of the heart. Examples of these interventions include minimizing metabolic needs by providing a neutral thermal environment to avoid stress to the infant, treating infections, reducing the infant's efforts or breathing, administering sedative medication if extremely irritable, decreasing external stimuli, decreasing environmental stimuli, and providing uninterrupted rest (Delaney et al., 2015). Improving the function of the myocardium and lessening the tissue oxygen demand result in improved tissue oxygenation. Oxygen administration helps improve respiratory function and gas exchange.

Summary

Infants born with cardiac defects resulting in an increased pulmonary blood flow include PDA, ASD, VSD, and AV canal. Sustained pulmonary congestion from pulmonary overcirculation in the infant can lead to serious complications, including pulmonary hemorrhage, elevated pulmonary pressures, and irreversible lung damage. Patients are at risk for right-sided heart failure and poor weight gain. Understanding the anatomy and physiology of each specific patient's cardiac anatomy is imperative to caring for the infant effectively. Providing efficient and holistic nursing care to hospitalized infants with congenital heart disease results in increased survival and quality of life in this vulnerable patient population.

Capozzi, G., & Santoro, G. (2011). Patent ductus arteriosus: Patho-physiology, hemodynamic effects and clinical complications. *The Journal of Maternal-Fetal and Neonatal Medicine, 24*(Suppl. 1), 15–16. doi:10.3109/14767058.2011.607564

Delaney, A., Baker, A., Bastardi, H., & O'Brien, P. (2015). The child with cardiovascular dysfunction. In M. Hockenberry, D. Wilson, & C. Rodgers (Eds.), *Wong's nursing care of infants and children* (10th ed., pp. 738–744). St. Louis, MO: Elsevier Mosby.

Jone, P.-N., Darst, J., Collins, K., & Miyamoto, S. (2016). Cardiovascular diseases. In W. Hay, Jr., M. Levin, R. Deterding, & M. Abzug (Eds.), *Current diagnosis & treatment pediatrics* (23rd ed., pp. 550–610). New York, NY: McGraw-Hill. Retrieved from http://accessmedicine.mhmedical.com/content.aspx?bookid=1795&Section id=125741666

Nelson, J., Hirsch-Romano, J., Ohye, R., & Bove, E. (2015). Congenital heart disease. In G. M. Doherty (Ed.), *Current diagnosis & treatment: Surgery* (14th ed., pp. 423–454). New York, NY: McGraw-Hill.

Park, M. (2016). *The pediatric cardiology handbook* (pp. 99–115). Philadelphia, PA: Elsevier Saunders.

■ INFANT OF A DIABETIC MOTHER

Mary F. Terhaar

Overview

Globally, the number of people living with diabetes mellitus is expected to rise to 592 million by 2035 (Guariguata et al., 2014). Many mothers and infants will be impacted because every pregnancy complicated by maternal diabetes is a pregnancy at risk. Despite a benign history, insulin deficiency or resistance develops during pregnancy in some women. The prevalence of this condition, called *gestational diabetes*, is approximately 2% to 6% globally and as high as 9.2% in the United States (DeSisto, Kim, & Sharma, 2014; Mitanchez, Burguet, & Simeoni, 2014). In both diabetes mellitus and gestational diabetes, unstable and often excessive glucose levels are a defining characteristic and may be linked to adverse fetal and neonatal outcomes.

Background

The infant of a diabetic mother (IDM) is at risk for numerous complications and requires careful monitoring during the early neonatal period. Two distinct clinical pictures present: the first is associated with overnutrition and the second with teratogenesis.

Gestational diabetes is a frequent clinical presentation in the pregnant woman and occurs when maternal glucose intolerance develops. The mother lacks sufficient functioning insulin and develops a persistent excess of her own serum glucose. The glucose-rich serum is perfused to the fetus, which results in fetal hyperglycemia. The fetus adapts by producing higher-than-normal levels of insulin in order to maintain fetal glucose levels within normal range. The fetus then converts and stores excess glucose as fat. The result is an overnourished, hyperinsulinemic, macrosomic infant. Complications associated with overnutrition and macrosomia include difficult labor, cephalo-pelvic disproportion, possible cesarean section, shoulder dystocia, birth trauma, hemorrhage, glucose instability, temperature instability, and respiratory distress in the first few days of life. For these neonates, unstable maternal insulin and glucose levels are associated with increased rates of perinatal asphyxia (Riskin & Garcia-Prats, 2016).

The second clinical presentation occurs when unrecognized or poorly controlled diabetes precedes pregnancy or complicates the early weeks of pregnancy. High serum glucose levels can be teratogenic during early fetal development and result in cardiovascular and neural malformations. These defects can lead to first-trimester loss, fetal demise, or serious congenital anomalies. Referred to as *diabetic embryopathy*, these complications are the direct result of pregestational diabetes (Hay, 2012; Riskin & Garcia-Prats, 2016). Pregnancy complicated by diabetes can lead to intrapartum complications, preterm birth, altered glucose metabolism, respiratory problems, and difficulty transitioning to extrauterine life (Mitanchez et al., 2015).

Clinical Aspects

A careful history, including family history of diabetes, mother's health before and during this pregnancy as well as previous pregnancies (including birthweight of infants), are key to interpreting the clinical picture, evaluating risks, stabilizing glucose levels, and preventing complications.

ASSESSMENT

Head-to-toe assessment by the bedside nurse will aid in identifying risks for complications in the IDM. Any infant with a birth weight greater than 90% on the growth chart for gestational age or greater than 4,000 g birth weight is classified as macrosomic and at risk for potential complications as an IDM (Hay, 2012; Riskin & Garcia-Prats, 2016).

NURSING INTERVENTIONS, MANAGEMENT, AND IMPLICATIONS

IDMs who present as macrosomic, overnourished, or hyperinsulinemic face many challenges requiring careful monitoring and support by nursing. Chief among these are low serum glucose concentrations; respiratory distress; electrolyte imbalances; polycythemia, cardiomegaly, and hyperbilirubinemia; temperature instability; feeding difficulties; and poor state regulation (Mitanchez et al., 2014; Riskin & Garcia-Prats, 2016).

Low blood glucose levels are an issue in the IDM. Accustomed to high-circulating serum glucose levels provided by the mother through the placenta, the IDM has become efficient in producing insulin to normalize blood glucose. After cutting the umbilical cord, the glucose supply from the mother is terminated resulting in glucose levels in the newborn to fall precipitously. As a result, the formerly adaptive elevated insulin levels also cause glucose levels to drop. Frequent glucose monitoring starting between 1 and 3 hours of life is necessary until levels stabilize. Serum glucose levels below 47 mg/dL are considered hypoglycemic and require intervention. However, thresholds vary by institutions (Sweet, Grayson, & Polak, 2013).

Early feedings help prevent or attenuate low serum glucose levels. Breastfeeding can be initiated in the delivery room and sustained through the early neonatal period. However, robust research to support this practice is not available (East, Dolan, & Forster, 2014). Some infants will be jittery, lethargic, or too unstable to breastfeed or take oral fluids. For this group of infants, providing intravenous (IV) glucose fluids at 4 to 6 mg/kg/min will meet metabolic demands and will not stimulate insulin responses that further decrease serum glucose (Riskin & Garcia-Prats, 2016).

Fetal hyperinsulinemia can have two diametrically opposed outcomes on the lungs. In some cases, hyperinsulinemia acts as a stressor, which may cause fetal steroid levels to rise, and trigger lung maturation. Therefore, the pulmonary development may be more advanced than expected for gestational age. However, hyperinsulinemia may inhibit maturation of airways and production of surfactant, resulting in respiratory distress (Riskin & Garcia-Prats, 2016).

Careful monitoring of pulse oximetry and respiratory assessment is required. Supplemental oxygen, artificial surfactant, and ventilator support may be needed.

Hyperinsulinemia may lead to hypoparathyroidism, hypomagnesemia, and hypocalcemia, which may result in acidosis because of the release of intracellular phosphorous. The hypocalcemic IDM will present as jittery and irritable and may develop myocardial hypocontractility (Hay, 2012). When serum levels are found to be low, breast milk or formula feedings are indicated. Recalcitrant hypocalcemia may indicate underlying hypomagnesemia and require correction with IV replacement (Mimouni, Mimouni, & Bental, 2013).

Elevated maternal glucose levels and resultant glycation of hemoglobin can reduce the oxygen-carrying capacity of fetal hemoglobin, which then stimulates erythropoiesis and results in polycythemia (Mitanchez et al., 2015). Simultaneously, fetal hyperglycemia and hyperinsulinemia increase metabolic demands of the placenta and fetus leading to increased oxygen consumption by both (Hay, 2012). Diminished capacity accompanies increased demand. Although polycythemia increases the oxygen-carrying capacity of fetal blood and is adaptive for the hyperinsulinemic fetus, it can lead to both cardiomyopathy and hyperbilirubinemia. In IDMs with cardiomyopathy, the heart muscle of the fetus hypertrophies as a result of generating increased cardiac output to compensate for low oxygen-carrying capacity of the blood, and from the increased effort of pumping blood, which is high in hemoglobin. This infant requires careful monitoring of heart rate, blood pressure (BP), cardiac output, and fluid status.

Hyperbilirubinemia develops when the IDM breaks down the surplus red blood cells that characterize polycythemia, conjugate the waste as bilirubin, and then eliminate the bilirubin in urine and stool. Hyperbilirubinemia is also exaggerated by macrosomia, which can contribute to difficult labor and result in bruising of the head and face. As bruising resolves, blood is resorbed and broken down, producing bilirubin that exceeds the capacity of the liver to conjugate and the kidneys and gastrointestinal tract to eliminate. The result is elevated serum bilirubin levels, which present as jaundice to the skin, conjunctiva, and mucous membranes; reduce alertness in the infant; and may cause feeding difficulties. The jaundiced infant will require assessment of serum bilirubin levels at intervals, frequent feedings to facilitate elimination of bilirubin in urine and stool, and phototherapy to increase trans-epithelial elimination of bilirubin (Wong & Bhutani, 2016). Phototherapy is commonly required and, in severe cases, exchange transfusions may be indicated.

Thermoregulation may be an issue for the distressed IDM. Gestational diabetes and macrosomia predispose the IDM to intrapartum complications, which result in a fatigued infant with little reserve to maintain body temperature. Careful monitoring by nursing is key. The infant will benefit from skin-to-skin care or from external heat sources. Maintaining the newborn in a neutral thermal environment will decrease oxygen requirements and reduce the likelihood of chemical thermogenesis.

Low serum glucose levels, a stressful delivery, and immaturity of the infant can result in poor state regulation, decreased the alert time for feeding and socializing, and feeding difficulties. Until insulin levels normalize, infants require frequent small feedings (as frequently as every 2 hours). Colostrum is most precisely suited for metabolic needs and is thought to minimize rebound hyperinsulinemia following feedings. Formula feedings are initiated if breastfeeding is not planned, and for infants whose glucose levels fall below 40 mg/dL, IV fluids with glucose are initiated (Riskin & Garcia-Prats, 2016).

Shoulder dystocia may result when a macrosomic infant is delivered to a mother with cephalo-pelvic disproportion. A difficult and prolonged second phase of labor may occur in which forceps or vacuum extraction may be used to facilitate delivery. This places infants at increased risk for complications, including fractured clavicle, Erb's palsy, Klumpke's paralysis, diaphragmatic nerve paralysis, or laryngeal nerve damage (Hay, 2012). The affected infant will present with asymmetrical tone and flexion in the arms and shoulders, asymmetry in the face, or abnormal cry. Nursing care is taken to maintain and support the arm and shoulder in good alignment. The infant is positioned for comfort and support in the affected limb (Mitanchez et al., 2014). Pediatric neurology follow-up is recommended.

The macrosomic infant who experiences a difficult labor and delivery can be fatigued and distressed at birth. This infant requires supportive care and may have little energy for feeding and bonding with the mother. Skin-to-skin care can help promote thermal stability and facilitate frequent feedings. Surveillance of pulse oximetry, glucose levels, respiratory status, temperature, and nutritional intake is important (Hay, 2012).

The infant may have bruising especially of the head and face and may have a cephalohematoma, or other bruising from assisted delivery. The infant may experience pain or discomfort, fatigue, and may develop hyperbilirubinemia. Observation, supportive care, and management of hyperbilirubinemia should begin as soon as laboratory values are confirmed (Hay, 2012).

Every newborn must make many complex adaptations in the first few minutes and hours of life. The adaptation for an IDM depends on vigilant nursing care and monitoring of cardiovascular, respiratory, metabolic, and thermoregulatory functions, as well as behavior and infant bonding. Preventing complications and long-term sequelae are the goals.

OUTCOMES

In the short term, the weight of the IDM normalizes because surplus insulin levels normalize, allowing clearance of excess fluid and fat stores. As a consequence, the burden on the heart and lungs is reduced and the infant can capably assume the work of respiration, circulation, and perfusion. As polycythemia resolves, the liver, kidneys, and intestines are better able to remove waste, process bilirubin, and resolve jaundice.

Long-term implications of overnutrition include increased the risk for diabetes mellitus, heart disease, and renal problems (Mitanchez et al., 2014). The best treatment then is prevention, and the best care for the newborn is the management of the pregnancy and care for the other.

Summary

The IDM presents as a fatigued, distressed, and fragile newborn. Their large size may create the impression of a robust newborn. In reality, they are not and require careful attention as they transition to extrauterine life. Careful management of all the complexities of the disease can contribute to the resolution of the imbalances in many interrelated body systems. Best practices include preventive care, frequent assessment, monitoring of all systems affected, and skin-to-skin care to keep the infant in a supportive, comfortable environment with easy and timely access to breast milk or nutrition.

DeSisto, C. L., Kim, S. Y., & Sharma, A. J. (2014). Prevalence estimates of gestational diabetes mellitus in the United States, Pregnancy Risk Assessment Monitoring System (PRAMS), 2007-2010. *Preventing Chronic Disease, 11*, E104. doi:10.5888/pcd11.130415

East, C. E., Dolan, W. J., & Forster, D. A. (2014). Antenatal breast milk expression by women with diabetes for improving infant outcomes. *Cochrane Database of Systematic Reviews, 2014*(7), CD010408. doi:10.1002/14651858.CD010408.pub2

Guariguata, L., Whiting, D. R., Hambleton, I., Beagley, J., Linnenkamp, U., & Shaw, J. E. (2014). Global estimates of diabetes prevalence for 2013 and projections for 2035. *Diabetes Research and Clinical Practice, 103*(2), 137–149. doi:10.1016/j.diabres.2013.11.002

Hay, W. W., Jr. (2012). Care of the infant of the diabetic mother. *Current Diabetes Reports, 12*(1), 4–15. doi:10.1007/s11892-011-0243-6

Mimouni, F., Mimouni, G., & Bental, Y. (2013). Neonatal management of infant of diabetic mother. *Pediatrics and Therapeutics, 4*(1), 1–4. doi:10.4172/2161-0665.1000186

Mitanchez, D., Burguet, A., & Simeoni, U. (2014). Infants born to mothers with gestational diabetes mellitus: Mild neonatal effects, a long-term threat to global health. *The Journal of Pediatrics, 164*(3), 445–450. doi:10.1016/j.jpeds.2013.10.076

Mitanchez, D., Yzydorczyk, C., Siddeek, B., Boubred, F., Benahmed, M., & Simeoni, U. (2015). The offspring of the diabetic mother: Short- and long-term implications. *Best Practice & Research, Clinical Obstetrics & Gynaecology, 29*(2), 256–269. doi:10.1016/j.bpobgyn.2014.08.004

Riskin, A., & Garcia-Prats, J. A. (2016). Infant of a diabetic mother. In M. S. Kim (Ed.), *UpToDate*. Retrieved from https://www.uptodate.com/contents/infant-of-a-diabetic-mother#H12

Sweet, C. B., Grayson, S., & Polak, M. (2013). Management strategies for neonatal hypoglycemia. *The Journal of Pediatric Pharmacology and Therapeutics, 18*(3), 199–208. doi:10.5863/1551-6776-18.3.199

Wong, R. J., & Bhutani, V. K. (2016). Treatment of unconjugated hyperbilirubinemia in term and late preterm infants. In M. S. Kim (Ed.), *UpToDate*. Retrieved from https://www.uptodate.com/contents/treatment-of-unconjugated-hyperbilirubinemia-in-term-and-late-preterm-infants?source=see_link

■ INTRAVENTRICULAR HEMORRHAGE

Helene M. Lannon

Overview

Neonatal intracranial hemorrhage is a complication of premature birth. Intraventricular hemorrhage (IVH) is defined as bleeding in or around the ventricles of the brain with potential for extended bleeding into the white matter of the brain, periventricular leukomalacia (PVL). PVL is defined as injury and death of areas of white matter tissue around fluid-filled ventricles and usually results from an extension of IVH (Annibale, 2014). The incidence of IVH/PVL increases as birth weight and gestation decrease. Full-term infants rarely experience IVH, but may develop a subarachnoid hemorrhage as related to pregnancy risk factors or a complication of delivery. The most vulnerable infants are those born prematurely less than 34 weeks gestation, with a threefold risk for very-low-birth-weight infants (VLBW) born between 28 and 32 weeks gestation and of VLBW, 1,001 to 1,500 g (Blackburn, 2015). IVH may cause serious disabilities involving cognitive and motor deficits, vision, and hearing. The onset of IVH occurs in the majority of the time by 72 hours of life and 99.5% occur on day 7 of life (Annibale, 2014). Although the incidence of IVH has started to decline in recent years, IVH remains a significant cause of morbidity and mortality in premature infants (Annibale, 2014). Prevention of preterm birth is not always possible. Treatment after delivery depends on early diagnosis and demonstration of meticulous supportive nursing care.

Background

Brain formation and cerebral blood flow are factors that influence the incidence of IVH. Volpe (2009) notes that preterm infants are at risk for IVH because birth occurs during the time of peak brain synaptogenesis and developmental differentiation, with the migration of cells to match with specific receptor sites and organize the central nervous system. The subependymal germinal matrix (SEGM) is the prominent area of cell growth. It is an extremely vascularized area with high oxygen needs to nourish glial cell growth that strengthens membranes. It matures by 36 weeks of gestation (Blackburn, 2015).

After birth, cerebral blood flow increases to meet oxygen demands. A steady blood flow is maintained by the mechanism of autoregulation. Autoregulation is the ability to maintain cerebral blood flow regardless of changes in cerebral perfusion pressure from physiologic changes; cerebral vessels constrict when pressure rises and dilate when pressure decreases (Elser, Holditch-Davis, & Brandon, 2011). This mechanism is mature at term. However, in prematurity, flow is pressure-passive, and systemic blood pressure becomes the primary determinant of cerebral blood flow and pressure (Annibale, 2014). The absence of autoregulation or severe changes in cerebral blood flow is hypothesized to cause central nervous system IVH (Elser et al., 2011).

Papile (2006) established the first grading system to define IVH that is used today. Classified as a small IVH are grades I and II. Grade I IVH is limited to the SEGM, often localized at the Foramen of Monroe. Grade II IVH has a partial filling of the lateral ventricle(s) without ventricular dilation. Grade III IVH includes ventricular hemorrhage with dilation. Severe grade IV IVH includes ventricular dilation with the parenchymal extension of blood into the cerebral tissue. Extension into the white matter of the brain is PVL that consists of ischemic lesions and multicystic encephalomalacia (Scher, 2013).

Mortality from severe IVH/PVL ranges from 27% to 50%. Low-grade I IVH usually resolves with only a 5% mortality rate, and grade II IVH has a 10% mortality rate (Annibale, 2014). Morbidity depends on the extension of the bleed. Approximately 25% to 30% of premature infants with grade I to II IVH will be discharged without major sequelae.

Clinical Aspects

Optimal screening is by cranial ultrasound because of its easy availability, relatively low cost, and its high resolution to identify bleeding. The study is performed at the bedside at day 7 of life as most IVH will occur by this time. For those infants who are of VLBW and unstable after birth, the ultrasound may be done within the first 72 hours of life. Serial ultrasounds are warranted based on the clinical course; however, some institutions will do routine screening for IVH at 30 to 60 and 90 days of age as PVL may appear as late as 6 to 10 weeks (Volpe, 2008). Additional radiologic studies include MRI to help detect slowly progressing hemorrhage, as well as extracerebral or infratentorial hemorrhages (Hawkins, 2015). CT scan is not an appropriate screening tool for PVL because of the exposure to radiation and transfer of a fragile, preterm infant to the radiology department. It is typically used for diagnosing subarachnoid hemorrhage in full-term infants.

ASSESSMENT

IVH results from premature birth; therefore, assessment begins antenatally with good prenatal care. Identification of a high-risk pregnancy with potential for premature birth, such as pregnancy-induced hypertension, maternal drug use, sepsis, or clotting disorders, must be noted in the maternal history. Transporting the mother fetus dyad to deliver at a tertiary care center is essential.

Scar formation at the initial site of bleeding is seen on cranial ultrasound as porencephalic cysts. Cerebral infarction may initiate the fibrinolytic cascade causing bleeding that extends into the white matter of the brain leading to PVL. However, IVH may also be asymptomatic and found on routine ultrasound.

NURSING INTERVENTIONS, MANAGEMENT, AND IMPLICATIONS

Assessment of clinical signs that indicate potential IVH may be subtle, dramatic, or asymptomatic. Subtle symptoms are evidenced by changes in tone, movement, or changes in respirations. However, IVH may have a catastrophic presentation with sudden onset hypotension, apnea/bradycardia, desaturation, full or bulging fontanel, decerebrate posturing, or a sudden drop in hematocrit. Sudden desaturation, bradycardia, hypotonia, and metabolic acidosis on blood sampling may precede dramatic changes of apnea; increased ventilator support; a decrease in hematocrit; decreased level of consciousness/activity; full, tense fontanel; and possible seizures. Nursing care is based on prevention and correction of any of these signs.

Evidence-based nursing research is limited for interventions specific to IVH because signs and outcomes are limited to retrospective studies that are complicated by other morbidities associated with prematurity. Major components of nursing care are aimed to reduce activities that can lead to hypoxia or asphyxia events, or rapid alterations and fluctuations in systemic blood pressure (Blackburn, 2015).

Oxygenation and perfusion are assessed by vital signs, oxygen saturation, and blood gases to maintain acid–base balance and perfusion pressures (Ditzenberger & Blackburn, 2014). Coagulopathies are corrected to prevent shock, and infusions of blood products or fluid boluses are administered slowly.

Comfort measures to avoid rapid swings in blood pressure that also promote physiologic support include clustering care to decrease periods of stimulation; limiting crying; positioning the VLBW infant in a neutral position with head midline and supine, avoiding neck flexion; and swaddling. Also, raising the head of the bed slightly, avoiding raising legs above head level as with a diaper change; avoiding the use of constrictive head bands and constrictive bilirubin eye shields; as well as good nutritional support and maintaining the neutral thermal environment are important (Ditzenberger & Blackburn, 2014).

Parental bonding is facilitated by including the family in the plan of care and teaching the family developmentally supportive care of handling and positioning techniques that will reduce environmental stress for their infant (Blackburn, 2015). Neurology and/or neurosurgical consultations are necessary to monitor the progression of IVH/PVL that may be lifelong. A social service referral is made for family emotional and financial support, with the identification of available intervention programs in the family's community to facilitate the infant's growth and development.

OUTCOMES

Outcomes from neurological sequelae of IVH/PVL cannot be predicted. Studies rely on results from retrospective studies and reports from clinic follow-up data. The outcome depends on the extent and location of the injury. Severe hemorrhage accompanies an 80% chance for neurodevelopmental disabilities along with potential seizures, hydrocephalus, and cerebral palsy (Scher, 2013). Cognitive dysfunction in learning, memory, and language; attention and socialization; vision, hearing, motor issues, and behavioral issues can continue into school age and adulthood. These sequelae occur in 15% to 25% of those born weighing less than 1,500 g birth weight and more than 50% in those less than 750 g birth weight (Blackburn, 2015).

Summary

The primary risk for IVH/PVL is prematurity. Multiple interventions needed to support premature organ function and environmental factors of handling, sound, and temperature change affect cerebral blood flow and pressure and place the infant at risk for IVH. Once an IVH occurs, the treatment is to prevent extension through supportive nursing care. There is no cure for IVH. The incidence of IVH/PVL has decreased over the years because of improved prenatal care with treatment to prevent preterm birth. Retrospective studies and data from clinical follow-up reports show promising outcomes for those infants with a small IVH; however, severe IVH holds a high risk for neurodevelopment morbidities that can extend into adulthood. Therefore, nursing education in understanding the risks for developing IVH and subsequent bedside care are key in preventing IVH.

Annibale, D. (2014). Periventricular hemorrhage-intraventricular hemorrhage. In T. Rosenkrantz (Ed.), *Medscape*. Retrieved from http://emedicine.medscape.com/article/976654-overview

Blackburn, S. (2015). Brain injury in preterm infants: Pathogenesis and nursing implications. *Newborn and Infant Nursing Reviews, 16*(1), 8–12. doi:10.1053/j.nainr.2015.12.004

Ditzenberger, G. R., & Blackburn, S. T. (2014). Neurologic system. In C. Kenner & J. W. Lott (Eds.), *Comprehensive neonatal nursing care* (5th ed., pp. 392–437). New York, NY: Springer Publishing.

Elser, H. E., Holditch-Davis, D., & Brandon, D. H. (2011). Cerebral oxygenation monitoring: A strategy to detect intraventricular hemorrhage and periventricular leukomalacia. *Newborn and Infant Nursing Reviews, 11*(3), 153–159. doi:10.1053/j.nainr.2011.07.007

Hawkins, C. E. (2015). Perinatal intracranial hemorrhages: Pathology. In A. M. Adesina (Ed.), *Medscape*. Retrieved from http://emedicine.medscape.com/article/2059564-overview

Papile, L. (2006). Intracranial hemorrhage and vascular lesions. In A. A. Fanaroff, R. J. Martin, & M. C. Walsh (Eds.), *Fanaroff and Martin's neonatal perinatal medicine: Diseases of the fetus and infant* (8th ed., pp. 891–899). Philadelphia, PA: Elsevier Mosby.

Scher, M. S. (2013). Brain disorders of the fetus and neonate. In A. A. Fanaroff & J. M. Fanaroff (Eds.), *Klaus and Fanaroff's care of the high-risk neonate* (6th ed., pp. 476–524). Philadelphia, PA: Elsevier Saunders.

Volpe, J. J. (2008). *Neurology of the newborn* (5th ed.). Philadelphia, PA: Elsevier Saunders.

Volpe, J. J. (2009). Cerebellum of the premature infant: Rapidly developing, vulnerable, clinically important. *Journal of Child Neurology, 24*(9), 1085–1104. doi:10.1177/0883073809338067

■ LATE PRETERM INFANT

Donna A. Dowling

Overview

Over the past 10 years, the specific needs of infants born late preterm, between 34 0/7 and 36 6/7 weeks of gestation, have been identified. These infants, who constitute more than 70% of all preterm births, have increased morbidity and mortality when compared to infants born at term. This entry provides an overview of current assessment and management approaches for this unique group of infants.

Background

Until 2005, the late preterm infant (LPI), born between 34 and 36 6/7 weeks of gestation, was not recognized as a unique subset of preterm infants (Raju, Higgins, Stark, & Leveno, 2006). In 2014, LPIs constituted 72% of all preterm infants born before 37 weeks of gestation (Hamilton, Martin, Osterman, Curtin, & Mathews, 2015). These infants, who, owing to their weight and appearance, can seem to be full term, have an increased risk of morbidities and mortality when compared to term infants (Barfield & Lee, 2016). These risks include sepsis, respiratory (transient tachypnea and respiratory distress syndrome [RDS]), metabolic (thermoregulation and hypoglycemia) and gastrointestinal (hyperbilirubinemia and feeding issues) problems, as well as the long-term risk of developmental delay (Vohr, 2013). Consequently, approximately 50% of LPIs require admission to the neonatal intensive care unit (NICU), which results in significant family stress and increased health care cost. It is essential that health care providers be proactive in the identification and management of this group of high-risk neonates.

Clinical Aspects

ASSESSMENT

The morbidities associated with late preterm birth, which increase with decreasing gestational age (Horgan, 2015), reflect the critical phase of development of the fetus that is interrupted when the infant is required to transition to extrauterine life. Owing to a decreased store of heat-generating brown adipose tissue, increased body surface to weight ratio, less white adipose tissue for insulation, as well as an underdeveloped hormonal response to cold, LPIs cannot conserve heat or respond adequately to heat loss (Phillips et al., 2013). The subsequent cold stress can impact the transition to extrauterine life by increasing oxygen and glucose requirements which, in turn, contribute to the development of respiratory distress and hypoglycemia.

LPIs are at risk for respiratory morbidities such as transient tachypnea of the newborn (TTN) and RDS. These morbidities reflect functional immaturity of lung structures, resulting in inadequate reabsorption of intrapulmonary fluid that predisposes the infant to TTN and inadequate surfactant production that predisposes the infant to RDS (Horgan, 2015). Both TTN and RDS increase oxygen and glucose requirements and possibly the need for assisted ventilation. In addition, because of immature development of brain stem function, including upper airway control and chemical control of breathing, LPIs are at increased risk for apnea of prematurity.

LPIs are two to three times more likely to have an episode of hypoglycemia in the neonatal period (Horgan, 2015). All infants respond to the loss of the glucose supply that occurs with cord clamping through glucogenolysis. However, LPIs have low glycogen stores and reduced function of gluconeogenic and glycolytic enzymes (Barfield & Lee, 2016), putting them at risk for hypoglycemia, especially if the first feeding is delayed.

LPIs are at twice the risk for hyperbilirubinemia at 5 days of age compared to term infants because of poor elimination of bilirubin and an increased bilirubin load related to red blood cell breakdown (Barfield & Lee, 2016). Poor elimination of bilirubin is related to low intestinal motility and inadequate or delayed feeding and the resulting increase in bilirubin puts the infant at risk for kernicterus (bilirubin neurotoxicity; Horgan, 2015).

LPIs have poor muscle tone, fatigue easily, and have difficulty coordinating sucking, swallowing, and breathing (Horgan, 2015), putting them at risk for poor feeding outcomes. This is of particular concern for infants who are breastfeeding, as good muscle strength and stamina are needed to latch correctly onto the breast and suck adequately to initiate and maintain milk transfer. Failure to adequately empty the breast results in poor milk production, putting the infant at risk for dehydration and suboptimal weight gain, which can delay discharge or be a reason for rehospitalization (Baker, 2015). Consequently, mothers may discontinue breastfeeding prematurely, citing an inadequate milk supply and breastfeeding difficulty as the reasons (Kair & Colaizy, 2016).

A significant increase in brain growth occurs between 34 and 40 weeks of gestation (Horgan, 2015), making the brain of the LPI more vulnerable to increased stress and at increased risk for long-term injury (Barfield & Lee, 2013). LPIs have been found to have developmental delays, emotional and behavioral problems, and less optimal school outcomes at preschool and kindergarten (Vohr, 2013) compared to term infants.

The assessment of the LPI begins before birth with the recognition that gestational age assessment can have an error of ±2 weeks (Medoff-Cooper et al., 2012) except for women who have conceived following reproductive technology. Therefore, health care providers should assess all infants born before 37 weeks of gestation every 30 minutes until stable for 2 hours, then every 4 hours for the first 24 hours, and then routinely until discharge using a risk assessment plan (Phillips et al., 2013). As cold stress, glucose metabolism, and respiratory distress are interrelated, a proactive approach to the prevention or immediate identification of problems can reduce short-term morbidities. It is essential that nurseries develop their own evidence-based protocols or use the guidelines from the National Perinatal Association. Baker (2015) provides an example of a Clinical Practice Guideline for the management of LPIs.

NURSING INTERVENTIONS, MANAGEMENT, AND IMPLICATIONS

The thermoregulation of the neonate is a primary responsibility of the nurse.

The initial action is drying and putting a hat on the infant. Infants placed in birth kangaroo care (KC) are covered with a warmed blanket and carefully monitored. When not in KC, the infant should be swaddled. The infant's temperature should be monitored with routine assessments; if the infant's temperature is less than 36.0°C, warming approaches should be initiated (increasing the ambient temperature, swaddling) and the temperature should be monitored every 30 minutes until returning to normal. If the temperature remains less than 36.0°C after 30 minutes, the infant should be placed in a radiant warmer (Horgan, 2015) and monitoring should continue.

Nursing must observe the infant for signs of respiratory distress such as grunting, retracting, nasal flaring, retractions, and cyanosis. For infants in KC, the SpO_2 can be monitored (Tourneux et al., 2015). Glucose levels should be monitored following the unit policy. Breastfeeding should be initiated within the first hour of life and the infant should be fed frequently thereafter. Observe the infants for symptoms of hypoglycemia, including jitteriness, tremors, and tachypnea (Phillips et al., 2013). The infant's oral intake and urine output should be monitored closely. The infant should have bilirubin levels measured according to unit policy and should be assessed for jaundice.

The nurse or lactation consultant should be present at initial breastfeeding sessions to assess the infant's ability to latch onto the breast and maintain sucking to promote milk transfer. Mothers should be taught to understand and respond to the infant's feeding cues and feed the infant every 2 hours. Infants should be weighed daily to monitor for excessive loss of birth weight.

The immature immune system of the LPIs puts them at higher risk for infection compared to term infants. Maternal risk factors include Group B Strep positive or unknown status, prolonged rupture of membranes, and fever during labor. LPIs should be monitored closely for signs of infection, which can be nonspecific (temperature instability, lethargy, and feeding problems) and septic workups should be initiated when symptoms appear (Phillips et al., 2013).

Detailed discharge teaching by the nursing staff is essential to promote family adaptation after discharge and to reduce the possibility of rehospitalization. In addition to the standard discharge teaching for all preterm infants, parents need to understand the specific risks for the LPI, particularly concerning inadequate feeding, dehydration, and hyperbilirubinemia, as these are the most common problems that lead to rehospitalization shortly after discharge (Baker, 2015). It is essential that parents be taught to assess the adequacy of the infant's feeding, including urine and stool output, and to assess for jaundice.

OUTCOMES

The anticipation of the birth of an LPI, which allows for the determination of the adequacy of the resources available, especially in terms of well-trained health care providers, is the first step in preventing or minimizing risks for these infants. Evidence-based multidisciplinary guidelines developed by the National Perinatal Association (www.nationalperinatal.org/Resources/LatePretermGuidelinesNPA .pdf) provide a foundation for providing safe care. An international collaborative organization, the Vermont Oxford Network, has the mission to improve the quality, safety, and efficiency of health care for newborns and has developed regional perinatal quality initiatives so the focus of the groups can reflect the health care systems in the region (Trembath, Iams, & Walsh, 2013). Projects have been aimed at reducing preterm births and reducing the morbidities and mortalities related to preterm birth. However, quality initiatives focusing on the care of LPIs have been impacted by both the lack of evidence-based practices and the wide variation in care practices among hospitals (Trembath et al., 2013), such as the definition and management of hypoglycemia.

Summary

The focus on the increased risk of morbidities and mortality for LPIs has recently expanded to the identification of the increased risk for moderately preterm (born between 31 and 33 6/7 weeks) and early term (born between 37 and 38 6/7 weeks; Baker, 2015). The recognition and proactive management of these infants of the ongoing risks by nursing and other health care providers are essential to improve short- and long-term outcomes for these infants and their families.

Baker, B. (2015). Evidence-based practice to improve outcomes for late preterm infants. *Journal of Obstetric, Gynecologic, and Neonatal Nursing, 44*(1), 127–134.

Barfield, W. D., & Lee, K. G. (2016). Late preterm infants. In M. S. Kim (Ed.), *UpToDate*. Retrieved from http://www.uptodate.com/contents/late-preterm-infants

Hamilton, B. E., Martin, J. A., Osterman, M. J., Curtin, S. C., & Matthews, T. J. (2015). Births: Final data for 2014. *National Vital Statistics Reports, 64*(12), 1–64. Retrieved from https://www.cdc.gov/nchs/data/nvsr/nvsr64/nvsr64_12.pdf

Horgan, M. J. (2015). Management of the late preterm infant: Not quite ready for prime time. *Pediatric Clinics of North America, 62*(2), 439–451. doi:10.1016/j.pcl.2014.11.007

Kair, L. R., & Colaizy, T. T. (2016). Breastfeeding continuation among late preterm infants: Barriers, facilitators, and any association with NICU admission? *Hospital Pediatrics, 6*(5), 261–268. doi:10.1542/hpeds.2015-0172

Medoff Cooper, B., Holditch-Davis, D., Verklan, M. T., Fraser-Askin, D., Lamp, J., Santa-Donato, A., . . . Bingham, D. (2012). Newborn clinical outcomes of the AWHONN late preterm infant research-based practice project. *Journal of Obstetric, Gynecologic, and Neonatal Nursing, 41*(6), 774–785. doi:10.1111/j.1552-6909.2012.01401.x

Phillips, R. M., Goldstein, M., Hougland, K., Nandyal, R., Pizzica, A., Santa-Donato, A., ... Yost, E. (2013). Multidisciplinary guidelines for the care of late preterm infants. *Journal of Perinatology, 33*(Suppl 2), S5–S22. doi:10.1038/jp.2013.53

Raju, T. N. K., Higgins, R. D., Stark, A. R., & Leveno, K. J. (2006). Optimizing care and outcome for late-preterm (near-term) infants: A summary of the workshop sponsored by the National Institute of Child Health and Human Development. *Pediatrics, 118*(3), 1207–1214. doi:10.1542/peds.2006-0018

Tourneux, P., Dubruque, E., Baumert, A., Carpentier, E., Caron-Lesenechal, E., Barcat, L., ... Fontaine, C. (2015). Skin-to-skin care in the delivery room: Impact of SpO$_2$ monitoring. *Archives de Pédiatrie: Organe Officiel de la Société Française de Pédiatrie, 22*(2), 166–170. doi:10.1016/j.arcped.2014.10.021

Trembath, A. N., Iams, J. D., & Walsh, M. (2013). Quality initiatives related to moderately preterm, late preterm, and early term births. *Clinics in Perinatology, 40*(4), 777–789. doi:10.1016/j.clp.2013.07.011

Vohr, B. (2013). Long-term outcomes of moderately preterm, late preterm, and early term infants. *Clinics in Perinatology, 40*(4), 739–751. doi:10.1016/j.clp.2013.07.006

◼ MECONIUM ASPIRATION SYNDROME

Rae Jean Hemway

Overview

Meconium represents the early passage of stool in the fetus. It is a material that accumulates in the intestines of a fetus and forms the first stools of an infant in the first few days after birth. Meconium is thick, sticky, odorless, and greenish to black in color (O'Toole, 2009). Water is the major component constituting 85% to 95% of meconium; the remaining 5% to 15% primarily includes secretions of the intestinal glands, amniotic fluid, and intrauterine debris, such as bile pigments, fatty acids, epithelial cells, mucus, lanugo, and blood. Meconium is sterile and free of bacteria, differentiating it from subsequent postnatal stools (Geis, 2017). Meconium is found in the intestinal tract as early as 12 weeks gestation (Meerkov & Weiner, 2016). Because meconium is seldom found in the amniotic fluid before the 34th week of gestation, aspiration into the airways before, during labor, and/or at the time of delivery generally affects term and post-term infants. Intrauterine distress may facilitate the passage of meconium into the amniotic fluid and increase the potential for meconium aspiration syndrome (MAS).

Background

MAS is defined as respiratory distress in an infant, usually term, born through meconium-stained amniotic fluid (MSAF) with symptoms that cannot otherwise be attributed to other causes such as infection or retained lung fluid (Fanaroff, 2008). MSAF occurs in 8% to 10% of term deliveries and approximately 2% to 3% of meconium-stained infants will develop MAS, translating to an incidence of one to two per 1,000 live term births per year (Meerkov & Weiner, 2016). Infants, born depressed, through thick MSAF are more likely to develop MAS (Chettri, Adhisivam, & Bhat, 2015). There is a significant correlation in the incidence of MSAF with gestational age, increasing almost linearly from 37 to 42 weeks of gestation (Fischer, Rybakowski, Ferdynus, Sagot, & Gouyon, 2012). Thus, MAS continues to remain a major clinical concern for obstetricians and neonatologists. The presence of meconium in the amniotic fluid under normal circumstances is thought to be a result of increased peristalsis associated with maturation of fetal intestinal function. However, there is enhanced passage of meconium in utero under certain high-risk conditions. Although the mechanisms affecting meconium passage are not fully explained, animal studies have demonstrated increased parasympathetic activity, resulting in increased peristalsis and relaxation of the anal sphincter following episodes of cord compression and fetal hypoxia (Meerkov & Weiner, 2016).

Factors that increase the passage of meconium in utero, often as a consequence of interruption of placental blood flow, include placental insufficiency, maternal hypertension, preeclampsia, oligohydramnios, infection, acidosis, and maternal drug abuse, particularly tobacco and cocaine (Geis, 2017). Irrespective of the mechanism of how it reaches the amniotic fluid, the presence of MSAF poses the threat of aspiration. The majority of infants who pass meconium are either term or post-term, with the latter exhibiting peeling skin, overgrown fingernails, and a decrease in the amount of vernix. MAS is a common cause of severe respiratory distress in this population and is associated with significant morbidity and mortality. The pathophysiology will vary to a large degree on the amount of meconium aspirated as well as the underlying pulmonary vascular development. For example, in the postmature infant, there is the potential for smooth muscle hypertrophy and pulmonary artery hypertension independent of the effects of the aspirated meconium. Meconium, when aspirated into the lungs of an infant, may result in mechanical obstruction of the small airways during the first few breaths and in addition may stimulate the release of cytokines (Swarnam, Soraisham, & Sivanandan, 2012). As a result, aspirated meconium interferes with normal breathing in a number of ways, including acute airway obstruction (partial or complete) dependent on the quantity and consistency of the aspirated meconium; inactivation or dysfunction of endogenous surfactant, particularly proteins A and B; altering compliance, functional residual capacity, and inducing alveolar edema; inducing chemical pneumonitis that may potentiate the release of cytokines and other vasoactive substances leading to cardiovascular and inflammatory responses and persistent pulmonary hypertension of the newborn (PPHN) with left to right shunting (Swarnam et al., 2012). These effects singularly or in combination can result in hypoxia, hypercarbia, and acidosis (Crowley, 2015).

Clinical Aspects

ASSESSMENT

Clinical signs and symptoms include tachypnea, nasal flaring, grunting, subcostal and intercostal retractions, cyanosis or desaturation, rhonchi on auscultation, and meconium staining of the umbilical cord, nails, and or skin. Meconium staining may be noted in the oropharynx. Infants with air trapping secondary to obstruction in the alveoli may have a barrel-shaped chest because of trapped gas in the lungs, which may result in a pneumothorax, pneumopericardium, and/or pneumomediastinum. Green urine may be noted in some newborns with MAS less than 24 hours after birth, related to meconium pigments that can be absorbed by the lung and then excreted in urine.

NURSING INTERVENTIONS, MANAGEMENT, AND IMPLICATIONS

About 10% of all infants require some assistance to begin breathing after birth, and approximately 1% requires extensive resuscitation (Wyckoff et al., 2015). Knowledge of potential high-risk situations and providers skilled in the Neonatal Resuscitation Program (NRP) guidelines is critical to the successful resuscitation of infants. Collaboration between obstetric and neonatal teams is also essential, particularly when a history reveals MSAF with a potential risk for MAS. Availability of a neonatal resuscitation team (where possible) before the delivery is vital, and allows the team to pre-brief and discuss potential problems and potential corrective actions, as well as define the role of each team member. The key to management of labor complicated by MSAF lies in the early identification of fetal distress, often indicated by changes in fetal heart rate patterns and/or whether the meconium is thin or thick. This should be identified immediately and corrective actions be taken, which may include delivering the infant in a timely manner if warranted.

Initial interventions are targeted at preventing aspiration by assisting in removing the meconium from the infant's oropharynx and nasopharynx before the initial breath. Recent evidence suggests that routine tracheal suctioning of neonates delivered with meconium-stained fluid has not been shown to improve outcome (Wyckoff et al., 2015). However, if the neonate's breathing appears obstructed, endotracheal suctioning should be immediately done. Early identification and treatment of meconium aspiration are critical. When this occurs, the primary goals of therapy are to maintain appropriate gas exchange and minimize complications.

Specific treatment strategies include judicious ventilator management, a surfactant for mechanically ventilated neonates with high O_2 requirements, and inhaled nitric oxide. High-frequency ventilation may be required if refractory hypoxemia develops, and extracorporeal membrane oxygenation (ECMO) if medical management fails.

Nursing strategies following resuscitation should include maintaining adequate oxygenation, maintaining temperature, monitoring glucose levels to avoid hypoglycemia, closely observing intravenous fluids administration, and administering intravenous antibiotic therapy. Signs of recovery include resolving respiratory distress and achieving metabolic homeostasis. There should be a focused strategy on providing parental support, which should include allowing parents to verbalize concerns regarding their infant's health and understanding the usual progression and resolution of MAS (London, Ladewig, Ball, & Bindler, 2006).

OUTCOMES

Outcomes have greatly improved in recent years because of improved obstetric and neonatal care, including the use of high-frequency ventilation, use of nitric oxide, and ECMO as indicated. The risk of death is increased in the presence of early thick meconium (Meis, Hall, Marshall, & Hobel, 1978).

Summary

Management of infants with MAS has evolved over the years such that infants who were routinely suctioned in the presence of MSAF are now suctioned, even when depressed, only when there are signs of airway obstruction. The management includes a team approach involving both the obstetrician and the neonatal providers coupled with a targeted neonatal management approach; the overwhelming majority of infants survive with a normal long-term outcome.

Chettri, S., Adhisivam, B., & Bhat, B. V. (2015). Endotracheal suction for nonvigorous neonates born through meconium stained amniotic fluid: A randomized controlled trial. *The Journal of Pediatrics, 166*(5), 1208–1213.e1. doi:10.1016/j.jpeds.2014.12.076

Crowley, M. (2015). Neonatal respiratory disorders. In R. J. Martin, A. A. Fanaroff, & M. C. Walsh (Eds.), *Fanaroff and Martin's neonatal-perinatal medicine* (10th ed.). St. Louis, MO: Elsevier Saunders.

Fanaroff, A. A. (2008). Meconium aspiration syndrome: Historical aspects. *Journal of Perinatology, 28*(Suppl 3), S3–S7. doi:10.1038/jp.2008.162

Fischer, C., Rybakowski, C., Ferdynus, C., Sagot, P., & Gouyon, J. B. (2012). A population-based study of meconium aspiration syndrome in neonates born between 37 and 43 weeks of gestation. *International Journal of Pediatrics, 2012*, 321545. doi:10.1155/2012/321545

Geis, G. M. (2017). Meconium aspiration syndrome treatment & management. In T. Rosenkrantz (Ed.), *Medscape*. Retrieved from http://emedicine.medscape.com/article/974110-treatment

London, M. L., Ladewig, P. W., Ball, J. W., & Bindler, R. C. (2006). *Maternal & child nursing care* (2nd ed.). Upper Saddle River, NJ: Pearson. Retrieved from www.prenhall.com/london2e/pages/london_final_ch31.pdf

Meerkov, M., & Weiner, G. (2016). Management of the meconium-stained newborn. NeoReviews, 17(8), e471–e477. doi:10.1542/neo.17-8-e471

Meis, P. J., Hall, M., III, Marshall, J. R., & Hobel, C. J. (1978). Meconium passage: A new classification for risk assessment during labor. *American Journal of Obstetrics and Gynecology, 131*(5), 509–513. doi:10.1016/0002-9378(78)90111-4

O'Toole, M. T. (Ed.). (2009). *Mosby's medical dictionary* (9th ed.). St. Louis, MO: Elsevier Mosby.

Swarnam, K., Soraisham, A. S., & Sivanandan, S. (2012). Advances in the management of meconium aspiration syndrome. *International Journal of Pediatrics*, 359571. doi:10.1155/2012/359571

Wyckoff, M. H., Aziz, K., Escobedo, M. B., Kapadia, V. S., Kattwinkel, J., Perlman, J. M., . . . , Zaichkin, J. G. (2015). Part 13: Neonatal resuscitation: 2015 American Heart Association guidelines update for cardiopulmonary resuscitation and emergency cardiovascular care. *Circulation, 132*(18 Suppl. 2), S543–S560. doi:10.1161/CIR.0000000000000267

■ NECROTIZING ENTEROCOLITIS

Charlene M. Deuber

Overview

Necrotizing enterocolitis (NEC) is the most common gastrointestinal emergency in the neonatal period. Involving ischemic necrosis of the bowel wall, or intestinal mucosa, gas-producing enteric organisms invade the mucosal lining of the intestine (pneumatosis intestinalis) potentially resulting in focal or widespread bowel perforation.

NEC occurs in one to three per 1,000 live births and occurs predominantly in preterm infants, with an incidence of approximately 6% to 7% in very-low-birth-weight (VLBW) infants (birth weight less than 1,500 g; Stoll et al., 2015). Secondary disease is most often seen in full-term infants with comorbid conditions, including birth asphyxia, trisomy 21, congenital heart disease, rotavirus infection, and Hirschsprung's disease. In neonatal intensive care units (NICUs) alone, NEC occurs in 1% to 5% of patients, accounting for nearly 20% of NICU costs annually (Gephart, McGrath, Effken, & Halpern, 2012). The overall incidence in the United States is approximately 3,000 infants annually with 1,000 infants succumbing to the disease.

Variations in the severity of this disorder occur, but all cases result in substantial short- and long-term morbidity in survivors. Morbidity and mortality rates associated with NEC have not improved in decades despite other substantial advances in neonatal care. The average mortality from NEC is 20% to 30%, with mortality as high as 50% for those infants requiring surgical intervention (Fitzgibbons et al., 2009). Characterized by host intestinal immaturity and multifactorial influences, reduction in the incidence and severity of NEC has focused on the identification and elimination of risk factors.

Background

The Centers for Disease Control and Prevention (CDC) defines NEC as a condition occurring in infants less than or equal to 1 year of age and meeting one of the two criteria: (a) at least one clinical sign (bilious aspirate, vomiting, abdominal distension, or occult/gross blood in stools without rectal fissure) and one imaging test finding (pneumatosis intestinalis, portal venous gas, or pneumoperitoneum or (b) one surgical finding (surgical evidence of extensive bowel necrosis, more than 2 cm of bowel affected, or surgical evidence of pneumatosis intestinalis with or without intestinal perforation; CDC, 2018).

Although the pathogenesis of NEC is complex and multifactorial, three major risk factors have been implicated in its development: prematurity, bacterial colonization of the gut, and formula feeding (Hackam, Afrazi, Good, & Sodhi, 2013). NEC is characterized by inflammation and initiated by impaired mesenteric perfusion with loss of mucosal integrity followed by necrosis. Disrupted, abnormal colonization of the intestine, mucosal barrier dysfunction, and an exaggerated, immune response contribute to the potential devastating consequences of the disease. Subsequent perforation of the bowel may occur at any location, allowing free air to migrate beyond the intestinal lumen to the peritoneum or venous portal system, progressing to peritonitis, sepsis, and death. The terminal ileum and colon are often affected, and, in its most severe form, the entire intestine may be involved.

Clinical manifestations vary and can be insidious or catastrophic in the presentation. Commonly, the infant who presents with NEC has been thriving and suddenly presents with clinical instability. Symptoms are typically nonspecific and suggestive of general instability, including temperature instability, apnea and bradycardia, hypotension, thrombocytopenia, abdominal tenderness or distension, abdominal wall erythema or discoloration, gastric residuals, absent bowel sounds, emesis, or blood in the stool.

Although NEC may occur as late as 3 months of age in VLBW infants, it typically presents in the second or third week of life. The greatest single risk factor for NEC is prematurity, with the rate of NEC decreasing after 32 weeks postmenstrual age. The majority of patients have received enteral feedings before diagnosis. Additional risk factors for the development of NEC include immaturity of the host immunologic system, luminal factors, intestinal epithelial barrier, and gut motility. Bacterial overgrowth in the context of low gastric–hydrogen ion output in the neonate contributes to the colonization of enteric pathogens (Carrion & Egan, 1990).

Effective treatment depends on a multisystem approach, including bowel rest, gastric decompression, supportive hydration, and correction of hypotension, hyponatremia, and metabolic acidosis. Antibiotic surveillance is warranted for potential overwhelming sepsis, with concurrent antifungal therapy if bowel perforation is suspected. Surgical consultation should be initiated when NEC is suspected and there are concerning findings of fixed dilated loops of bowel or evidence of pneumoperitoneum (free peritoneal air or portal venous gas) present on abdominal radiographs. Surgical management may include placement of a peritoneal drain or laparotomy with bowel resection for the removal of necrotic bowel.

Clinical Aspects

ASSESSMENT

NEC is a progressive disease necessitating serial laboratory testing, radiographic surveillance, and keen clinical assessment. The most significant single predictor of outcome following NEC is gestational age. When controlled for gestational age, whether or not the infant needs surgery is predictive of outcome; however, mortality and morbidity are highest in those infants requiring surgical intervention (Henry & Moss, 2008). There are also poorer long-term developmental outcomes in infants requiring surgical intervention versus medical management of NEC.

NURSING INTERVENTIONS, MANAGEMENT, AND IMPLICATIONS

Nursing care focuses on surveillance for NEC in populations at risk, with early recognition of clinical symptoms, serial clinical assessments, and preparation for surgery or transport to a tertiary care center. A high index of suspicion in any infant meeting the identified risk factors during the prenatal, intrapartum, or postpartum course should prompt intensive surveillance of signs and symptoms; serial radiographs, measurement of abdominal girth, analysis of blood pressure, intake, output, and acid–base balance are important indicators of severity of disease. Optimal outcome following the diagnosis of NEC rests on early recognition, treatment, and access to a tertiary care center when progressive disease or bowel perforation is suspected.

Research has identified strategies to reduce the incidence of NEC. Prenatal strategies for prevention include maternal administration of antenatal corticosteroids (ANCS). A Cochrane review has suggested that maternal treatment with a single course of antenatal steroids reduced NEC by 46% (Brownfoot, Gagliardi, Bain, Middleton, & Crowther, 2013).

The use of human milk has been shown to be protective against NEC in multiple randomized controlled trials. Donor breast milk for enteral feedings is protective when maternal breast milk is not available (Quigley & McGuire, 2014). Nursing support of maternal breast feeding or pumping of breast milk is influential in the prevention of NEC, especially in preterm infants.

Standardized, unit-specific feeding protocols guiding slow advancement of feeding volume and caloric density, avoidance of hypertonic formulas and medications, and prompt treatment of polycythemia are additional preventive measures suggested in the literature, although with less scientific rigor. In a recent meta-analysis (Morgan, Young, & McGuire, 2015), the slow advancement of enteral feedings delays the establishment of full enteral feedings but did not show a statistically significant effect on the risk of NEC in very preterm or VLBW infants.

Ibuprofen treatment as an alternative to indomethacin for closure of a patent ductus arteriosus, which is a common complication in very preterm infants, has been associated with a reduction in the incidence of NEC (Ohlsson, Walia, & Shah, 2015). Also of note, probiotics have been cited as having a protective effect in the prevention of NEC in premature infants, and in the reduction of severity as well as the mortality (Neu, 2014). Ongoing research is focused on the safest preparation and administration of probiotics.

Summary

Early recognition and aggressive treatment of this disorder have improved clinical outcomes, yet NEC accounts for substantial long-term morbidity and mortality, especially in VLBW infants. Effective preventive strategies include the feeding of breast milk and the use of standardized feeding guidelines. Nurses play a critical role in recognizing signs and symptoms of NEC to facilitate early diagnosis and treatment in infants at highest risk, and in encouraging mothers to provide breast milk.

Brownfoot, F. C., Gagliardi, D., Bain, E., Middleton, P., & Crowther, C. (2013). Different corticosteroids and regimens for accelerating fetal lung maturation for women at risk of preterm birth. *The Cochrane Database of Systematic Reviews, 2013*(8), CD006764. doi:10.1002/14651858.CD006764.pub3

Carrion, V., & Egan, E. A. (1990). Prevention of neonatal necrotizing enterocolitis. *Journal of Pediatric Gastroenterology and Nutrition, 11*(3), 317–323. Retrieved from http://journals.lww.com/jpgn/Fulltext/1990/10000/Prevention_of_Neonatal_Necrotizing_Enterocolitis.6.aspx

Centers for Disease Control and Prevention. (2018). NEC-necrotizing enterocolitis. *CDC/NHSN surveillance definitions for specific types of infections.* Retrieved from https://www.cdc.gov/nhsn/pdfs/pscmanual/17pscnosinfdef_current.pdf

Fitzgibbons, S. C., Ching, Y., Yu, D., Carpenter, J., Kenny, M., Weldon, C., . . . Jaksic, T. (2009). Mortality of necrotizing enterocolitis expressed by birth weight categories. *Journal of Pediatric Surgery, 44*(6), 1072–1076; discussion 1075. doi:10.1016/j.jpedsurg.2009.02.013

Gephart, S. M., McGrath, J. M., Effken, J. A., & Halpern, M. D. (2012). Necrotizing enterocolitis risk: State of the science. *Advances in Neonatal Care, 12*(2), 77–87; quiz 88. doi:10.1097/ANC.0b013e31824cee94

Hackam, D. J., Afrazi, A., Good, M., & Sodhi, C. P. (2013). Innate immune signaling in the pathogenesis of necrotizing enterocolitis. *Clinical & Developmental Immunology, 2013,* 475415. doi:10.1155/2013/475415

Henry, M. C., & Moss, R. L. (2008). Neonatal necrotizing enterocolitis. *Seminars in Pediatric Surgery, 17*(2), 98–109. doi:10.1053/j.sempedsurg.2008.02.005

Morgan, J., Young, L., & McGuire, W. (2015). Slow advancement of enteral feed volumes to prevent necrotizing enterocolitis in very low birth weight infants. *Cochrane Database of Systematic Reviews, 2015*(10), CD001241. doi:10.1002/14651858.CD001241.pub6

Neu, J. (2014). Probiotics and necrotizing enterocolitis. *Clinics in Perinatology, 41*(4), 967–978. doi:10.1016/j.clp.2014.08.014

Ohlsson, A., Walia, R., & Shah, S. S. (2015). Ibuprofen for the treatment of patent ductus arteriosus in preterm or low birth weight (or both) infants. *Cochrane Database of Systematic Reviews, 2015*(2), CD003481. doi:10.1002/14651858.CD003481.pub6

Quigley, M., & McGuire, W. (2014). Formula versus donor breastmilk for feeding preterm or low birth weight infants. *Cochrane Database of Systematic Reviews, 2014,* CD002971. doi:10.1002/14651858.CD002971.pub3

Stoll, B., Hansen, N., Bell, E., Walsh, M., Carlo, W., Shankaran, S., . . . Higgins, R.; the Eunice Kennedy Shriver National Institute of Child Health and Human Development Neonatal Research Network. (2015). Trends in care practices, morbidity and mortality of extremely preterm neonates, 1993-2012. *Journal of the American Medical Association, 314*(10), 1039–1051. doi:10.1001/jama.2015.10244

■ RESPIRATORY DISTRESS SYNDROME

Mary Ann Blatz

Overview

Respiratory distress is the most common diagnosis for infants admitted to the neonatal intensive care unit (NICU; Stoll et al., 2010). The term *neonatal respiratory distress* refers to hypoventilation and/or hypoxia in the neonate (Reuter, Moser, & Baack, 2014). Neonatal respiratory distress syndrome (RDS) is a surfactant-deficient state that is most frequently associated with infants born prematurely (Lozano & Newnam, 2016). However, RDS occurs much less frequently in term infants related to inactivation of surfactant in a variety of other conditions, including asphyxia, history of maternal diabetes, infection, and/or meconium aspiration (Reuter et al., 2014). Increased incidence of RDS has been noted if there was a sibling with RDS, cesarean delivery, or induction of labor before 37 weeks of gestation; a compromised infant at delivery decreasing adequate circulation; multiple pregnancy or a precipitous delivery; history of gestational or chronic diabetes, chorioamnionitis; or those of European descent (Newman, 2016; Wambach & Hamvas, 2015). Neonatal nurses are essential for the immediate and ongoing collaborative care for the infant with RDS that requires continuous, meticulous monitoring, management, and support to attain and maintain physiologic stability.

Background

RDS was previously called *hyaline membrane disease* (Wambach & Hamvas, 2015). It is difficult to analyze statistics related to incidence, mortality, and neonatal outcomes because a consensus definition of RDS has not been agreed on by clinical experts (Wambach & Hamvas, 2015). RDS is a broad term that generally includes respiratory symptoms that appear at birth or shortly thereafter, primarily in preterm neonates. RDS encompasses worsening atelectasis, hypoventilation, and/or hypoxia (Newman, 2016; Polin & Carlo, 2014).

In the United States, almost 40,000 infants are diagnosed with RDS every year. Males are affected twice as often as females. There is an inverse relationship between the gestational age of the infant and the incidence of RDS. It is found in almost 98% of 23-week infants, 86% of 28-week infants, 29% of 35-week infants, and 7% of term infants (Newman, 2016). Approximately 1 out of every 100 infants born will suffer from RDS (Coe, Jamie, & Baskerville, 2014).

It is essential for nurses to have a basic understanding of fetal lung structure, function, and development to appreciate the impact of prematurity on the respiratory system and to collaborate with members of the health care team in providing optimally effective ventilation management and nursing care for neonates. At approximately 4 to 5 weeks of gestation, lung development begins to advance in a sequential predetermined order. Lung maturation is finished in late childhood. The stages of fetal lung development are: embryonic, or formation of the proximal airway (gestational age of weeks 4–6); psuedoglandular or formation of conducting airways (gestational age of weeks 7–16); canalicular or formation of acini (gestational age of weeks 17–28); secular or development of gas-exchange sites (gestational age of weeks 29–35); and alveolar that allows expansion of surface area (gestational age of weeks 36–childhood; Lozano & Newnam, 2016; Newman, 2016). Neonatal survival becomes possible in the canalicular stage as gas-exchanging acinar units emerge. At approximately 23 to 24 weeks of gestation, the surfactant is evident in amniotic fluid, with gas exchange and surfactant production starting (Lozano & Newnam, 2016).

RDS starts with compromised or delayed production and secretion of surfactant that increases surface tension in alveoli to allow alveolar expansion thus enabling adequate oxygenation and ventilation (Wambach & Hamvas, 2015). Insufficient surfactant causes diffuse atelectasis, cell injury, and pulmonary edema. Surfactant is a complex liquid comprising lipids and proteins in the lining of the alveoli of the lungs that inhibits alveolar collapse and allows bronchioles to remain open during respiration. Surfactant also protects the lungs from injuries and infections from inhaled particles and microorganisms (Griese, 1999). Surfactant production is an active process influenced by pH, temperature, and perfusion and negatively affected by cold stress, hypovolemia, hypoxia, and acidosis (Wambach & Hamvas, 2015).

On microscopic examination in neonates with RDS, the most prominent characteristic is diffuse atelectasis, or collapse of alveoli (Wambach & Hamvas, 2015). Pulmonary edema contributes to the pathogenesis of RDS. In premature infants, extra lung fluid causes epithelial injury, changes in the lung epithelium, and subsequently, oliguria in the first 2 days after birth. Generally, by the fourth day, premature infants get better after a normal physiologic diuresis (Reuter et al., 2014).

Efforts to prevent RDS and its consequences include prevention of premature birth. Antenatal corticosteroids administration is another preventive measure that pharmacologically accelerates pulmonary maturation. Antenatal corticosteroids administered to the expectant mother at least 24 to 48 hours before delivery decrease the incidence and severity of RDS most effectively for infants between 24 weeks and 34 weeks gestation or with a birth weight of less than 1,250 g, as well as the occurrence of comorbidities linked to prematurity (Polin & Carlo, 2014; Wambach & Hamvas, 2015).

Clinical Aspects

ASSESSMENT

Clinical indications that lead to the diagnosis of RDS include physical examination findings, laboratory data, blood gas analysis, and radiographic findings (Newman, 2016). Comprehensive assessment of the neonate's condition includes evaluating work of breathing, vital signs, oxygen needs, pulse oximetry readings, a detailed maternal, prenatal, and birth history, and the course of respiratory illness (Coe et al., 2014; Newman, 2016). Symptoms usually appear immediately after birth, but sometimes they may not be evident for several hours after delivery. Symptoms may include cyanosis, apnea, decreased urinary output, nasal flaring, rapid (tachypnea is more than 60 breaths/min), irregular and or shallow breathing, shortness of breath, grunting, retractions, and increased oxygen requirement (Newman, 2016; Wambach & Hamvas, 2015). If RDS progresses, the neonate may experience alterations in central nervous system status such as lethargy, decreased responsiveness, and decreased muscle tone. If RDS advances, changes in cardiac function may lead to decreased perfusion, pallor, tachycardia, and bradycardia (Newman, 2016). Nurses need to observe for possible complications such as pneumothorax, pneumomediastinum, or pneumopericardium (Wambach & Hamvas, 2015).

Tests that help to diagnose and manage RDS include blood gas analysis that may indicate high carbon dioxide levels, low oxygen levels, low pH, and increased lactic acid levels related to altered cardiac function; complete blood count to test for anemia or polycythemia; blood typing and screen; and a blood culture to rule out infection (Newman, 2016). Chest radiograph, preferably the anterior–posterior view, may reveal a "ground glass" appearance in the lung fields typically associated with RDS and is generally evident about 6 to 12 hours after birth (Newman, 2016; Wambach & Hamvas, 2015).

NURSING INTERVENTIONS, MANAGEMENT, AND IMPLICATIONS

Collaboration is essential among nurses, neonatologists, and respiratory therapists to optimize health outcomes for neonates diagnosed with RDS. Neonatal nurses are in a strategic position to monitor infant status and response to administered therapies thereby optimizing neonatal short- and long-term health outcomes. Infants with RDS require continuous monitoring and meticulous attention to care and treatment to avoid complications or sequelae such as chronic lung disease (CLD) or retinopathy of prematurity (ROP; Newman, 2016). Nursing actions include the provision of vital signs monitoring, physical assessment, a quiet atmosphere, gentle handling, a neutral thermal environment, adequate fluid and nutrition, prescribed medications, venous and or arterial access, and parental support and education.

Treatments include respiratory support such as surfactant administration, warmed humidified oxygen, continuous positive airway pressure, synchronized intermittent airway pressure, or noninvasive positive pressure ventilation or mechanical ventilation. However, assisted ventilation may harm lung tissue, so use should be judicious. Nurses need to monitor oxygen levels and maintain levels in a therapeutic range to avoid potentially harmful side effects (Newman, 2016; Wambach & Hamvas, 2015). Nurses should monitor and collaborate to manage comorbidities such as patent ductus arteriosus, sepsis, and apnea of prematurity. Nurses must be familiar with pharmacologic treatments, such as caffeine and antibiotic use (Newman, 2016). The innovative practice of selective use of animal-derived or synthetic surfactants has been the most influential intervention to decrease severity, mortality rates, and comorbidities associated with RDS (Polin & Carlo, 2014; Wambach & Hamvas, 2015).

OUTCOMES

Nurses may employ interventions to minimize effects and complications of RDS by monitoring neonatal status and trends in neonatal oxygenation, assuring administration of recommended treatments, providing infant comfort measures, and educating families. Nurses can also participate in multidisciplinary systematic reviews, randomized controlled trials, or nursing research that may yield new information to optimize neonatal health outcomes related to RDS.

Summary

RDS is a pathologic disease process that involves decreased or lack of surfactant production and primarily affects premature infants. New treatments have evolved that have decreased the incidence, severity, occurrence of complications, and long-term sequelae. Neonatal nurses can offer important interventions and prescribed treatments that will enhance neonatal health outcomes as well as support and education for families in the NICU.

Coe, K. L., Jamie, S. F., & Baskerville, R. M. (2014). Managing common neonatal respiratory conditions during transport. *Advances in Neonatal Care, 14*(Suppl. 5), S3–S10. doi:10.1097/ANC.0000000000000120

Griese, M. (1999). Pulmonary surfactant in health and human lung diseases: State of the art. *The European Respiratory Journal, 13*(6), 1455–1476. Retrieved from http://erj .ersjournals.com/content/erj/13/6/1455.full.pdf

Lozano, S. M., & Newnam, K. M. (2016). Modalities of mechanical ventilation: Volume-targeted versus pressure-limited. *Advances in Neonatal Care, 16*(2), 99–107. doi:10.1097/ANC.0000000000000272

Newman, K. (2016). Respiratory system. In C. Kenner & J. W. Lott (Eds.), *Neonatal nursing care handbook* (2nd ed., pp. 3–54). New York, NY: Springer Publishing.

Polin, R. A., & Carlo, W. A. (2014). Surfactant replacement therapy for preterm and term neonates with respiratory distress. *Pediatrics, 133*(1), 156–163. doi:10.1542/ peds.2013-3443

Reuter, S., Moser, C., & Baack, M. (2014). Respiratory distress in the newborn. *Pediatrics in Review, 35*(10), 417–428; quiz 429. doi:10.1542/pir.35-10-417

Stoll, B. J., Hansen, N. I., Bell, E. F., Shankaran, S., Laptook, A. R., Walsh, M. C., . . . & Higgins, R. D.; Eunice Kennedy Shriver National Institute of Child Health and Human Development Neonatal Research Network. (2010). Neonatal outcomes of extremely preterm infants from the NICHD Neonatal Research Network. *Pediatrics, 126*(3), 443–456. doi:10.1542/peds.2009-2959

Wambach, J. A., & Hamvas, A. (2015). Respiratory distress syndrome in the neonate. In R. J. Martin, A. A. Fanaroff, & M. C. Walsh (Eds.), *Fanaroff and Martin's neonatal–perinatal medicine* (10th ed., pp. 1072–1086). Philadelphia, PA: Elsevier Saunders.

■ RETINOPATHY OF PREMATURITY

Mary Ann Blatz

Overview

Retinopathy of prematurity (ROP) results from the aberrant growth of retinal blood vessels that may cause blindness in premature infants. ROP generally resolves without producing permanent retinal injury. However, severe ROP may force the retina to separate from the edge of the eye and potentially produce blindness. Infants who are born weighing 1,250 g or less and are less than 31 weeks of gestation are at greatest risk for developing ROP (American Association for Pediatric Ophthalmology and Strabismus, 2016). Nurses play a critical role in the monitoring, management, and screening of premature infants in the neonatal intensive care unit (NICU), thereby directly impacting the occurrence of ROP (Jefferies & Canadian Paediatric Society, Fetus and Newborn Committee, 2016).

Background

It is estimated 15 million babies are born prematurely, before 37 completed weeks of gestation, throughout the world annually (World Health Organization, 2017). Approximately 3.9 million infants are born in the United States annually, with 28,000 of these infants weighing 1,250 g or less. Approximately 14,000 to 16,000 of these infants develop ROP (National Eye Institute, 2014). ROP contributes to visual damage in 1,300 children and significant visual loss in 500 children in the United States yearly. The rate of ROP for premature infants is almost 16% (Ozsurekci & Aykac, 2016). Minor cases of ROP resolve without residual damage and 90% of infants with ROP are in the milder category and do not need treatment. However, infants with more severe disease may develop impaired vision or even blindness. About 1,100 to 1,500 infants annually develop ROP that is severe enough to require medical treatment. Each year in the United States 400 to 600 infants are diagnosed as legally blind from ROP (National Eye Institute, 2014).

The incidence of ROP is higher in preterm infants with lower birth weights and decreased gestational age. Premature infants who are born before retinal vessels complete normal growth may develop ROP. Ischemia in the ocular region contributes to this disease. In the underdeveloped retina, hyperoxia leads to obliteration of the tiny blood vessels in the eye. Research has found that maintaining oxygen saturation at lower levels from birth decreases the occurrence of the severe form of this disease (American Academy of Ophthalmology, 2015).

Hyperoxia is a significant contributing factor to retinal changes and ROP. Extremely preterm infants generally require long-term mechanical ventilation and high levels of oxygen, which may lead to inflammation and oxidative stress that contributes to an increased risk of incurring lung, brain, and retinal injury

(Poon et al., 2016). ROP occurs as blood vessels grow abnormally and proliferate throughout the retina. These blood vessels are delicate and may bleed, damaging and shifting the alignment of the retina, which results in retinal detachment, the chief cause of visual loss and blindness from ROP.

The eye begins to grow at approximately 16 weeks of gestation, and retinal blood vessels emerge from the optic nerve in the posterior ocular region. Oxygen and nutrients are delivered by the neovascularization that develops and stretches toward the periphery of the developing retina. The eye matures quickly in the last 12 weeks of gestation and is almost complete when a full-term infant is born. Retinal maturation is completed within the first month after delivery. However, if an infant is born prematurely before the blood vessels have extended to the retinal edge, abnormal blood vessel development may occur (National Eye Institute, 2014). These new blood vessels are fragile and may bleed, contributing to retinal scarring. As the scars contract, they pull on the retina, leading it to separate from the back of the eye (National Eye Institute, 2014).

Numerous reasons contribute to the onset of ROP. Factors that influence the development of ROP in addition to prematurity and lower birth weight include anemia, blood transfusions, respiratory distress, neonatal infections, and general neonatal health status (National Eye Institute, 2014). Additional ROP triggers include depression of retinal vascularization; placental nutrients and growth factor deficiencies; interrupted vascularization with ensuing hypoxia because of retinal growth and increasing metabolic requirements; hypoxic retina stimulating structure of the oxygen-regulated components that drive retinal vascularization by utilizing erythropoietin and vascular endothelial growth factor (VEGF); and variations in oxygen stimulating cells to cause endothelial cell death, which causes avascular retinal development (Ozsurekci & Aykac, 2016).

Clinical Aspects

ASSESSMENT

The International Committee for Classification of Retinopathy of Prematurity created a diagnostic classification system. ROP is evaluated by location or concentric zones of retinal vascularization, incomplete or immature stage and extent of the disease. A qualified ophthalmologist should provide an indirect ophthalmoscopic examination based on the gestational age of the premature infant. Examinations may need to be repeated at intervals or surgical treatment with argon or diode lasers may need to be utilized based on findings (National Eye Institute, 2014). Neonatal nurses need to be familiar with screening protocols, treatment modalities, and pathogenesis of the diagnosis.

The American Academy of Pediatrics issued a policy statement (Fierson, 2013) to guide screening practices to detect the presence and severity of ROP in premature infants. These guidelines remain the current standard to drive screening protocols. The Canadian Paediatric Society released an update on screening and management to minimize visual losses in preterm infants (Jefferies & Canadian

Paediatric Society, Fetus and Newborn Committee, 2016). Classification of stages of ROP is necessary for consistency of treatment, so interventions can be provided at designated stages when the visual loss is likely. Researchers evaluated ROP screening guidelines for extremely premature infants and concluded that additional research is essential to identify the best time frame for ROP screening for infants born at less than 24 weeks or more than 27 weeks of gestation (Kennedy et al., 2014). Nurses and other health care professionals should be familiar with ROP screening and management guidelines as well as treatment options for severe ROP in this high-risk neonatal population.

NURSING INTERVENTIONS, MANAGEMENT, AND IMPLICATIONS

Nurses can collaborate with neonatologists, respiratory therapists, and ophthalmologists to optimize results for infants who require treatment. Neonatal nurses are in a key position to minimize ROP in the NICU population. Continuous monitoring of administered oxygen to assure that infant oxygen saturation levels remain within prescribed therapeutic ranges may reduce the risk and severity of ROP. As premature infants are screened for ROP, nurses must carefully administer prescribed dilating ophthalmic and topical anesthetic drops before the examination and monitor for side effects such as apnea. As the ROP examination begins, the nurse needs to assure the infant is comfortable using techniques such as swaddling and offering 24% sucrose with a pacifier. Cardiorespiratory monitoring and pulse oximetry should continue to assure an immediate response if physiologic instability occurs (Jefferies & Canadian Paediatric Society, Fetus and Newborn Committee, 2016). The neonatal nurse is the first link to providing increased assistance, as well as additional interventions and support to the infant as necessary during the ROP examination. Nurses can provide parent education by explaining ROP in terms that parents can understand as well as offering education-appropriate reading materials or directing them to suitable Internet resources. Nurses can give support related to ROP screening and treatment if needed, by linking families to social workers, early childhood intervention programs, financial assistance, and support groups. Therapeutic management for severe ROP includes laser ablation, cryotherapy, bevacizumab injection, which is a monoclonal antibody for VEGF, scleral buckle, which is a procedure to repair a retinal detachment or vitrectomy in which there is removal of small portions of the vitreous humor from the front structures of the eye (Kennedy et al., 2014).

OUTCOMES

Strategies nurses may use to minimize the incidence and severity of ROP include monitoring trends in neonatal oxygenation, assuring compliance with standardized screening recommendations, observing physiologic stability during ROP screening examinations and treatments, providing infant comfort measures, and educating families. Nurses can also participate in multidisciplinary large-scale research activities or nursing studies that may produce new information to enhance neonatal health outcomes related to ROP.

Summary

ROP is a pathologic disease process that affects premature infants and may lead to a permanent visual loss. Many factors interact to stimulate abnormal retinal blood vessel growth. Improved screening guidelines and treatments have helped to reduce permanent visual losses. Neonatal nurses can provide important interventions that will enhance neonatal health outcomes.

American Academy of Ophthalmology. (2015). Retinopathy of prematurity. *EyeWiki*. Retrieved from http://eyewiki.aao.org/Retinopathy_of_Prematurity

American Association for Pediatric Ophthalmology and Strabismus. (2016). Retinopathy of prematurity. Retrieved from https://www.aapos.org/terms/conditions/94

Fierson, W. M.; American Academy of Pediatrics Section on Ophthalmology; American Academy of Ophthalmology; American Association for Pediatric Ophthalmology and Strabismus; American Association of Certified Orthoptists. (2013). Screening examination of premature infants for retinopathy of prematurity. *Pediatrics, 131*(1), 189–195. doi:10.1542/peds.2012-2996

Jefferies, A. L., & Canadian Paediatric Society, Fetus and Newborn Committee. (2016). Retinopathy of prematurity: An update on screening and management. *Paediatrics and Child Health, 21*(2), 101–104. Retrieved from https://www.ncbi.nlm.nih.gov/pmc/articles/PMC4807789

Kennedy, K. A., Wrage, L. A., Higgins, R. D., Finer, N. N., Carlo, W. A., Walsh, M. C., . . . Phelps, D. L. (2014). Evaluating retinopathy of prematurity screening guidelines for 24- to 27-week gestational age infants. *Journal of Perinatology, 34*(4), 311–318. doi:10.1038/jp.2014.12

National Eye Institute. (2014). Facts about retinopathy of prematurity (ROP). Retrieved from https://nei.nih.gov/health/rop/rop

Ozsurekci, Y., & Aykac, K. (2016). Oxidative stress related diseases in newborns. *Oxidative Medicine and Cellular Longevity, 2016*, 2768365. doi:10.1155/2016/2768365

Poon, A. W. H., Ma, E. X. H., Vadivel, A., Jung, S., Khoja, Z., Stephens, L., . . . Wintermark, P. (2016). Impact of bronchopulmonary dysplasia on brain and retina. *Biology Open, 5*(4), 475–483. doi:10.1242/bio.017665

World Health Organization. (2017). Preterm birth fact sheet. Retrieved from http://www.who.int/mediacentre/factsheets/fs363/en

■ SEPSIS

Karla Phipps

Overview

Neonatal sepsis is a systemic infection with a positive blood or spinal fluid culture, occurring in the first 28 days of life and is either early onset or late onset in the neonatal population. This differentiation is based on the timing of the infection and likely mode of transmission. Most commonly caused by bacteria, both fungi and some viruses can also lead to sepsis with the infection in the blood and or spinal fluid. Early-onset sepsis (EOS) is variably defined by bacteremia occurring in the first 3 days of life in preterm infants and before 7 days of life in full-term infants. EOS usually has multisystem involvement and has a rapid onset, often fulminate, with a high mortality rate. Late-onset sepsis (LOS) occurs after 3 days in preterm or hospitalized infants and after 7 days in term infants. LOS can be acute but often have a slower onset and is usually focal with meningitis being common (Fanaroff & Fanaroff, 2013). Nurses must have the critical knowledge and skills to identify the patient with developing sepsis and provide competent care to prevent complications.

Background

Historically, before treatment with antibiotics, sepsis was almost always fatal. Mortality has decreased over the last two decades because of advancements in technology and specific preventive measures. Before antibiotics, the predominant organism was *Streptococcus*, which decreased after the introduction of antibiotics and gram-negative organisms became prominent. In the 1960s, Group B *Streptococcus* (GBS) replaced *Staphylococcus aureus* as the most common cause of neonatal sepsis. A study done by the National Institute of Child Health and Human Development (NICHD) Neonatal Research Network (NRN) estimates the overall incidence of EOS to be 0.98 cases per 1,000 live births, with increased rates in premature infants (Camacho-Gonzalez, Spearman, & Stoll, 2013). GBS and *Escherichia coli* have been associated with approximately 70% of all EOS infections combined, and the most common cause of mortality is from *E. coli* sepsis (Bizzarro et al., 2015; Simonsen, Anderson-Berry, Delair, & Davies, 2014). EOS is often seen with preterm delivery, premature rupture of membranes, maternal peripartum infection, infants of low birth weight or asphyxia (Fanaroff & Fanaroff, 2013). In the early 1990s, it was estimated that EOS caused by GBS infection was 1.7 cases per 1,000 live births.

In 1996, the Centers for Disease Control and Prevention (CDC) published the first set of guidelines for the prevention of perinatal GBS infection, by using intrapartum antibiotic (IPA) treatment for maternal GBS colonization. After IPA, a reduction in the incidence of EOS with GBS was evident; however, by 2001, the rate had plateaued. With the adoption of universally screening of mothers for

GBS and the use of IPA treatment in 2002, the incidence of EOS–GBS decreased to 0.3/1,000 live births. The prevalence of GBS has declined dramatically over the past 15 years. However, as a result of screening and early IPA, there has been an increase in the rate of gram-negative infections. *E. coli* is the second leading cause of EOS accounting for 24% of all cases (Simonsen et al., 2014).

LOS is a significant cause of morbidity and mortality because of the longer survival of very-low-birth-weight, lower gestational age infants. LOS is an important cause of neurodevelopmental delays and bronchcopulmonary dysplasia (BPD) in preterm infants (Shah, Jefferies, Yoon, Lee, & Shah, 2015). The pathogens most commonly seen are those that colonize the skin and mucous membranes: coagulase negative *Staphylococcus* (CONS), *S. aureus*, *E. coli*, *Klebsiella*, and *Candida* species, each of which is transmitted from the environment or vertically transmitted during the peripartum period. IPA prophylaxis has not impacted LOS. Instead, LOS is often seen with prolonged hospitalization, use of indwelling catheters, and endotracheal tubes as well as other invasive procedures (Fanaroff & Fanaroff, 2013). CONS is the most common cause of LOS with death occurring in 0.9%. *S. aureus* accounts for approximately 17% of LOS cases (Bizzarro et al., 2015), with methicillin-resistant *S. aureus* seen in 28% of all infections in preterm infants (Camacho-Gonzalez et al., 2013).

Clinical Aspects

One of the most common neonatal problems in observation for infection or suspected sepsis is that the symptoms are often nonspecific. The clinician's ability to identify neonates with sepsis is difficult. Because various maternal, neonatal, and environmental factors are associated with risk for infection, it is important to recognize them early in order to identify high-risk neonates.

ASSESSMENT

Manifestations for sepsis may include respiratory distress, apnea, decreased level of activity, abdominal distention, vomiting, diarrhea, temperature instability, jaundice, loss of muscle tone, and seizures. These symptoms are associated with other inflammatory diseases seen in the neonatal population, which makes identifying infants with sepsis challenging. When the diagnosis is obvious, the infant is usually very ill (Polin & Committee on Fetus and Newborn, 2012). It is the nurse at the bedside who is often the first to observe these signs and symptoms and will identify changes in a newborn's examination. As the first professional to note these changes, the nurse can ensure timely diagnostic testing and the start of empiric antimicrobials that are essential in saving lives. With supportive care, the majority of infants with suspected sepsis will recover.

Maternal risk factors are most commonly associated with EOS. Because the infant is maintained in a relatively sterile environment in utero, infection usually occurs when pathogens reach the fetus or neonate after birth. Maternal chorioamnionitis and GBS colonization are associated with high rates of EOS. Nurses can identify infants at risk by reviewing maternal labor and delivery history with attention to these key factors.

NURSING INTERVENTIONS, MANAGEMENT, AND IMPLICATIONS

The neonatal risk factor most commonly associated with neonatal sepsis is preterm birth and is linked with both EOS and LOS. An infant's birth weight is inversely related to the risk of EOS with lower birth weight infants being at higher risk for sepsis (Camacho-Gonzales et al., 2013). A preterm infant's skin is underdeveloped and therefore more susceptible to nosocomial pathogens. Preterm infants have a large body mass to surface ratio, which plays a role in hydration, temperature stability, and a barrier against infection. Preventing hypothermia in preterm infants is a major nursing focus with direct impact on mortality. Because of evaporative loss, humidity is maintained by placing infants in incubators. Nurses are responsible for maintaining and monitoring the neutral thermal environment and are aware of the tiny changes in status that can reflect temperature instability and early sepsis.

Skin care in neonates is essential in preventing skin breakdown. Nurses can individualize bathing and care to prevent infections. Studies show daily bathing with soap and water is important; however, bathing with antiseptics like chlorhexidine can affect the skin's normal microflora (Dong & Speer, 2015). Frequent exposure to skin-disrupting procedures, such as heel sticks and intravenous (IV) placements, increases the risk for LOS. It is the nurse who can cluster blood draws, prevent multiple blood sampling, and suggest long-term intravascular access for infants, thus preventing skin breakdown where pathogens can enter.

The preterm infant's gut is essential in the development of the innate immune defenses against infection. Term infants are colonized with anaerobes after breastfeeding is initiated. Many premature infants may not receive breast milk for the first few days after birth, leading to abnormal gut microflora and delayed colonization. This may then promote bacterial translocation into the bloodstream causing LOS (Dong & Speer, 2015).

The need for slow-feeding advances and use of intravascular access devices for parenteral nutrition put infants at higher risk for LOS. Attention must be paid to feeding intolerance. The nurse must monitor the abdominal girth, residuals, emesis, and weight closely for any subtle sign of sepsis. Initiation of small-volume feeds within the first few days of life has shown to be beneficial in the prevention of nosocomial infection (Dong & Speer, 2015).

The two principal influences in LOS are the hospital setting and invasive procedures. Neonates are prone to being colonized by organisms from their environment. Meticulous cleaning of equipment and handwashing help keep colonization risk low. Continued invasive interventions, such as mechanical ventilation and intravascular catheterization, lead to the disruption of the normal neonatal flora and allow hospital-acquired pathogens to colonize infants (Dong & Speer, 2015). By following ventilator-associated and central lines–related bacterial bundles (grouping of evidence-based, high-impact interventions), nurses play the most important role in minimizing the incidence of pneumonia and central line–associated infections.

Many clinicians use the CDC (2009) and American Academy of Pediatrics Committee on the Fetus and the Newborn (Polin & Committee on Fetus and Newborn, 2012) algorithms for evaluation and management of infants at risk for EOS (Polin & Committee on Fetus and Newborn, 2012). The neonatal EOS calculator, a means for predicting risk of EOS combining both maternal risk factors with objective measures of a newborn's clinical exam, is being adopted in many NICUs and has demonstrated to be beneficial (Escobar et al., 2014). This has resulted in a decrease of prolonged hospitalizations and antibiotic exposure in infants.

Complete blood counts (CBCs) and acute phase reactants, such as C-reactive protein, provide diagnostic markers that help determine the length of antibiotic therapy. Other laboratory studies, such as lumbar puncture for evaluation of CSF, urine culture, and blood culture, may be indicated to determine a specific pathogen. A limitation for early diagnosis of sepsis is the length of time it may take for a culture to be read as positive. However, treatment with antimicrobials needs to begin immediately after the sepsis evaluation is completed.

OUTCOMES

Mortality rates are lower in term infants compared to preterm infants in both early and late onset sepsis. Mortality estimates vary depending on gestational age of the infant and if there is a defined pathogen.

Prevention, rather than treatment, improves clinical outcomes. With the implementation of bundles, there are reduced episodes of LOS. Bundles available include hand hygiene, full-barrier precautions, prompt removal of central lines, and avoidance of femoral route for IV access.

Summary

EOS and LOS continue to be an issue for neonates. Diagnostic tests help with the decisions to begin and stop treatment but do not have the high diagnostic accuracy or validity that can aid in early detection of sepsis in neonates. Antibiotics awareness and stewardship are important in preventing issues in the future. Standard contact precautions and care with good hand hygiene are essential in keeping sepsis risks low. The use of bundles of intravascular lines and tubes is now vital in the prevention of LOS.

It is the astute nurse at the bedside who can be the guide to early detection. With strict adherence to assessment skills, infection control policies (e.g., strict hand washing, catheter, and ventilator management), nurses can reduce and possibly eliminate infections in neonates, thus improving morbidity and mortality.

Nursing can mandate best practices to prevent infections. Nurses need to understand causes, clinical manifestations, and the risk factors for neonatal sepsis. With this knowledge and with a continued assessment of interventions, nurses can play a vital role in preventing mortality and limiting morbidity from neonatal sepsis.

Bizzarro, M. J., Shabanova, V., Baltimore, R. S., Dembry, L.-M., Ehrenkranz, R. A., & Gallagher, P. G. (2015). Neonatal sepsis 2004-2013: The rise and fall of coagulase-negative staphylococci. *The Journal of Pediatrics, 166*(5), 1193–1199. doi:10.1016/j .jpeds.2015.02.009

Camacho-Gonzalez, A., Spearman, P. W., & Stoll, B. J. (2013). Neonatal infectious diseases: Evaluation of neonatal sepsis. *Pediatric Clinics of North America, 60*(2), 367–389. doi:10.1016/j.pcl.2012.12.003

Centers for Disease Control and Prevention. (2009). Trends in perinatal group B streptococcal disease—United States, 2000–2006. *Morbidity and Mortality Weekly Report, 58*, 109–112. Retrieved from https://www.cdc.gov/mmwr/preview/mmwrhtml/ mm5805a2.htm#top

Dong, Y., & Speer, C. P. (2015). Late-onset neonatal sepsis: Recent developments. *Archives of Disease in Childhood—Fetal and Neonatal Edition, 100*(3), F257–F263. doi:10.1136/archdischild-2014-306213

Escobar, G. J., Puopolo, K. M., Wi, S., Turk, B. J., Kuzniewicz, M. W., Walsh, E. M., . . . Draper, D. (2014). Stratification of risk of early-onset sepsis in newborns ≥ 34 weeks' gestation. *Pediatrics, 133*(1), 30–36. doi:10.1542/peds.2013-1689

Fanaroff, A., & Fanaroff, J. (2013). *Klaus and Fanaroff's care of the high-risk neonate* (6th ed., pp. 346–367). Philadelphia, PA: Elsevier Saunders.

Polin, R. A., & Committee on Fetus and Newborn. (2012). Management of neonates with suspected or proven early-onset bacterial sepsis. *Pediatrics, 129*(5), 1006–1015. doi:10.1542/peds.2012-0541

Shah, J., Jefferies, A. L., Yoon, E. W., Lee, S. K., & Shah, P. S. (2015). Risk factors and outcomes of late-onset bacterial sepsis in preterm neonates born at <32 weeks' gestation. *American Journal of Perinatology, 32*(7), 675–682. doi:10.1055/s-0034-1393936

Simonsen, K. A., Anderson-Berry, A. L., Delair, S. F., & Davies, H. D. (2014). Early-onset neonatal sepsis. *Clinical Microbiology Reviews, 27*(1), 21–47. doi:10.1128/ CMR.00031-13

■ SUBSTANCE ABUSE/OPIOID WITHDRAWAL

Helene M. Lannon

Overview

Substance abuse during pregnancy has increased substantially over the past 10 years and has reached national, epidemic proportions. In the United States, approximately 225,000 infants yearly are exposed to illicit substances (MacMullen, Dulski, & Blobaum 2014). Retrospectively, by 2011, 1.1% of pregnant women abused opioids, pain relievers, and heroin; 12.9% were dispensed an opioid at some time during the pregnancy, and the incidence of infant withdrawal rose from 1.2 to 5.8 per 1,000 births (Hall et al., 2016). From the years 2000 to 2009, the number of infants in the United States diagnosed with neonatal abstinence syndrome (NAS) grew threefold, accounting for $720 million in national health care expenditures (Patrick et al., 2015). In response to the growth and variable treatment for infants, the American Academy of Pediatrics requested the medical community to standardize care delivered to infants withdrawing from opioids (Patrick et al., 2016).

Background

NAS is a drug-withdrawal syndrome experienced by opioid-exposed infants shortly after birth (Patrick et al., 2016), with clinical signs that affect the central nervous system, as well as the autonomic, gastrointestinal, and respiratory systems. Legal use of tobacco and alcohol alone is harmful to the growing fetus, yet, when coupled with illicit drugs or opiates, it is difficult to extrapolate what substance or drug combinations are causing withdrawal. Because of the potential for multiple exposures, the data outcomes for infants are not conclusive and may be impossible to predict. In response to the increased incidence of infants experiencing NAS and a desire to optimize infant outcomes, collaborative neonatal groups combined strategies to develop evidence-based guidelines to treat NAS pharmacologically (Hall et al., 2014, 2016).

The health care team can anticipate withdrawal signs to develop if the mother is enrolled in a methadone clinic or substance abuse program and is receiving methadone or buprenorphine to treat her own withdrawal. However, it is difficult to anticipate infant withdrawal when there is no prenatal care or a poor maternal history. Pregnancy may be the first time a woman finds help for her addiction. Despite these challenges, most drugs and substances are known to cross the placenta and affect the fetus.

The effects of infant exposure to chemical substances were recognized more than 50 years ago, but fetal development has only been seriously studied in the past 30 years. Nicotine has been studied since 1960, alcohol since 1970, and illicit drugs since 1980. Marijuana is the most commonly used illicit substance during pregnancy with approximately 2.5% of women using during pregnancy, often concurrently with tobacco and alcohol. Therefore, isolated effects alone are difficult to study (Jaques et al., 2014). It is unknown whether the long-term effects of prenatal exposure to medicinal cannabis used in a controlled manner differ from the effects of cannabis used as a legal, recreational drug during pregnancy. However, follow-up developmental growth data report school-age children exposed to in utero marijuana exhibited decreased attention, hyperactivity, and impulsivity. Reading, spelling, and math skills were lacking particularly for those children who were heavily exposed to marijuana during the first trimester of pregnancy (Metz & Stickrath, 2015).

The exact mechanism by which nicotine produces adverse effects are unknown, but it is believed the vasoconstrictive effects on the placenta and umbilical vessels lead to fetal hypoxia resulting in poor infant growth and brain development (Behnke & Smith, 2013). Maternal excessive ingestion of alcohol during pregnancy may cause fetal alcohol syndrome. Infants may demonstrate neurodevelopmental deficits of poor habituation, subtle language delays, low levels of arousal with motor abnormalities, growth restriction, and potential for congenital anomalies (Behnke & Smith, 2013). Methamphetamine and cocaine long-term effects as potent vasoconstriction agents are unclear but suggest an association with prematurity and intrauterine growth restriction. Animal studies have shown disruptions in neural and glial cell organization, migration, and altered nucleic acid and protein production in the brain suggestive of overall compromise in brain growth (Behnke & Smith, 2013).

Of critical concern is maternal substance use on the developing fetal brain. During the embryonic stage, drugs can have significant teratogenic effects that persist as subtle effects of abnormal growth and maturation. Jaques et al. (2014), studied animal–cannabis-exposed models and suggested that during the animal embryonic stage, neurotransmitter pathways and receptors, particularly dopamine receptors, were disrupted. Disturbances in dopamine function have been associated with an increased risk of neuropsychiatric disorders such as drug addiction, schizophrenia, and depression. However, whether these changes are implicated in the future risk of addictive behaviors in the human is yet unknown (Jaques et al., 2014).

Acute narcotic withdrawal usually begins 24 to 48 hours after birth; however, symptoms may not appear until 3 to 4 days after birth. Methadone exposure symptoms may appear within 48 to 72 hours or may not be exhibited until 3 weeks of age. Readmission is common as infants are often discharged before symptoms appear. Opiate withdrawal develops in 55% to 94% of exposed infants (Hall et al., 2014). The infant with opiate NAS may exhibit hyperactivity; irritability; sleep disturbances; hypertonia and tremors; potential seizures; exaggerated Moro reflex; increased muscle tone; exaggerated sucking; high-pitched cry; diaphoresis; poor feeding; diarrhea; vomiting; poor weight gain; and overall poor orientation for self-regulation with autonomic signs of yawning, sneezing, nasal stuffiness, mottling of skin, and fever (Hudak, Tan, Committee on Drugs, & Committee on Fetus and Newborn, 2012). Nursing interventions alone for these symptoms often are not adequate treatment. The most commonly used therapeutic, opioid treatment for withdrawal is morphine, although some centers use methadone with emerging use of buprenorphine and clonidine as an adjunct therapy (Kraft & van den Anker, 2012).

Clinical Aspects

The Finnegan Neonatal Abstinence Scoring System (NASS) is a tool initially established by Finnegan in 1975, modified, published in the standardized form, and used by nursing staff to assess an infant's withdrawal symptoms and need for pharmacologic intervention (Asti, Magers, Keels, Wispe, & McClead, 2015). It is an easy, comprehensive scoring system composed of 21 items relating to signs of neonatal withdrawal and the predominant tool used in the United States.

ASSESSMENT

The nursing assessment of interventions for nonpharmacologic therapy was gathered from systematic reviews of literature based on nursing case reports, descriptive or retrospective studies, nursing articles and reviews, or sometimes, based on the tradition of what seemed to work. A systematic literature review published by MacMullen et al. (2014) lists nursing interventions based on a level of evidence scale. Levels I to II have high-level evidence based on randomized control trials; level III evidence is based on retrospective cohort studies; and level IV evidence is based on case studies or observational reports.

The nursing assessment begins with a thorough maternal history to identify infants at risk. Maternal drug history and screening should be conducted for all pregnant women. Nurses use their center's NAS scoring tool to identify infant signs and symptoms of withdrawal and closely monitor scores per protocol to determine initiation, escalation, weaning, or discontinuation of pharmacological therapy.

NURSING INTERVENTIONS, MANAGEMENT, AND IMPLICATIONS

Nonpharmacologic nursing therapies based on the level of evidence are as follows: supportive care measures of swaddling, decreased stimulation, low-lighted environment, limiting noise; cluster care, sucrose pacifier, and cuddling or infant massage; swaying or rocking as appropriate based on evidence score, level IV, case series. Auditory and eye-to-eye contact in a randomized-control trial received a high level of evidence, levels I to II. Rooming-in as a retrospect, cohort study scored a level III. Nutritional deficiencies from increased energy expenditure, or vomiting, diarrhea, or loose stools require a high-calorie formula; poor oral skills, which may require intravenous therapy or gavage feedings, received an evidence level IV.

Nurses must record intake and output and serum electrolytes to indicate dehydration and/or deficiencies. Daily weight is an important indicator of nutritional status. Breastfeeding may be contraindicated in some instances; however, breastfeeding provides optimal nutrition and promotes maternal–infant bonding. Mothers on methadone therapy may breastfeed, which is supported by the American Academy of Pediatrics and per most institutions, as evidence levels III–IV. Skin care for any breakdown areas may require topical ointments, barrier shields of clear, transparent dressings over reddened areas, and positioning for comfort, as evidence level IV. Pharmacologic therapy is indicated for moderate-to-severe signs of NAS and is used to prevent complications of fever, weight loss, and seizures, or if the infant is not responding to nonpharmacologic therapies.

OUTCOMES

An infant born to a mother on a low-dose prescription opiate with a short half-life may be safely discharged if there are no signs of withdrawal by 3 days of age, whereas an infant born to a mother on an opiate with a prolonged half-life should be observed for a minimum of 5 to 7 days after cessation of pharmacologic therapy. Methadone withdrawal signs may continue for months, but late signs are often subtle and only require comfort measures as treatment. Because initiation of the 2012 American Academy of Pediatrics calls for an evidence-based protocol for NAS, outcomes to date are favorable. Use of a stringent protocol for pharmacological therapy has reduced the duration of opioid exposure and length of hospital stay, with continued research to refine the pharmacological weaning protocol in progress (Hall et al., 2014).

Nursing protocols based on evidence-based research versus systematic reviews are valuable in refining nonpharmacological therapies to treat NAS. Family-centered, rooming-in models of care are showing favorable outcomes in shortening opioid treatment for NAS and thus decreasing the length of stay. Nurses must continue to be active participants in NAS protocol development through participation in committees to evaluate literature, and create policies and procedures to refine nonpharmacologic treatment for NAS. Therapy for NAS begins at the bedside with the nursing assessment and is the integral component that determines therapy and, ultimately, the outcome.

Summary

There is a need to disentangle the many variables of substances and drugs associated with newborn exposure, withdrawal, and follow-up care. The harmful effects of any substance or drug use on the fetus and newborn are well documented. The short- and long-term effects of drug use on infant growth and development are uncertain. Health care has responded by researching pharmacological and nonpharmacological interventions to minimize withdrawal, minimize the risk of adverse outcomes, and shorten the length of hospital stay to minimize health care costs. Until there is a significant decrease in drug abuse during pregnancy, hopeful outcomes rely on health care's dedication to research that results in effective methods and therapies to treat NAS.

Asti, L., Magers, J. S., Keels, E., Wispe, J., & McClead, R. E., Jr. (2015). A quality improvement project to reduce length of stay for neonatal abstinence syndrome. *Pediatrics, 135*(6), e1494–e1500. doi:10.1542/peds.2014-1269

Behnke, M., Smith, V. C., Committee on Substance Abuse, & Committee on Fetus and Newborn. (2013). Prenatal substance abuse: Short- and long-term effects on the exposed fetus. *Pediatrics, 131*(3), e1009–e1024. doi:10.1542/peds.2012-3931

Hall, E. S., Wexelblatt, S. L., Crowley, M., Grow, J. L., Jasin, L. R., Klebanoff, M. A., . . . Walsh, M. C. (2014). A multicenter cohort study of treatments and hospital outcomes in neonatal abstinence syndrome. *Pediatrics, 134*(2), e527–e534. doi:10.1542/peds.2013-4036

Hall, E. S., Wexelblatt, S. L., Crowley, M., Grow, J. L., Jasin, L. R., Klebanoff, M. A., . . . Walsh, M. (2016). Implementation of a neonatal abstinence syndrome weaning protocol: A multicenter cohort study. *Pediatrics, 136*(4), 803–810. doi:10.1542/peds.2015-1141

Hudak, M. L., Tan, R. C., Committee on Drugs, & Committee on Fetus and Newborn (2012). Neonatal drug withdrawal. *Pediatrics, 129*(2), e540–e560. doi:10.1542/peds.2011-3212

Jaques, S. C., Kingsbury, A., Henshcke, P., Chomchai, C., Clews, S., Falconer, J., . . . Oei, J. L. (2014). Cannabis, the pregnant woman and her child: Weeding out the myths. *Journal of Perinatology, 34*(6), 417–424. doi:10.1038/jp.2013.180

Kraft, W. K., & van den Anker, J. N. (2012). Pharmacologic management of the opioid neonatal abstinence syndrome. *Pediatric Clinics of North America, 59*(5), 1147–1165. doi:10.1016/j.pcl.2012.07.006

MacMullen, N. J., Dulski, L. A., & Blobaum, P. (2014). Evidence-based interventions for neonatal abstinence syndrome. *Pediatric Nursing, 40*(4), 165–172, 203. Retrieved from https://www.pediatricnursing.net/ce/2016/article40051.pdf

Metz, T. D., & Stickrath, E. H. (2015). Marijuana use in pregnancy and lactation: A review of the evidence. *American Journal of Obstetrics & Gynecology, 213*(6), 761–778. doi:10.1016/j.ajog.2015.05.025

Patrick, S. W., Dudley, J., Martin, P. R., Harrell, F. E., Warren, M. D., Hartmann, K. E., . . . Cooper, W. O. (2015). Prescription opioid epidemic and infant outcomes. *Pediatrics, 135*(5), 842–850. doi:10.1542/peds.2014-3299

Patrick, S. W., Schumacher, R. E., Horbar, J., Buus-Frank, M., Edwards, E., Morrow, K., . . . Soll, R. (2016). Improving care for neonatal abstinence syndrome. *Pediatrics, 137*(5), 1–8. doi:10.1542/peds.2015-3835

■ THERMOREGULATION

Paula Forsythe

Overview

In utero, the fetus is dependent on the mother as the source of heat. At birth, the neonate transitions from a warm environment to one that is much colder. After delivery, the neonate must assume self-regulation of body temperature. This is one of the most significant challenges faced by every newborn. Failure to regulate temperature has serious implications for many body systems and may cause even healthy newborns to experience respiratory, metabolic, and cardiovascular complications, all of which can be prevented by diligent nursing care.

Background

Thermoregulation is the ability to regulate heat production and loss to maintain normal body temperature between 36.5°C to 37.5°C (American Heart Association and American Academy of Pediatrics, 2015; Brand & Boyd, 2015; Knobel-Dail, 2014). It is a key physiologic requirement for survival. In utero, fetal body heat is the result of the infant's rapid metabolic rate and heat transferred from the mother via the placenta and uterus. The result is a body temperature 0.3°C to 0.5°C higher than the mother (Asakura, 2004; Knobel-Dail, 2014). Heat loss and cold stress, which often occurs during delivery and in the minutes that follow, stimulate the newborn's skin and thermal receptors, especially the trigeminal area of the face, to signal the hypothalamus to conserve or produce heat (Brand & Boyd, 2015; Karlson, 2013). The hypothalamus activates the sympathetic nervous system and norepinephrine is released triggering several adaptations vital to maintaining body temperature (Brand & Boyd, 2015; Chaplain Maternal Newborn Regional Program [CMNRP], 2013; Karlson, 2013). Norepinephrine increases metabolism, respiratory rate, oxygen consumption, and the utilization of glucose. Norepinephrine also vasoconstricts peripheral blood vessels to minimize environmental heat loss and retain core body heat, as well as vasoconstricts pulmonary vessels, increases pulmonary vascular pressure, and shunts deoxygenated blood away from the lungs through the ductus arteriosus to the aorta. It also stimulates brown fat metabolism (Brand & Boyd, 2015; Karlson, 2013). This constellation of physiologic reactions places the newborn, especially those born premature and/or ill at risk for hypoxemia, hypoxia, hypoglycemia, anaerobic metabolism, and acidosis, which can lead to cell damage and even death (Brand & Boyd, 2015; CMNRP, 2013; Karlson, 2013).

Neonates rely on nonshivering thermogenesis to metabolize brown adipose fat (BAT) and release energy. BAT contains mitochondria, fat vacuoles, sympathetic nerve endings, and an abundant blood supply (Asakura, 2004; Brand & Boyd, 2015). BAT develops primarily during the third trimester of pregnancy and is deposited around the kidneys, adrenal glands, mediastinum, scapulae, and axilla. BAT serves as the primary source for heat generation during the perinatal and postnatal period. Metabolism of brown fat requires oxygen and glucose and is stimulated by nerve endings that activate lipase, resulting in lipolysis, fatty acid oxidation, and the generation of heat, which warms circulating blood, transferring heat throughout the body (Brand & Boyd, 2015; CMNRP, 2013; Karlson, 2013).

Although central thermoregulatory mechanisms are present at birth, they are developmentally deficient and not well differentiated (Asakura, 2004; Knobel-Dail, 2014) placing neonates, particularly the smallest and most critically ill, at great risk for heat loss or hypothermia. Heat loss occurs by evaporation, conduction, convection, and radiation. Factors that impact the rate of body heat transfer or loss in the neonate include a large surface area to body mass ratio; decreased amounts of subcutaneous fat and BAT; high body water content; immature, non-keratinized skin that allows transepidermal water and heat loss; vasoconstrictive, motor and metabolic function; and differences in temperature between the neonate and environment. Without appropriate environmental modifications and nursing care interventions, the newborn loses body heat at a rate of up to 1°C per minute (Brand & Boyd, 2015; Karlson, 2013).

Hyperthermia, a condition in which the body temperature higher than 37.5°C (Karlson, 2013), is less common in the neonatal period but can result in deleterious effects. Neonates are at high risk for hyperthermia because of their inability to dissipate heat (Brand & Boyd, 2015). The most frequent causes are environmental such as overheating from incubators, radiant warmers or high room temperatures, phototherapy, or excessive clothing or bundling. Hyperthermia may, however, be a sign of infection, dehydration, narcotic withdrawal, or central nervous system disorders such as asphyxia and neonatal encephalopathy. Efficient differentiation between environmental causes and illness-related causality is required for appropriate care and interventions (Brand & Boyd, 2015; CMNRP, 2013).

Clinical Aspects

ASSESSMENT

Thermal regulation begins at delivery. Gestational age and risk factors for both newborn and mother determine what is needed for a safe delivery. The delivery room temperature should be set at 25°C to 26°C (75°–77°F) and a radiant warmer, preheated should be available. Immediately following delivery, the infant is evaluated by Apgar (appearance, pulse, grimace, activity, and respiration) scoring. A stable newborn with Apgar scores greater than 6, showing no signs of complications, is dried, the head is covered with a hat, and is placed on mother's chest for warmth and bonding. Both are covered with a warmed blanket (Brand & Boyd, 2015; CMNRP, 2013). A very ill, immature, or compromised newborn with Apgar scores less than or equal to 6 is stabilized, resuscitated if needed, and transferred to the neonatal intensive care unit (NICU) in a transport incubator. A polyethylene body wrap or thermal mattress is used to promote thermal stability (Brand & Boyd, 2015; Knobel-Dail, 2014).

Assessment for signs of hypothermia includes frequent, continuous monitoring of body temperature and respiratory status; observing for signs of distress such as apnea, bradycardia, tachypnea, or irregular breathing patterns; acrocyanosis; cool, mottled, or pale skin; hypoglycemia; lethargy; and poor feeding (CMNRP, 2013). Axillary temperatures are used for assessment as they correlate well with core temperatures and are noninvasive. Rectal temperatures are not recommended because of the risk for intestinal trauma or injury (Brand & Boyd, 2015).

NURSING INTERVENTIONS, MANAGEMENT, AND IMPLICATIONS

Temperature control is a primary concern for nursing. Nursing care must focus on preventing temperature instability, as well as resultant metabolic and respiratory acidosis. The goal is to manage the newborn in an environment that does not expend calories and oxygen to maintain a normal body temperature.

Interventions to prevent heat loss begin at birth. Healthy, normothermic newborns are lightly dressed. If an axillary temperature falls below 36.3°C, the head is covered with a hat, and skin-to-skin contact with the mother in a warm room, covered with blankets, is practiced (CMNRP, 2013; Knobel-Dail, 2014).

A care bundle, a set of interventions used together to improve patient outcomes, is initiated to maintain body warmth for newborns who are premature, ill, or requiring resuscitation. This includes increasing the delivery room air temperature to 25°C to 26°C; head coverings and body wrap for the neonate; a thermal mattress if needed; heated humidified respiratory gases; and skin–skin care when feasible (CMNRP, 2013; Karlson, 2013; Knobel-Dail, 2014). Applying polyethylene body wraps immediately after birth, while neonates are wet with amniotic fluids, creates a warm, humid environment that improves body temperatures in the immediate postnatal period. Covering the head with a hat or plastic wrap minimizes heat loss associated with the neonate's large head-to-body size ratio. A thermal mattress placed under the infant provides a source of heat for short periods of time (Karlson, 2013; Knobel-Dail, 2014). Caution must be used when combining interventions to avoid idiopathic hyperthermia (Knobel-Dail, 2014).

A radiant warmer is preferred during the admission, stabilization, and procedure process before the infant is placed in an incubator. Hybrid incubators provide both environments without moving the neonate (Brand & Boyd, 2015; Knobel-Dail, 2014). The temperature of the radiant warmer or incubator is regulated by feedback from a probe placed on the neonate's abdomen in the right upper quadrant, avoiding the liver or any bone. Temperature is either regulated by automatic feedback from the probe to maintain a set skin temperature (servo-control mode) or regulated by caregivers controlling the desired environmental temperature (manual, air control mode). Skin temperature monitoring is continuous and correlates well with axillary core temperatures.

Heated humidity is added to incubators of very-low-birth-weight neonates to prevent transepidermal water loss. High humidity (greater than 70%) is used during the first week of life, then decreased to standard humidity levels to minimize bacterial growth and the risk of infection (Brand & Boyd, 2015; Knobel-Dail, 2014). Humid environments also minimize weight loss and hypernatremia but delay maturation of the skin barrier (Knobel-Dail, 2014). Neonates are undressed, the servo-control mode is used and oxygen, if required, is heated and humidified to minimize insensible water loss (Karlson, 2013; Knobel-Dail, 2014).

Transitioning neonates to open cribs occurs sequentially with continuous monitoring of body temperature and weight. Humidity is removed incrementally, guided by the neonate's weight progression. The neonate remains in the incubator to gain weight, is lightly dressed, head covered, and managed in air control mode. The incubator temperature is then incrementally decreased until 28°C (room temperature) has been reached in the incubator and the neonate's temperature stabilized. Neonates are transitioned to an open crib at approximately 1,500 to 1,600 g who are feeding enterally and demonstrating consistent weight gain over several days (Brand & Boyd, 2015). Additional layers of blankets are applied the first day to maintain temperature stability.

Transitioning medically stable neonates to open cribs, who are approximately 32 weeks gestational age and 1,500 g, can begin with a thermal challenge (applying a blanket and decreasing the incubator temperature by 1.5°C). Early transition to open cribs is associated with higher weight accrual and shortened hospital stays (CMNRP, 2013; Knobel-Dail, 2014).

Rewarming hypothermic neonates occurs slowly in an incubator, increasing the neonate's temperature 0.5°C per hour to avoid physiologic instability such as apnea. However, significant hypothermia, less than 35°C, requires rapid rewarming: the incubator temperature is set 1°C to 1.5°C greater than the body temperature, readjusting the set temperature as the neonate warms, until 36.5°C is attained. Careful monitoring of the neonate's respiratory and cardiac status, blood pressure, oxygen requirement, and blood glucose levels provide evidence whether the neonate is successfully managing the warming process or deteriorating, requiring an escalation of physiologic management (CMNRP, 2013; Karlson, 2013).

Neonates who are hyperthermic require cooling measures: adjustment of environment temperature, removal of clothing, and provision of fluids to prevent dehydration. With severe hyperthermia, the focus is on identification and management of the cause (CMNRP, 2013).

Quality and safety issues focus on successful temperature management of the newborn during the perinatal, postnatal processes. Through the implementation of evidence-based practice, delivery room temperatures have increased and skin-to-skin contact has increased for stable newborns. Polyethylene body wraps and thermal, chemical mattresses are standard practice and NRP Guidelines include temperature management as an integral part of resuscitation (American Heart Association and American Academy of Pediatrics, 2015; Brand & Boyd, 2015). Golden Hour protocols implemented in NICU settings to improve the efficiencies of admitting and stabilizing a newborn within 60 minutes of arrival stress the importance of temperature management (Brand & Boyd, 2015).

Summary

Successful thermoregulation is based on the identification of neonates at risk for temperature instability, rigorous control of environmental factors, utilization of additional heat sources, and vigilant nursing care to detect and manage hypothermia and hyperthermia. Prevention is preferable to management for successful newborn transitions and eliminates the incidence of associated sequelae and morbidities.

American Heart Association and American Academy of Pediatrics. (2015). Summary AAP/AHA 2015 guidelines for cardiopulmonary resuscitation and emergency cardiovascular care of the neonate. Retrieved from https://www.aap.org/en-us/Documents/nrp_guidelines_english.pdf

Asakura, H. (2004). Fetal and neonatal thermoregulation. *Journal of Nippon Medical School, 71*(6), 360–370. doi:10.1272/jnms.71.360

Brand, M. C., & Boyd, H. A. (2015). Thermoregulation. In M. T. Verklan & M. Walden (Eds.), *Core curriculum for neonatal intensive care nursing* (5th ed., pp. 95–109). St. Louis, MO: Elsevier Sanders.

Chaplain Maternal Newborn Regional Program. (2013). Newborn thermoregulation: Self-learning module. Retrieved from http://www.CMNRP.ca/uploads/documents/NEWBORN_THERMOREGULATION_SLM_2013_06.pdf

Karlson, K. (2013). *The S.T.A.B.L.E. program. Learner/provider manual* (6th ed., pp. 63–93). Park City, UT: American Academy of Pediatrics.

Knobel-Dail, R. B. (2014). Role of effective thermoregulation in premature neonates. *Research and Reports in Neonatology, 2014*(4), 147–156. doi:10.2147/RRN.S52377

Index

Printed in the United States
By Bookmasters